# Exercise testing and interpretation
## A practical approach

In *Exercise Testing and Interpretation: A Practical Approach*, Drs Christopher Cooper and Thomas Storer offer a practical and systematic approach to the acquisition, interpretation, and reporting of physiologic responses to exercise.

Pulmonologists, cardiologists, and sports physicians, as well as respiratory therapists and other allied health professionals, will find this book an indispensable resource when learning to select proper instruments, identify the most appropriate test protocols, and integrate and interpret physiologic response variables. The final chapter presents clinical cases to illuminate useful strategies for exercise testing and interpretation. Useful appendices offer answers to frequently asked questions, laboratory forms, algorithms, and calculations, and a glossary of terms, symbols, and definitions. *Exercise Testing and Interpretation: A Practical Approach* offers clearly defined responses (both normal and abnormal) to over 40 performance variables including aerobic, cardiovascular, ventilatory, and gas exchange variables.

Practical, portable, and easy-to-read, this essential guidebook can be used as a complement to more detailed books on the topic, or stand on its own.

**Christopher Cooper** is Professor of Medicine and Physiology at the UCLA School of Medicine and Medical Director of the Exercise Physiology Laboratories at the UCLA Medical Center. Dr. Cooper is a Fellow of the American College of Chest Physicians, Royal College of Physicians, and the American College of Sports Medicine. He has authored several research publications, reviews, and book chapters on the topics of exercise physiology and fitness, chronic obstructive pulmonary disease, pulmonary rehabilitation, and oxygen therapy.

**Thomas W. Storer** established the Exercise Science Laboratory programs for exercise physiology and fitness at El Camino College in 1979 and is now Professor, Division of Health Sciences and Athletics at El Camino College, serves as Director of the Exercise Science Laboratories and Pulmonary Exercise and Education Program at El Camino, and holds an appointment in the Department of Medicine at Charles R. Drew University of Medicine and Science in Los Angeles. He also teaches graduate and undergraduate exercise physiology and community fitness at El Camino College and was the 1998–99 recipient of their Distinguished Faculty Award.

# Exercise testing and interpretation

## A practical approach

**Christopher B. Cooper**
University of California Los Angeles

**Thomas W. Storer**
El Camino College

CAMBRIDGE
UNIVERSITY PRESS

PUBLISHED BY THE PRESS SYNDICATE OF THE UNIVERSITY OF CAMBRIDGE
The Pitt Building, Trumpington Street, Cambridge, United Kingdom

CAMBRIDGE UNIVERSITY PRESS
The Edinburgh Building, Cambridge CB2 2RU, UK
40 West 20th Street, New York, NY 10011-4211, USA
10 Stamford Road, Oakleigh, VIC 3166, Australia
Ruiz de Alarcón 13, 28014 Madrid, Spain
Dock House, The Waterfront, Cape Town 8001, South Africa

http://www.cambridge.org



First published 2001

Printed in the United Kingdom at the University Press, Cambridge

*Typeface* Utopia 8.5/12pt *System* Poltype® [VN]

*A catalogue record for this book is available from the British Library*

*Library of Congress Cataloguing in Publication data*

Cooper, Christopher B.
Exercise testing and interpretation; a practical guide / Christopher B. Cooper, Thomas W. Storer.
p. cm.
Includes bibliographical references and index.
ISBN 0 521 64842 4 paperback
I. Exercise tests. I. Storer, Thomas W. II. Title.
RC683.5.E94 C66 2001
613.7'1'0287–DC21 00–045509

ISBN 0 521 64842 4 paperback

---



---

**Dedicated to Nancy and Paula**

"Those who do not make time for exercise will eventually have to make time for illness"

The Earl of Derby (1863)

# Contents

Preface ix

1 **Purpose** 1

2 **Instrumentation** 15

3 **Testing methods** 51

4 **Response variables** 93

5 **Data integration and interpretation** 149

6 **Illustrative cases and reports** 181

Appendix A Glossary (terms, symbols, definitions) 204
Appendix B Calculations and conversions 211
Appendix C Reference values 220
Appendix D Protocols and supplemental materials 241
Appendix E Frequently asked questions 261

Index 265

# Preface

Exercise is fundamental to human existence. For most men and women exercise is essential for quality of life and for many it is the essence of their livelihood. Some have a competitive instinct for athletic performance in the pursuit of individual human achievement. We now understand that the maintenance of physical fitness throughout life is crucial if we are to remain healthy and live to an advanced age. In these contexts, the assessment of exercise ability is of considerable importance to humanity. Exercise testing becomes the means of assessing ability to perform specific tasks, quantification of athletic performance, diagnosis of disease, assessment of disability, and evaluation of responses to physical training, therapeutic intervention, and rehabilitation.

Recent years have indeed witnessed widespread applications of exercise testing that range from clinical uses in assessing debilitated patients to sports medicine venues and the testing of élite athletes. Some exercise tests are appropriately performed with a minimum of equipment, such as a watch and a measured course. Others involve more sophisticated instrumentation enabling more detailed assessments. Advances in technology have rendered all exercise tests more accessible and more affordable, although not necessarily easier to perform with accuracy and reliability. Wireless heart rate monitors give instantaneous and reliable heart rates in the field or in the laboratory. Bi-directional, light-weight, mass flow sensors have obviated the need for cumbersome valves and tubing and, together with miniaturized and fast-responding gas analyzers, enable the calculation of oxygen uptake with every breath. Computer technology has revolutionized the real-time acquisition and analysis of data, although not necessarily made exercise tests any easier to interpret.

We have both practiced and taught in the field of exercise testing and interpretation for many years. We saw the need for a practical text that succinctly explains the physiology of exercise and also gives detailed advice regarding the conduct and interpretation of exercise tests in a variety of settings. We have included clinical and sports medicine applications because we are convinced that these disciplines will merge in the future. We have addressed technical considerations, pitfalls, and solutions. We have placed emphasis on creative figures and diagrams to offer systematic explanations and schemata for interpretation. We have also attempted to address the confusion that surrounds terminology in this diverse field. We have done so through a systematic, logical, and critical examination of the concepts and applications of the field. We hope our approach is enlightening and not a mere addition to the plethora of terms and symbols already in use.

*Exercise testing*, which we abbreviate to XT, can be conducted for several purposes, in a variety of settings. *Performance* exercise tests (PXT) can be performed in the *field* or *laboratory* using a selection of protocols, depending upon the purpose of the test. Typicaly, PXT are conducted to establish exercise-training guidelines and to monitor progress. *Clinical* exercise tests (CXT) have a somewhat different emphasis and are almost exclusively conducted in a laboratory setting. CXT can be *diagnostic*, seeking an explanation for exercise impairment; for *risk assessment*, such as from coronary artery disease or surgery; or alternatively for *monitoring*, for example to quantify the response to therapeutic or surgical interventions or to document progress in rehabilitation. Exercise capacity can be measured by different protocols ranging from the time required to complete a measured course to the acquisition of a wide range of cardiovascular, ventilatory, and gas exchange variables. *Functional* exercise tests focus on ability to perform a specific task whereas *integrative* exercise tests compile an array of variables with which to study the underlying physiology of the exercise response.

Several features of this book are unique. The core of the book describes instrumentation and protocols for exercise testing followed by response variables and their interpretation. The book is laid out so that the reader can easily locate a piece of equipment or response variable for ready reference. Chapter 2 (Instrumentation) describes apparatus for exercise testing explaining, succinctly, the principles of operation and essential facts about calibration and maintenance of the equipment. Chapter 3 (Testing methods) describes protocols for exercise testing with many important details, gleaned from years of experience, that facilitate a successful test. Chapter 4 (Response variables) expands on the many physiological variables that can be derived from exercise testing, ranging from simple timed distances to the complex integrated cardiovascular and gas exchange variables which underlie the exercise response. Each variable has its own section including a definition, derivation, and units of measurement, along with examples of the normal and abnormal responses. Chapter 5 (Data integration and interpretation) presents a novel and systematic approach to help the reader develop a confident and meaningful interpretation of the data. There is an emphasis here on integrative exercise testing because interpretation of this type of XT has often presented more problems to the exercise practitioner. Chapter 6 illustrates the principles expounded in Chapters 2 through 5 with a selection of real cases. Finally, the appendices are designed to be a valuable resource for the exercise practitioner. They include a glossary of proper terms and symbols as adopted by exercise physiologists, simplified algorithms to help explain the derivation of secondary variables, predicted normal values with appropriate critique, examples of worksheets that facilitate testing, and a section on frequently asked questions.

Finally, a few words about the units of measurement incorporated in this book. Our goal has been to write a book that will be of practical value to persons throughout the world who are involved in exercise testing and interpretation. As such we have had to deal with certain inconsistencies in currently accepted units of measurement. Some countries, including the USA, continue to use imperial rather than metric units for certain measurements. The *Système International d'Unités* attempts to bring everyone into concordance with a metric system. However, some traditional units do not lend themselves comfortably to this conversion. We have used SI units wherever possible but referred to traditional units as well when conversion was not straightforward. Readers will undoubtedly find some inconsistencies and discrepancies but hopefully these can always be resolved by reference to Table B1 in Appendix B which explains any necessary conversions.

This book is intended to be a practical text which exercise practitioners would want readily available in their clinical or research laboratories, rehabilitation facilities, and sports clubs. The book may prove useful for chest physicians, cardiologists, exercise physiologists, occupational health physicians, sports physicians, sports scientists, laboratory technicians, physical or respiratory therapists, medical students, and postgraduate students in the exercise sciences. The material for the book has evolved over many years of teaching exercise physiology, exercise testing, and interpretation. Parts of the book reflect a syllabus that we have developed and refined over the past eight years for an annual symposium that has taken place at UCLA as well as several national and international venues. Reflecting our own careers and experiences, we have tried to approach the topic simultaneously from the perspectives of exercise science and clinical medicine. By doing so we have attempted to develop a comprehensive and balanced view of a complex subject which we hope will appeal to, and draw together, a broad range of disciplines with a common purpose – that of understanding the human exercise response.

**CBC, TWS**
Los Angeles, California

## Acknowlegments

This book has evolved from what we have learnt from our mentors, students, and patients. However, its production owes much to the support of others. We wish to thank the staff at Cambridge University Press, particularly Jocelyn Foster who was involved at the conception of the project and Liz Graham who undertook the formidable task of copyediting. We are especially indebted to Judy Valesquez for her meticulous preparation of the figures. Finally, we must acknowledge our families for accepting the many hours we were not with them.

**CBC, TWS**

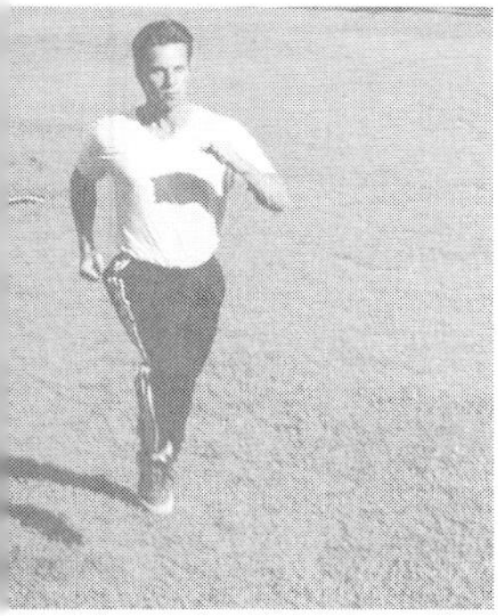

# 1

# Purpose

## Introduction

The human body is designed for the performance of exercise. Habitual patterns of exercise activity are known to be linked to health, well-being, and risk of disease. In fitness and athletics, exercise capacity is linked to performance and achievement. In clinical medicine, exercise performance is intricately related to functional capacity and quality of life. Hence the importance of exercise testing and interpretation as a means of determining exercise capacity and identifying factors which might limit exercise performance. Exercise professionals, whether concerned with physical fitness and sports or clinical medicine and rehabilitation, should be well versed in methods of exercise testing and interpretation. Hence the need for a practical guide to assist in this undertaking.

A wide variety of methods have evolved for the purpose of assessing exercise capacity and identifying specific limiting factors. Field tests are commonly used in fitness and sports to assess athletic performance, but can be used to assess progress in clinical or rehabilitative settings. Laboratory exercise protocols are also used to assess fitness and are often combined with electrocardiography to diagnose coronary artery disease. Symptom-limited, incremental exercise testing, including measurement of ventilation and gas exchange, has proven to be an important diagnostic, clinical, prescriptive, and rehabilitative tool. These more complex laboratory tests evaluate the integrated human cardiovascular, ventilatory, and musculoskeletal responses to exercise. Whether the assessment is conducted in the field or in the laboratory, all of these exercise tests require careful attention to detail if meaningful information is to be derived.

This book provides a detailed examination of the instruments, methods, proper conduct, and interpretation of a variety of exercise tests. This is meant to be a practical guide, assisting the reader in every step of the process with fundamental information, examples, and practice using a time-tested methodology. The next section of this chapter reviews the basic exercise physiology that underlies exercise testing and interpretation. It is included not as a primer, but rather to illustrate the important concepts involved.

## Basic exercise physiology

### Coupling of cellular respiration to external work

During the performance of most types of exercise, it is well known that oxygen uptake ($\dot{V}o_2$) is tightly coupled to external work rate ($\dot{W}$) or power output. The essential components of this coupling are illustrated in Figure 1.1. Central to our understanding of exercise physiology is the measurement of alveolar oxygen uptake ($\dot{V}o_{2alv}$) by collection and analysis of exhaled gases. $\dot{V}o_{2alv}$ provides the systemic arterial oxygen content for delivery to exercising muscles. Hence, the extent to which $\dot{V}o_{2alv}$ matches muscle oxygen consumption ($\dot{Q}o_{2mus}$) is in part a reflection of the effectiveness of oxygen delivery via the

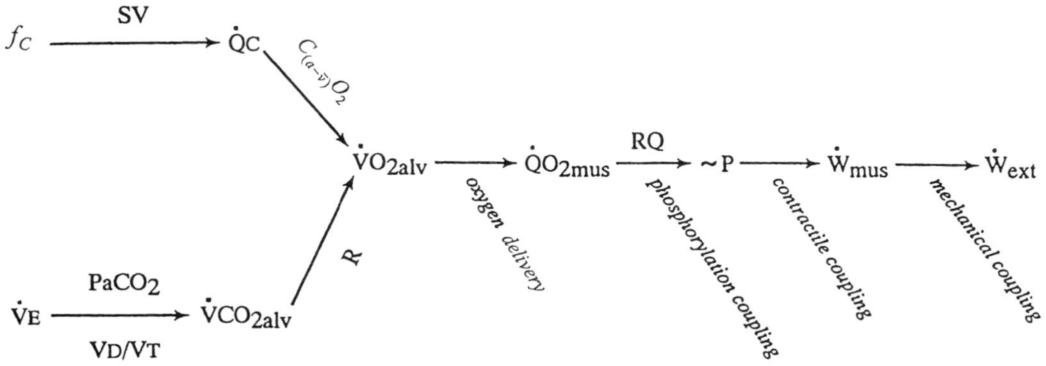


**Figure 1.1** Cardiovascular and ventilatory coupling to external work. See the accompanying text and Appendix A for definitions of the symbols.

circulation. In steady-state conditions $\dot{V}o_{2alv}$ should reflect the oxygen consumption of all tissues, including $\dot{Q}o_{2mus}$. However, in unsteady-state conditions, such as during an incremental exercise test or during the transition from rest to constant work rate exercise, changes in $\dot{V}o_{2alv}$ typically lag behind changes in $\dot{Q}o_{2mus}$. In exercising muscle oxygen is utilized in the production of high-energy phosphate compounds (*~P*). The yield of *~P* per oxygen molecule is dependent on the substrate being utilized for energy generation, which in turn dictates the respiratory quotient (RQ) of the muscle tissue. The conversion of chemical energy in the form of *~P* to intrinsic muscle work ($\dot{W}_{mus}$) depends on contractile coupling and mechanisms that result in actin–myosin cross-bridge formation and muscle shortening. Finally comes the conversion of $\dot{W}_{mus}$ to external work ($\dot{W}_{ext}$), which can be measured by an ergometer. This last stage has a significant effect on work efficiency, being influenced by musculoskeletal coordination and undoubtedly incorporating a skill factor. Aside from the choice of substrate and the skill factor, it can be appreciated that the sequence of mechanisms described above is largely defined by immutable metabolic reactions and ultrastructural properties of human skeletal muscle. Not surprisingly, therefore, when a short-duration exercise protocol which utilizes carbohydrate as the predominant metabolic substrate is performed on a cycle ergometer which minimizes the skill factor, the relationship between $\dot{V}o_{2alv}$ and $\dot{W}_{ext}$ demonstrates linearity and remarkable consistency among normal subjects (see Chapter 4).

## Cardiopulmonary coupling to external work

Integrated exercise testing usually attempts to study the simultaneous responses of the cardiovascular and pulmonary systems. Commonly the cardiovascular response is judged by changes in heart rate ($f_C$) with respect to measured $\dot{V}o_2$ whereas the pulmonary response is judged in terms of minute ventilation ($\dot{V}_E$). Figure 1.1 illustrates how each of these variables is coupled to $\dot{V}o_2$.

Cardiac output ($\dot{Q}_C$) is of central importance in the cardiovascular coupling. The Fick equation (see Chapter 4) reminds us that the relationship between $\dot{Q}_C$ and $\dot{V}o_2$ is determined by the difference in oxygen content between systemic arterial blood and mixed systemic venous blood ($C_{(a-\bar{v})}o_2$). Obviously $\dot{Q}_C$ and $f_C$ are linked through cardiac stroke volume (SV).

Carbon dioxide output ($\dot{V}co_2$) is of central importance in ventilatory coupling. The Bohr equation (see Chapter 4) reminds us that the relationship between $\dot{V}co_2$ and $\dot{V}_E$ is determined by the level at which arterial carbon dioxide tension ($P$aco$_2$) is regulated and the ratio of dead space to tidal volume ($V_D/V_T$). Obviously alveolar $\dot{V}co_2$ and $\dot{V}o_2$ are linked by the respiratory exchange ratio, *R*.

## Metabolic pathways

This book will not attempt a detailed description of all of the metabolic pathways involved in exercise. However, a simplified description of cellular energy generation follows and is illustrated in Figures 1.2 and 1.3.

Whilst fat and protein degradation can sometimes be important in the metabolic response to exercise, undoubtedly the principal substrate for muscle metabolism is carbohydrate in the form of muscle glycogen. The degradation of glycogen to pyruvate occurs in the cytosol and is termed anaerobic glycolysis or the Embden–Meyerhof pathway (Figure 1.2). Firstly, glycogen must be split into glucose units by a glycogen phosphorylase. Each molecule of glucose is then converted to two molecules of pyruvate, with the net generation of two ATP molecules and four hydrogen ions. The hydrogen ions are taken up by the coenzyme NAD to form $NADH + H^+$.

Pyruvate undergoes oxidative decarboxylation that irreversibly removes carbon dioxide and attaches the remainder of the pyruvate molecule to coenzyme A (CoA), forming acetyl-CoA. Note that acetyl-CoA is also the product of fatty acid $\beta$-oxidation. Acetyl-CoA enters the mitochondrion and combines with oxaloacetate to become citrate. In this way acetyl-CoA becomes fuel for the tricarboxylic acid (TCA) cycle, otherwise known as the Krebs cycle or citric acid cycle (Figure 1.2). This sequence of enzymatic reactions dismembers acetyl-CoA, yielding carbon dioxide and hydrogen atoms. Once again the hydrogen ions are accepted by coenzymes. For every acetyl unit consumed in the cycle, there are two carbon dioxide molecules produced along with three $NADH + H^+$ and one $FADH_2$. In addition there is one directly produced molecule of GTP which contains an equivalent amount of energy to ATP. Note that by accepting hydrogen ions the coenzymes NAD and FAD play a vital role in trapping energy.

The main engine for cellular energy generation is the mitochondrial pathway for oxidative phosphorylation, which is shown in Figure 1.3. This pathway is also called the respiratory chain or electron transport chain. The chain is a complex device consisting of lipoproteins with different cytochromes, metals, and other cofactors. Essentially, the chain facilitates the flow of electrons from coenzymes $NADH + H^+$ and $FADH_2$ releasing energy for the phosphorylation of ADP to ATP at three sites. Finally, two electrons are combined with two protons ($H^+$) and oxygen to form water. $NADH + H^+$ enters the first stage of the chain, giving rise to NAD and three ATP, whereas $FADH_2$ enters the second stage of the chain, giving rise to FAD and two ATP. The oxidized coenzymes are released and become available to catalyze dehydrogenase reactions further.

Summarizing all of the pathways described above, the usual process of cellular energy generation can be described by two equations:

$$NADH + H^+ + \tfrac{1}{2}O_2 + 3Pi + 3ADP \rightarrow 3ATP + NAD + H_2O \quad (1.1)$$

$$FADH_2 + \tfrac{1}{2}O_2 + 2Pi + 2ADP \rightarrow 2ATP + NAD + H_2O \quad (1.2)$$

Complete combustion of one molecule of glucose in the presence of sufficient oxygen leads to the generation of approximately 36 molecules of ATP. This number varies depending on how one views the degradation of glycogen and to what extent energy is consumed transporting protons from anaerobic glycolysis into the mitochondrion. $NADH + H^+$ does not cross the mitochondrial membrane and therefore its protons are transferred by a "shuttle" to FAD which enters the electron transport chain at the second rather than the first stage.

When oxygen is not available in sufficient quantity for complete oxidative phosphorylation, then several important changes ensue:

1. The mitochondrial pathways, including the TCA cycle and electron transport chain, are ineffective.
2. Pyruvate accumulates in the cytosol and is converted to lactate.
3. The regeneration of ATP from ADP slows by a factor of approximately 18.
4. Muscle glycogen is more rapidly consumed.

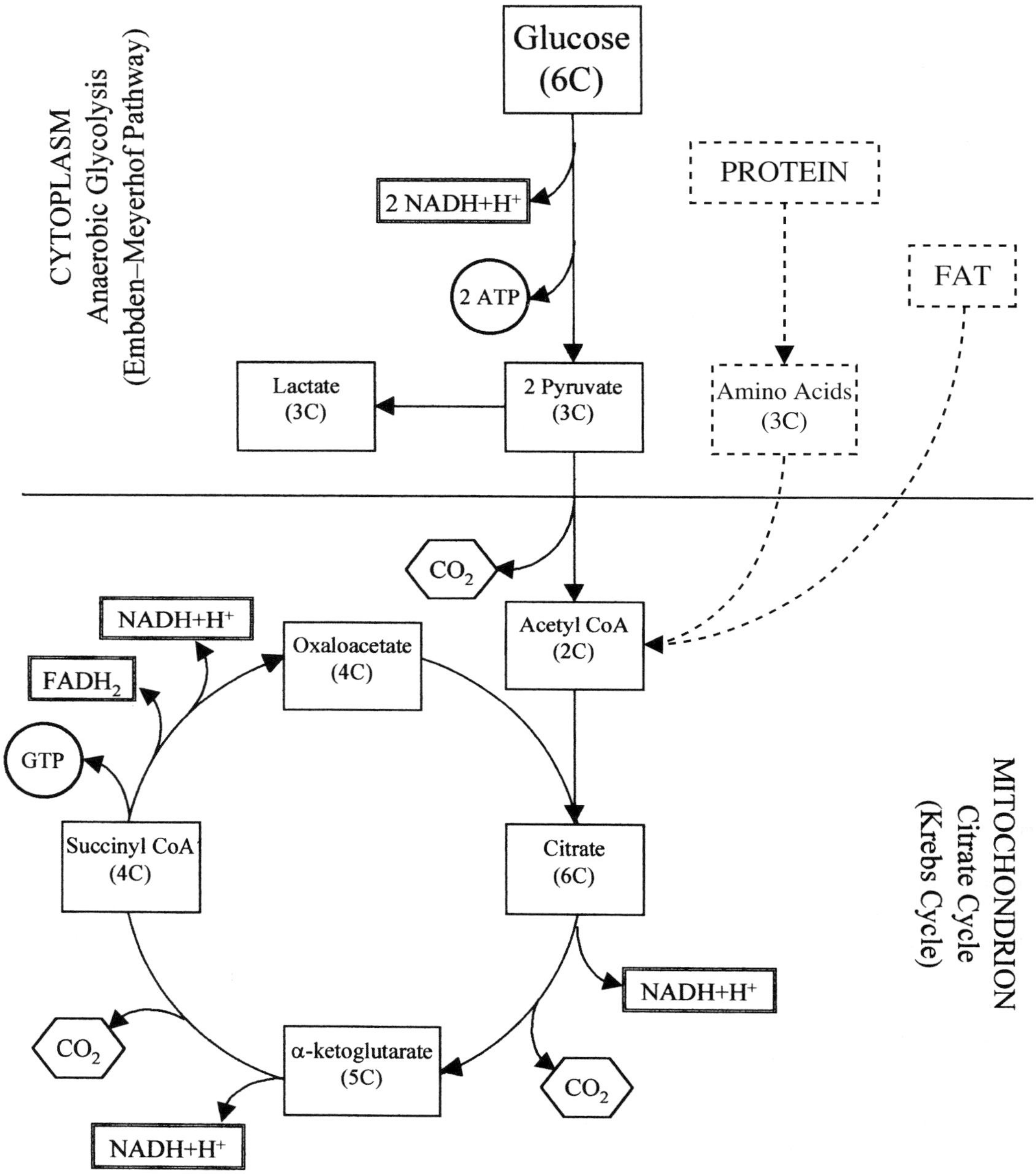


**Figure 1.2** Metabolic pathways for cellular energy generation showing anaerobic glycolysis in the cytoplasm and the citrate cycle in the mitochondrion.

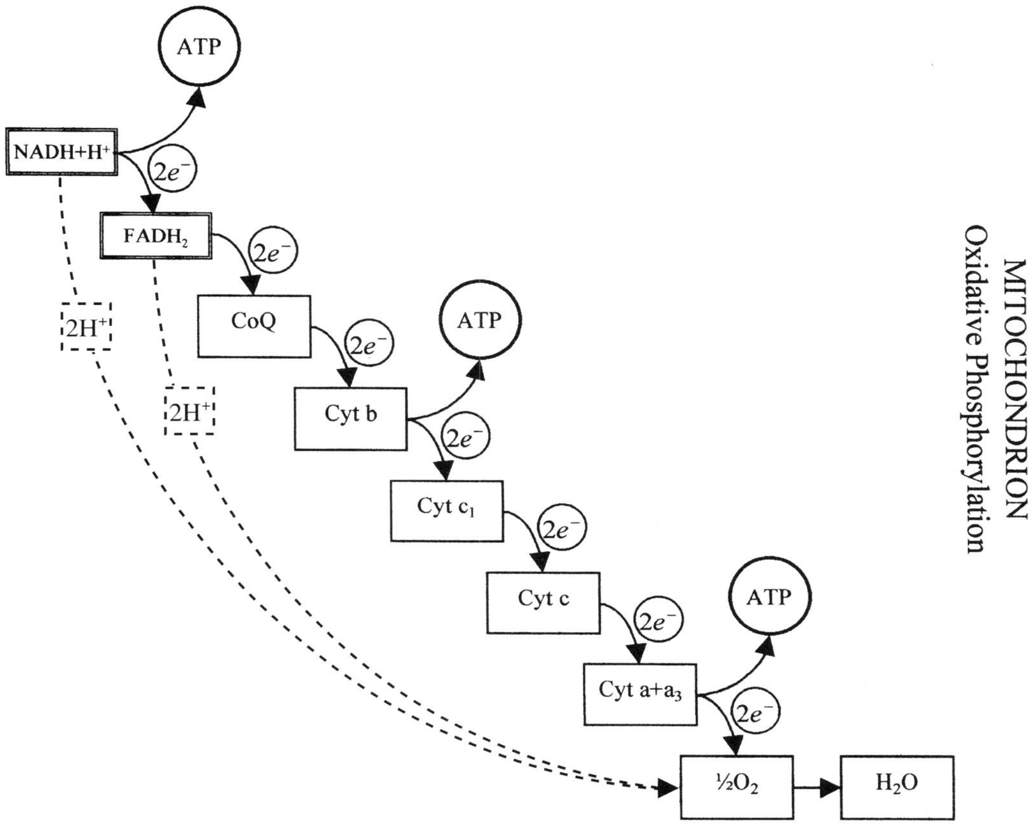


**Figure 1.3** Schematic representation of the mitochondrial electron transport chain.

5. Lactate effluxes into the plasma where bicarbonate buffering generates carbon dioxide.
6. Gas exchange and ventilatory changes occur in response to the need to eliminate the additional carbon dioxide.

A compromised ability to regenerate ATP from ADP by oxidative phosphorylation leads to the accumulation of ADP. In these circumstances the myokinase reaction can combine two ADP molecules to create one ATP molecule and one AMP molecule (see Equation 1.3). AMP is then degraded by the action of the enzyme myoadenylate deaminase to create inosine and ammonia (see Equation 1.4).

$$2ADP \rightarrow ATP + AMP \qquad (1.3)$$

$$AMP \rightarrow Inosine + NH_3 \qquad (1.4)$$

These secondary pathways of ATP regeneration seem to be invoked in various clinical conditions which result in cellular energy deprivation.

## Aerobic and anaerobic metabolism

Considerable controversy surrounds the use of the terms aerobic and anaerobic to describe the physiological responses to exercise because of the temptation to associate anaerobic metabolism simplistically with insufficient oxygen uptake by the body. During incremental exercise there is not a sudden switch from aerobic metabolism to anaerobic

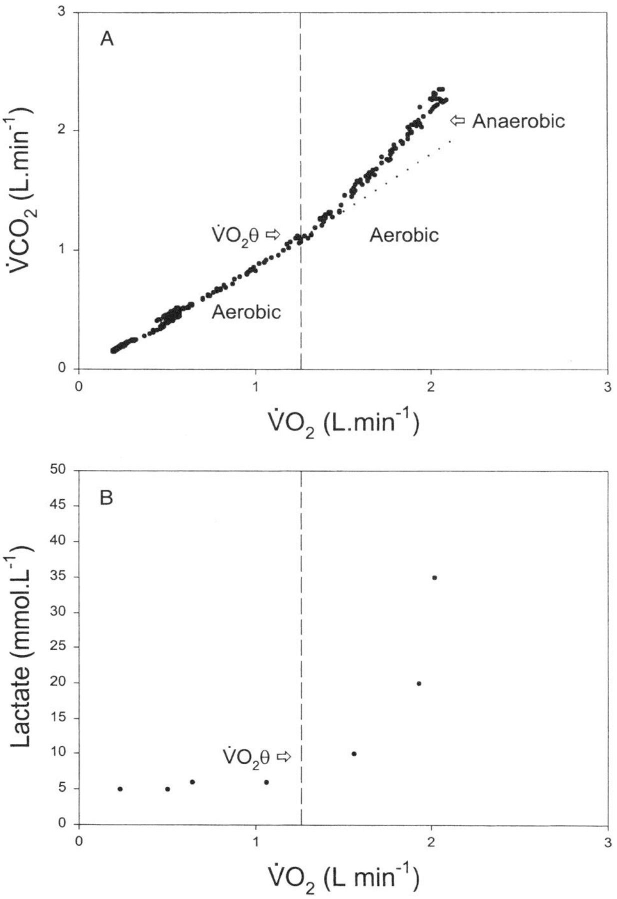


**Figure 1.4** Physiological domains of exercise showing the contribution of aerobic and anaerobic metabolism to gas exchange. (A) Changes in $\dot{V}CO_2$ with increasing $\dot{V}O_2$. (B) Corresponding increase in blood lactate. $\dot{V}O_2\theta$ is the metabolic threshold separating the aerobic from the aerobic plus anaerobic domains.

metabolism when the supply of oxygen runs short. Nevertheless, it is possible to distinguish two different domains of exercise intensity.

Lower-intensity exercise predominantly utilizes aerobic metabolic pathways, including oxidative phosphorylation for the regeneration of ATP. A small amount of lactate is formed in exercising muscle but blood lactate levels remain low and stable due to effective lactate disposal in other tissues. Constant work rate exercise of this intensity can be performed for long periods without fatigue and the physiological parameters of the exercise response exhibit a steady state.

By contrast, higher-intensity exercise utilizes a combination of aerobic and anaerobic metabolism in order to produce sufficient quantities of ATP. A sustained increase in blood lactate occurs, resulting in a measurable increase in carbon dioxide output derived from bicarbonate buffering, as illustrated in Figure 1.4. In other words, the physiological parameters of the exercise response do not achieve a steady state. A distinction between these two physiological domains of exercise intensity can often be made using noninvasive gas exchange measurements.

In summary, two domains of exercise intensity can be identified and, for the purposes of exercise testing and interpretation, it is helpful to consider the transition between these domains as a metabolic threshold. At the same time the terms aerobic and anaerobic should be used strictly to describe metabolic processes which respectively use oxygen or do not use oxygen regardless of its availability.

## Threshold concepts

Incremental exercise testing in a variety of circumstances is likely to reveal not only limitations to maximal performance but also certain thresholds of exercise intensity below or above which different physiological or pathological factors influence the exercise response. Some of these thresholds might be clear-cut. Others will be represented by more gradual transitions. The preceding discussion indicates that the transition from an exercise domain where metabolism is predominantly aerobic to a domain where anaerobic metabolism plays an increasing role is not necessarily clear-cut. However, for the purposes of exercise test interpretation, definition of this threshold has practical value. This is true for exercise tests that assess physical performance in apparently healthy subjects as well as tests which attempt to define exercise limitations in pa-

**Table 1.1.** Energetic properties of different metabolic substrates relevant to the exercise response

| Substrate | Respiratory quotient | Efficiency of energy storage ($kcal \cdot g^{-1}$) | Caloric equivalent for oxygen ($kcal \cdot l^{-1}$) | Caloric eqivalent for carbon dioxide ($kcal \cdot l^{-1}$) |
|---|---|---|---|---|
| Carbohydrate | 1.00 | 4.1 | 5.05 | 5.05 |
| Fat (e.g., palmitate) | 0.71 | 9.3 | 4.74 | 6.67 |
| Protein | 0.81 | 4.2 | 4.46 | 4.57 |

tients with illness. Other clinical thresholds of practical importance in patients with cardiovascular or pulmonary diseases undergoing exercise rehabilitation are described below in the section on exercise prescription.

## Energetics and substrate utilization

This section on basic exercise physiology concludes with a brief consideration of cellular energetics and substrate utilization. Whatever the substrate being used for muscle metabolism during exercise, it is important to consider the related processes of cellular energy generation both in terms of their efficiency and also the gas exchange and ventilatory consequences for the exercise response. Firstly, let us consider the chemical equations that define the complete oxidation of carbohydrate (glucose) and a fat (palmitate) in the presence of sufficient oxygen, to carbon dioxide and water.

For glucose:

$$C_6H_{12}O_6 + 36ADP + 36Pi + 6O_2 \rightarrow 6CO_2 + 6H_2O + 36ATP \quad (1.5)$$

For palmitate:

$$C_{15}H_{31}COOH + 129ADP + 129Pi + 23O_2 \rightarrow 16CO_2 + 16H_2O + 129ATP \quad (1.6)$$

These equations enable calculations of the respiratory quotient (RQ, or $\dot{V}CO_2$ divided by $\dot{V}O_2$), the efficiency of energy storage, and the caloric equivalents for oxygen and carbon dioxide of each metabolic substrate, as shown in Table 1.1. The corresponding values for protein are also included.

These different respiratory quotients are well known. Table 1.1 shows that fat is almost twice as efficient as a storage medium for energy as compared with both carbohydrate and protein. The caloric equivalents for oxygen indicate that carbohydrate is the most efficient substrate in terms of energy generation for every liter of oxygen used in its combustion. Work efficiency during an incremental exercise test, as illustrated by the relationship between external work rate ($\dot{W}$) and $\dot{V}O_2$ is clearly related to the caloric equivalent for oxygen of the substrate or substrates being metabolized during the study. Finally, the caloric equivalents for carbon dioxide serve as a reminder that fat generates less carbon dioxide than carbohydrate and should therefore demand a smaller ventilatory response.

## Exercise test nomenclature

Many terms have been used to describe exercise tests leading to some confusion with the nomenclature. However, exercise testing can be conveniently partitioned into two general disciplines, two principal settings and numerous specific protocols (Figure 1.5). The discipline, setting, and protocol of the exercise test should be appropriate for the purpose of the test with the intention of deriving the desired information with the greatest ease and fidelity. The two general exercise test disciplines are performance exercise testing (PXT) and clinical exercise testing (CXT). A PXT is usually performed on apparently healthy individuals for the purposes of quantification of aerobic capacity or fitness assessment, exercise prescription, and response to training or

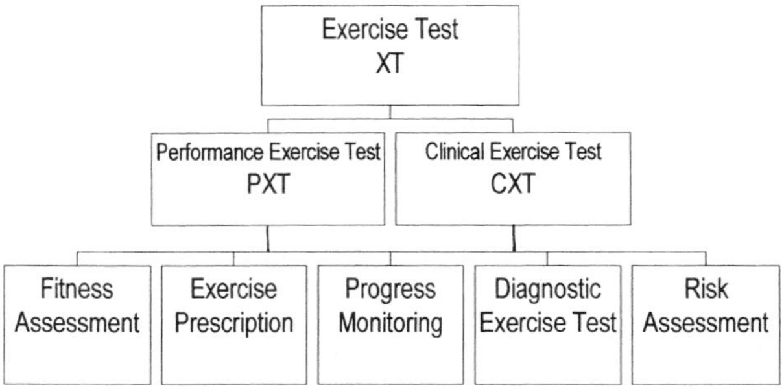


**Figure 1.5** A classification for exercise testing distinguishing performance exercise tests for healthy individuals from clinical exercise tests used for the evaluation and management of patients.

lifestyle modification. A CXT is performed on subjects presenting with symptoms and signs of disease for the purposes of diagnosis, risk assessment, progress monitoring, and response to therapeutic interventions. The setting for both PXT and CXT can be in the field or in the laboratory. The convention displayed in Figure 1.5 will be used throughout this book. Chapter 3 describes detailed methods for a variety of field and laboratory exercise tests within these categories.

## Evaluation of the exercise response

An exercise response might be judged normal or abnormal on the basis of one or more specific variables or based on a range of variables, which together constitute a physiological response pattern. The extent of this analysis clearly depends on what type of exercise test has been performed, how much data is available, and what the normal response would be expected to resemble. A normal response can be identified in the context of a true maximal or submaximal effort. On the other hand, when abnormalities are identified they need to be characterized according to certain recognized abnormal exercise response patterns (Table 1.2).

A detailed analysis of abnormal exercise response patterns is illustrated in Chapter 5. Cardiovascular limitation is normal, but when it is associated with an abnormal cardiovascular response pattern or impaired oxygen delivery, this points to diseases of the heart or circulation, or perhaps the effects of medications. Ventilatory limitation is usually abnormal and points to diseases of the lungs or respiratory muscles. Occasionally, one sees failure of ventilation due to abnormal control of breathing. With more sophisticated types of exercise testing, abnormalities of pulmonary gas exchange can be identified. This type of abnormality generally points to diseases of the lungs or pulmonary circulation. Reduced aerobic capacity and impairments of the metabolic response to exercise can be due to abnormalities of muscle metabolism due to inherited or acquired muscle disease. Finally, abnormal symptom perception can be associated with malingering or psychological disturbances. Figure 1.6 summarizes the principal categories of exercise limitation and indicates how many common conditions and diseases impact cardiovascular and ventilatory coupling to external work.

## Specific applications

Exercise testing has wide applications in health and disease. This section proffers several ways in which exercise testing may be employed, including assessment of physical fitness, evaluation of exercise intolerance, diagnosis of disease, exercise prescription both in sports and clinical rehabilitation, and evaluation of therapeutic interventions. These broad categories, along with more specific applications of exercise testing, are listed in Table 1.3.

### Assessment of physical fitness

Aerobic performance is one of the essential elements of physical fitness, along with muscle strength, flexibility, and body composition. Aerobic performance is defined by certain parameters that can be measured using carefully selected exercise-testing protocols. The best known of these parameters is maximum oxygen uptake ($\dot{V}O_{2max}$). The

**Table 1.2.** Recognizable exercise response patterns which assist in exercise test interpretation

| Normal response | Abnormal response |
|---|---|
| Maximal effort | Abnormal cardiovascular response pattern |
| Cardiovascular limitation | Impaired oxygen delivery |
| Suboptimal effort | Ventilatory limitation |
| | Abnormal ventilatory response pattern |
| | Abnormal ventilatory control |
| | Impaired gas exchange |
| | Abnormal muscle metabolism |
| | Abnormal symptom perception |

other parameters are the metabolic threshold ($\dot{V}o_2\theta$), work efficiency ($\eta$), and the time constant for oxygen uptake kinetics ($\tau\dot{V}o_2$). Each of these parameters is described in detail in Chapter 4. They can be derived with accuracy provided the appropriate instrumentation and testing methods are used, as described in Chapters 2 and 3. Determination of one or more of the parameters of aerobic performance for a given individual facilitates the prescription of exercise based on meaningful physiological data. Furthermore, the identification of the important metabolic markers such as $\dot{V}o_{2max}$, $\dot{V}o_2\theta$ and the ventilatory threshold ($\dot{V}_E\theta$) defines the physiological domains of exercise intensity for a given individual. These domains can in turn be used to prescribe an exercise program logically based on knowledge of the metabolic profile of that individual.

Exercise testing, with repeated determination of certain parameters, e.g., timed walking distance, $\dot{V}o_{2max}$ (directly measured or estimated), the relationship between $f_C$ and $\dot{W}$, and $\dot{V}o_2\theta$ can be used to track individual progression in response to exercise training or a program of rehabilitation. Properly conducted field tests using appropriate instruments (see Chapter 2) generally provide reliable results. Field tests are valuable for progress monitoring, even though absolute accuracy may be less than desired. This latter point is particularly applicable to estimations of $\dot{V}o_{2max}$.

## Evaluation of exercise intolerance

In the clinical laboratory specially designed exercise-testing protocols can be used to study the wide range of physiological variables during incremental exercise. Applied to a symptom-limited maximal exercise test, this approach facilitates the identification of specific physiological limitations for a given individual. Hence, when an individual complains of exercise intolerance, the physiological responses can be carefully examined to see if they offer a plausible explanation for the subject's symptoms.

A special application in the evaluation of exercise intolerance is disability evaluation. A successful disability claim often has important financial implications for the claimant. Thus, it needs to be supported by objective measures of exercise incapacity. The symptom-limited incremental exercise test identifies those with genuine exercise limitation, those who deliberately give a submaximal effort, and those who have normal exercise capacity despite their symptoms.

## Differential diagnosis of disease

### Cardiovascular diseases

One of the most valuable applications of clinical exercise testing is the ability to distinguish cardiovascular from pulmonary causes of exercise limitation. In the arena of clinical exercise testing, particularly with older subjects, cardiovascular and pulmonary diseases frequently coexist. The symptom-limited incremental exercise test helps identify which of these conditions is the limiting factor. This can have important implications in terms of the direction and goals of treatment.

A variety of incremental treadmill protocols have been used for the detection of myocardial ischemia due to coronary artery disease. These protocols are usually limited to measurement of heart rate, blood pressure, and a detailed recording of the electrocardiogram. The incremental exercise test can also identify early cardiovascular disease such as cardiomyopathy. However, it is often difficult to distinguish early cardiovascular disease from physical

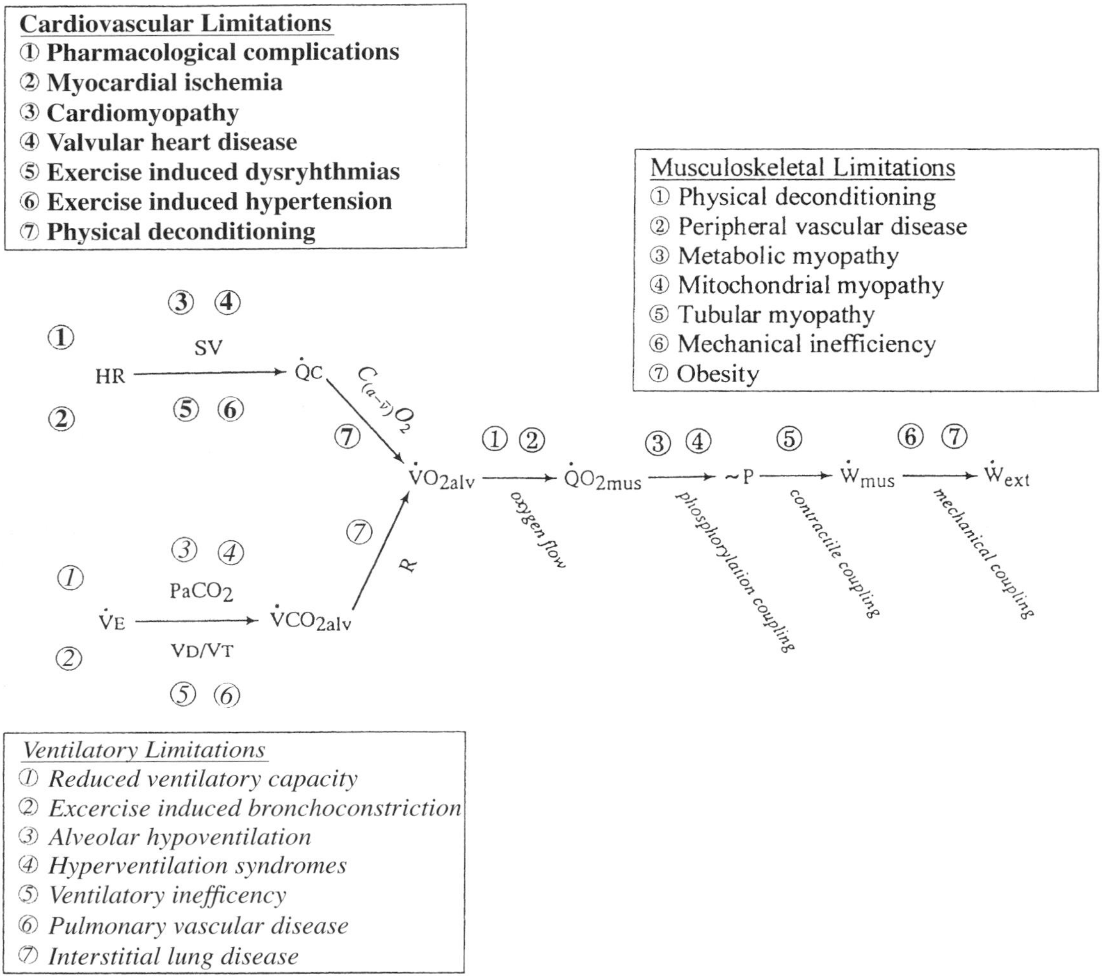


**Figure 1.6** Cardiovascular, ventilatory, and musculoskeletal limitations which affect the performance of external work.

deconditioning. This dilemma will always exist in the field of exercise assessment because the physiological consequences of these two conditions are similar. The best way to resolve this dilemma is by using exercise prescription and repeated testing to reveal how much of the physiological abnormality is reversible.

### Disorders of ventilation

Diseases of the lungs and respiratory muscles are usually characterized by pulmonary function testing as being either obstructive (e.g., asthma and chronic bronchitis) or restrictive (e.g., pulmonary fibrosis or respiratory muscle weakness). Unfortu-

**Table 1.3.** Specific applications of exercise testing

| Specific applications of exercise testing |
| --- |
| **Assessment of physical fitness** |
| Baseline fitness evaluation |
| Exercise training prescription |
| Demonstration of training response |
| **Evaluation of exercise intolerance** |
| Identification of specific physiological limitations |
| Disability evaluation |
| **Differential diagnosis of disease** |
| *Cardiovascular diseases* |
| Cardiomyopathy |
| Distinguishing cardiovascular from pulmonary disease |
| Screening for coronary artery disease |
| *Disorders of ventilation* |
| Obstructive pulmonary disease |
| Restrictive pulmonary disease |
| Hyperventilation syndrome |
| *Disorders of pulmonary gas exchange* |
| Interstitial lung disease |
| Pulmonary vascular disease |
| *Diseases of muscle* |
| Distinguishing myalgia from myopathy |
| *Psychological disorders* |
| Malingering |
| Anxiety |
| Secondary gain |
| **Exercise prescription** |
| Physical training |
| Clinical rehabilitation |
| **Evaluation of other therapeutic interventions** |
| *Lifestyle modifications* |
| Nutritional |
| Weight management |
| Smoking cessation |
| *Pharmacological interventions* |
| Ergogenic drugs |
| Oxygen therapy |
| *Surgical interventions* |
| Preoperative risk assessment |
| Coronary artery bypass grafting (CABG) |
| Valve replacement |
| Cardiac transplantation |
| Lung volume reduction surgery (LVRS) |
| Lung transplantation |

nately, this categorization does not predict what physiological limitations or inefficiencies these types of disease impose during exercise. Symptom-limited incremental exercise testing reveals those individuals with true ventilatory limitation dictated by mechanical factors and those with abnormalities of ventilatory control. Furthermore, a detailed study of breathing pattern can be undertaken at various stages of exercise intensity.

### Disorders of pulmonary gas exchange

Incremental exercise remains the best method for challenging the mechanisms of pulmonary gas exchange and detecting early interstitial lung disease. By the same token, sequential exercise testing offers the most accurate means of assessing progression of interstitial lung disease and the response to treatment. Physiological abnormalities can be detected at maximal exercise when resting pulmonary function tests and arterial blood gases are normal. A specific situation where knowledge of whether or not someone has abnormal pulmonary gas exchange is important is the person who might have interstitial lung disease from an occupational exposure (e.g., asbestos).

### Diseases of muscle

Increasing numbers of patients complain of muscle soreness on exercise or one of the fatigue syndromes. Incremental exercise testing provides the means of determining whether exercise capacity is truly diminished, and again points to the specific physiological limitations. An exercise-testing laboratory can evaluate patients with myalgia to determine whether muscle biopsy is justifiable. When the pattern of the exercise response suggests myopathy, a muscle biopsy can be requested with special histochemical stains and electron microscopy. Thus, exercise testing finds a role in making the important distinction between myalgia and true myopathy.

### Psychological disorders

A variety of psychological conditions present with exercise intolerance. Exercise capacity may be surprisingly normal. More commonly, exercise capacity is reduced. This may be due to simple deconditioning from inactivity. Alternatively, it may appear that the physiological responses to submaximal exercise are normal and that exercise capacity is consciously or subconsciously reduced for nonphysiological reasons. Observation of the pattern of submaximal effort is particularly helpful in this type of evaluation.

Experienced exercise laboratory staff often find they have the ability to detect when an individual is not genuinely limited. Discreet inquiry can reveal that these individuals receive secondary gains from their apparent disability. Other psychological problems such as anxiety and hyperventilation are readily observed in the setting of the exercise laboratory. Laboratories should develop reliable methods for reporting these types of observation (e.g., using psychometric scales).

## Exercise prescription

### Apparently healthy individuals

Increasing numbers of healthy individuals seek an exercise prescription for the maintenance of physical fitness. Individuals training for competition demand more intensive physical training. In both of these situations, the exercise prescription is best developed on the basis of formal exercise testing.

Traditional approaches have relied upon estimates of maximum heart rate to determine a "training zone." These methods, whilst unarguably effective to some extent, cannot be regarded as totally reliable. A preferred approach is to use exercise testing to define the metabolic domains of exercise intensity, which exist for a given individual. These domains can be anchored by heart rates or ratings of perceived exertion and linked to metabolic energy expenditure. Exercise programming can then be devised with a true scientific basis.

Given that baseline exercise testing is the most reliable method for establishing an exercise prescription, thereafter repeated exercise testing is necessary to document improvement in aerobic performance, or improved performance for a specific field event.

**Table 1.4.** Clinical exercise thresholds relevant to cardiac and pulmonary rehabilitation

| Cardiac rehabilitation | Pulmonary rehabilitation |
|---|---|
| Metabolic (lactate) | Metabolic (lactate) |
| Myocardial ischemia (angina) | Hypoxemic (desaturation) |
| Hypertension | Dyspneic (breathlessness) |
| Hypotension | Tachypneic (anxiety) |
| Dysrhythmia | |

### Individuals with recognized illness

Exercise prescription is widely used in the discipline of rehabilitation, whether this is after musculoskeletal injury, myocardial infarction, or exacerbation of chronic pulmonary disease. Again, baseline exercise testing establishes an appropriate exercise prescription and repeated testing documents progress. In the cases of individuals with known cardiovascular or pulmonary diseases, specific thresholds need to be identified so that the exercise prescription can be delivered effectively within documented margins of safety.

Table 1.4 illustrates the important pathophysiological thresholds that may exist in individuals with recognized cardiovascular or pulmonary disease. Identification of these thresholds assists in developing a safe and effective exercise prescription for patients undergoing cardiac or pulmonary rehabilitation and is thus an important outcome of exercise testing. Importantly, individuals with cardiovascular and pulmonary diseases, even severe, should not be denied the potential benefits of regular exercise participation. Rather, they should be encouraged to exercise within safe limits to overcome the otherwise inevitable consequences of inactivity that would lead to physical deconditioning and contribute to a worsening of their overall health and quality of life. In this regard, exercise testing is a valuable asset.

## Evaluation of other therapeutic interventions

### Lifestyle modifications

Every year in the USA, 40 million individuals seek to reduce their body weight by nutritional or other means. Dietary adjustment alone is inappropriate without an exercise regimen. Therefore proper exercise prescription plays an essential role in weight management. Sequential exercise testing, either by simple field tests or with determination of oxygen uptake, documents the anticipated improvement in exercise capacity which in turn serves as positive feedback to the individual.

Another lifestyle modification which is important for many individuals is smoking cessation. Coupled with a carefully programmed exercise regimen, smoking cessation should lead to significant physical reconditioning and improvement in exercise capacity.

### Pharmacological interventions

The sports industry has long been preoccupied with debate as to whether certain drugs have ergogenic properties, i.e. whether they themselves increase exercise capacity. Statements about the ergogenic capabilities of many drugs are exaggerated. However, the appropriate means of determining whether a drug itself is responsible for increased exercise capacity is to conduct field tests, maximal exercise tests, or comparison of key physiological variables for selected submaximal exercise protocols.

In the clinical arena, many pharmacological agents are prescribed with the intention, directly or indirectly, of improving exercise capacity and ability to perform the activities of daily living. These agents include drugs purported to improve skeletal muscle contractility, cardiac output, and ventilatory capacity or alternatively to reduce blood pressure, fatigue, breathlessness, or other limiting symptoms. Exercise testing is necessary to demonstrate objective evidence of such improvements.

### Surgical interventions

Several studies have attested to the usefulness of exercise testing in preoperative risk assessment, particularly in patients with moderate and severe cardiac or pulmonary disease. In the past, many surgeons relied on intuition or a simple exercise challenge like stair climbing to assess physical fitness before surgery. Often their judgments were accurate, although not necessarily based on objective measures. In the modern era, with the availability of a range of formal exercise tests, actual determination of exercise capacity is appropriate. Maximum oxygen uptake and also the metabolic threshold of lactate accumulation have been shown to have discriminatory value.

Exercise testing has been used to assess patients awaiting heart and lung transplantation. The information which formal testing provides has been successfully used to prescribe rehabilitative exercise and obtain surprising improvements in exercise capacity in these groups of patients. Indeed, the rehabilitative improvements in some cardiac patients have been sufficient to obviate the need for transplantation. A similar approach might be considered before other types of cardiac surgery.

A surgical approach is now advocated for certain patients with severe emphysema. One of the major claims of so-called lung volume reduction surgery is improvement in exercise capacity. Indeed, this should be a primary goal if such surgery is to become widely accepted. Consequently, this type of intervention needs to be evaluated by formal exercise testing before and after surgery.

## Conclusion

The ability to perform exercise is one of the most fundamental aspects of human existence. The ability to test exercise performance is therefore of utmost importance whether a subject desires athletic performance, exercise prescription, diagnosis of exercise limitation, or evaluation of a therapeutic intervention. This book attempts to bring a level of sophistication to exercise testing and interpretation that, if embraced, can greatly enhance the expertise of exercise professionals and increase the value of the information they provide.

## FURTHER READING

Åstrand, P.-O. & Rodahl, K. (1986). *Textbook of Work Physiology. Physiological Bases of Exercise*, 3rd edn. New York: McGraw-Hill.

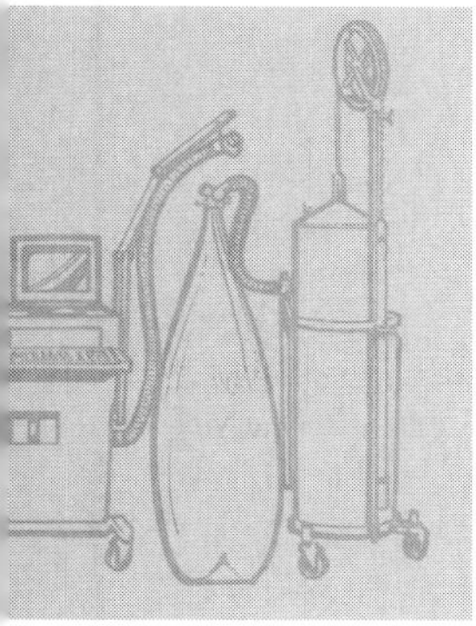

# 2

# Instrumentation

## Introduction

Before exercise tolerance is evaluated, the practitioner must carefully consider a number of factors that will ultimately influence the interpretation of results and ensuing interventions. These include the purpose of the test (Chapter 1), key variables required for accurate test interpretation (Chapter 4), and the best test available for the test objectives (Chapter 3). In considering which data will best serve these objectives, the practitioner should select the most appropriate instrumentation available for their collection. This chapter presents a number of instrumentation options in the context of test purposes and data desired for interpretation. These include relatively simple field tests, submaximal laboratory tests, and maximal effort tests. Details of actual application of these instruments will be presented in Chapter 3. Each instrument will be presented with its description and principle of operation followed by methods of calibration, its accuracy, and precision. Maintenance of the instrument is also discussed. This chapter begins with a brief review of important measurement concepts that influence instrument selection. Figure 2.1 illustrates these concepts.

## Measurement concepts

### Validation

An instrument is thought to be valid if it accurately measures the variable(s) it is said to measure. For example, a heart rate meter is valid if it accurately represents the true value of the heart rate. It is prudent for the practitioner to ensure the accuracy of measurement instruments. This requires periodic validation studies in which the instrument in question is compared against a "gold standard" or reference method in its ability to measure the variable in question. Unfortunately, absolute accuracy can only be determined if one is absolutely certain of the true value. This may be impossible. Thus, one must decide how much deviation from the true value (error) is acceptable. This decision should be made prior to the purchase of any instrumentation.

### Calibration

Calibration is a procedure in which an instrument is adjusted consequent to its measurement of values for a variable known to be true. For example, when a scale is being calibrated, known weights are placed on the scale that is then adjusted according to the scale's reading. It is important that calibrations be performed over the expected range of measurement for the variable of interest. Generally, this requires multiple trials with different known values. Again, using the scale example, if a laboratory scale was to be used for children, it might be reasonable to ensure calibration over a range of 20–50 kg, whereas in a sports medicine setting, a range of 80–180 kg may be more appropriate. Instrumentation should be purchased in consideration of the range of expected measurements. Calibration is not validation.

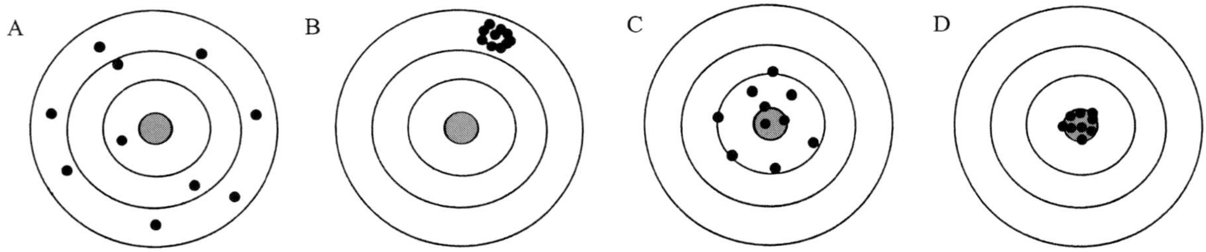


**Figure 2.1** Illustrations of accuracy and precision using the analogy of shots fired at targets. (A) Poor precision and poor accuracy. (B) Good precision and poor accuracy. (C) Improved precision and improved accuracy. (D) Good precision and good accuracy.

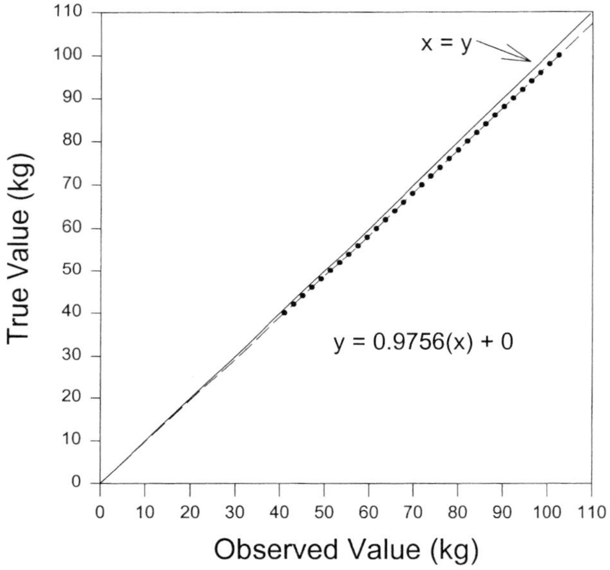


**Figure 2.2** A calibration curve using the example of data obtained from the calibration of a laboratory scale. The true value for the measurement is plotted on the *y*-axis while the corresponding observed value is plotted on the *x*-axis. The regression equation is used to correct future measurements.

### What to do with calibration data

In the event that the instrument cannot be physically adjusted to provide the true value, mathematical "adjustments" can be made in the form of a calibration curve. Suppose calibration is desired over the range of 40–100 kg, using the scale example suggested above. Known precision weights in 2-kg increments are set upon the scale and the observed value recorded from the scale's display. The true value (precision weight) is plotted against the observed value. A curve is then fitted to the data depending upon which model best fits the plotted data. A regression equation is obtained which is then applied to future observations. Figure 2.2 illustrates this method. Thus, if a subject is weighed on this scale with an observed value of 80 kg, applying the calibration curve would give the more accurate weight of $(80 \times 0.9756) + 0$ or 78 kg.

## Accuracy

Accuracy refers to the ability of an instrument to measure its true value. If an instrument is accurate it is also said to be valid and reliable (or precise). For example if an oxygen analyzer reads a calibration gas certified to be 16.00% as 16.00%, it is accurate for that value. The oxygen analyzer (or, by extension, any other instrument) may not be accurate at another value. Instruments should have the capability of acceptable accuracy over the range of values one expects to measure.

## Precision

Precision (reliability) indicates the ability of an instrument to yield the same measurement for a variable when that variable is measured repeatedly over time. Precision does not necessarily infer accuracy.

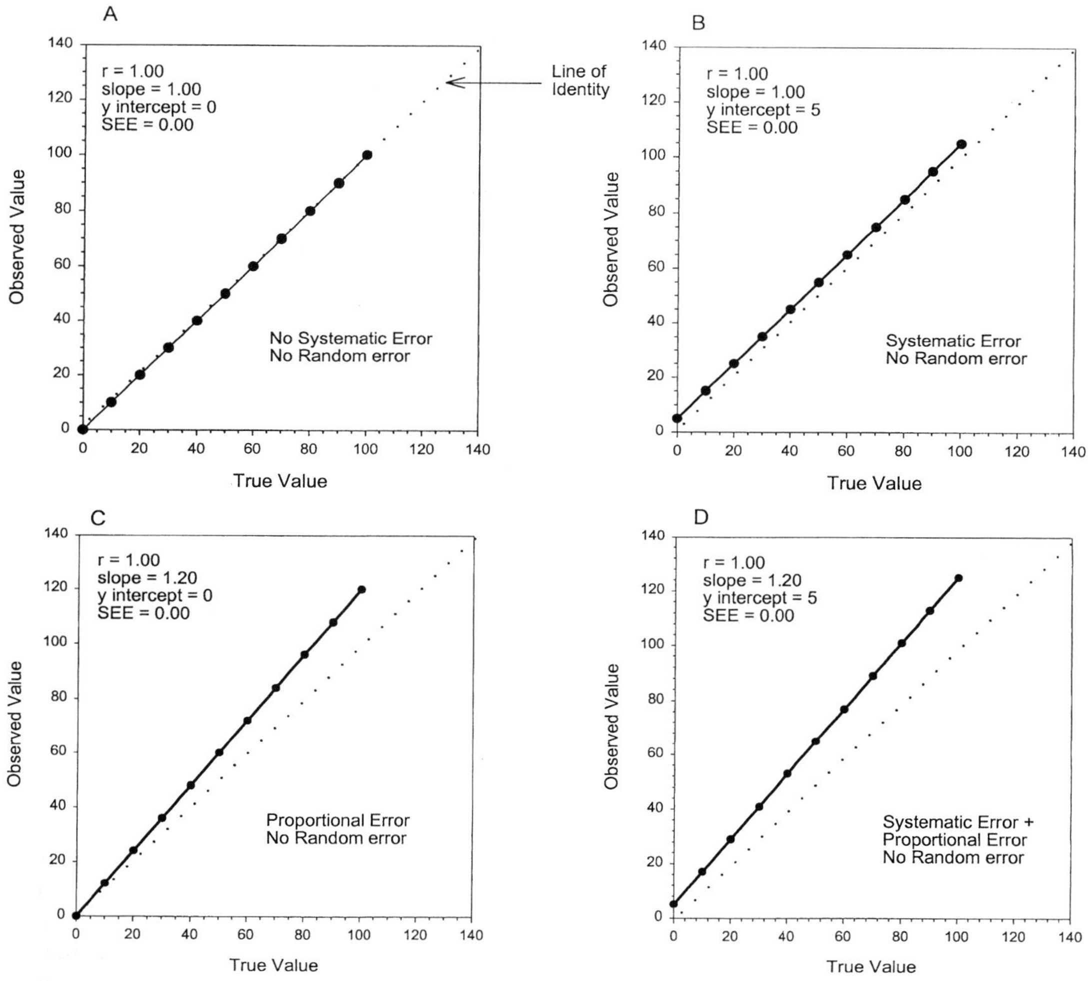


**Figure 2.3** Examples of systematic errors. Observed values are plotted on the *y*-axes with corresponding true values plotted on the *x*-axes. Each of the four panels represents a different type of systematic error.

## Error

Error reflects deviations from the true value and can be separated into random and systematic errors (Figure 2.3). Thus, for any measurement, the observation is equal to the true value plus the random error and the systematic error. Random errors (often referred to as noise) are unpredictable deviations from the true value. In Figure 2.1A, the sum of all the random errors is zero (i.e., there would be as many negative errors as positive ones). Random error adds variability to the data but does not affect the mean score.

Systematic error is caused by factors that have definite value and direction. As such, they tend to result in observations that are consistently either greater than or lesser than the true value. Presumably, these errors can be identified and corrected. Systematic errors may derive from the instrument itself (e.g., gas analyzer drift), from the manner in which the instrument is used including methods (e.g., failure to change the Nafion® gas sample line regularly) or from the technician performing the measurement (e.g., terminal digit bias in reading blood pressure). Systematic error is often called bias in measurement.

## Measured courses

### Introduction

The use of an established route with a known distance for exercise can be of value in settings where more sophisticated measurements are either inappropriate or unavailable. Severely limited patients may be able to walk for only short distances before they are forced to stop because of shortness of breath, claudication, or severely compromised oxygen delivery, such as in patients with chronic heart failure. Apparently healthy individuals are often able to complete the measured course by running.

The practitioner may wish to consider whether the measured course should be one with distance or time as the criterion variable. For example, will the patient respond best, and are conditions better controlled, when the patient covers a specified distance (e.g., 400 m) with time as the criterion measurement? Or, is it more desirable if the patient exercises for a specific period of time (e.g., 12 min) with distance covered as the criterion variable?

Both approaches are frequently used, but the measurement of time to complete a premeasured distance is preferable as both time and distance can be known more precisely. When a patient walks for a fixed period of time, distance can be measured, but often with less precision, and usually with more difficulty. Additionally, knowing, and when possible, being able to see the distance to be covered seem to set a more easily interpreted endpoint for the participant.

Walking and running courses should be chosen so that barriers and hazards are kept clear. A busy hospital corridor is clearly an inappropriate place. However, underutilized corridors, or other areas in medical or rehabilitation facilities, parking lots, school tracks, or sports facilities are ideal.

### Indoor courses

#### Description and principle of operation

Indoor walking courses are typically shorter due to space limitations and may be appropriate for more severely disabled individuals. Indoor courses have the advantage of controlling for temperature, wind, and air-borne pollutants that might adversely affect the test outcome. Additionally, patient monitoring may be easier to perform. Indoor courses should be chosen with care not to include too many turns (which slows down the pace) or distractions that may influence test performance. This latter point is especially important for the elderly, in whom multitasking may lead to falls. This may even include attempting to attend to the task of walking while attention is diverted to a changing floor pattern.

Measured courses used for walking should have few turns (especially U-turns) and distances of 100–400 m. Courses established for shuttle walking or running tests require only 10 or 20 m, respectively, plus turn areas of 5 m at each end. See Chapter 3 for an illustration and description of the shuttle course.

#### Calibration, accuracy, and precision

A measuring wheel provides the easiest way to measure a walking or running course accurately. Alternatively, careful measurement with a 30-m tape measure would be acceptable. The accuracy of such courses need not be perfect. However, reproducible starting and ending points, as well as a reproducible route, are of primary importance. Marks along the baseboard on a wall or on the floor are useful for tallying distance covered. The walking or running path should be clearly delineated so that the patient is sure of the route.

#### Maintenance

Measured courses should be kept clear of obstacles (including other people), with care taken to ensure a flat, regular surface.

### Outdoor courses

#### Description and principle of operation

Because of fewer space constraints, outdoor courses may be longer, more wide-open, and contain fewer turns. Eighth-mile (220-yd or about 200-m) and longer courses are ideal. The 20-m shuttle test may also be administered outdoors (see Figure 2.4). Good outdoor courses can be established in controlled parking lots, schoolyards, running tracks, or any open space. The longer outdoor courses are especially useful for less limited individuals, including those who are able to run. Variables to be considered, however, include climatic conditions and the need to monitor patients closely.

#### Calibration, accuracy, and precision

As with the indoor courses, a measuring wheel allows the easiest and most accurate way to measure outdoor walking or running courses. Careful measurement with a 30-m tape measure is an acceptable alternative. The accuracy of such courses need not be perfect. Reproducible start, finish, and the walking or running path should be clearly delineated. For example, walking on the inside curb of a 400-m track will result in walking 400 m per lap. However, walking in the outside lane of a nine-lane track will increase the distance. Cones or other similar markers are useful in identifying the limits of the shuttle course.

#### Maintenance

See the section on indoor courses, above.

## Timing devices

### Introduction

The accurate measurement of time is basic to exercise testing and provides the construct of rate. Since many measurements are expressed as a rate such as the work rate ($\dot{W}$), the oxygen uptake rate, and speed, accurate measurements of time are import-

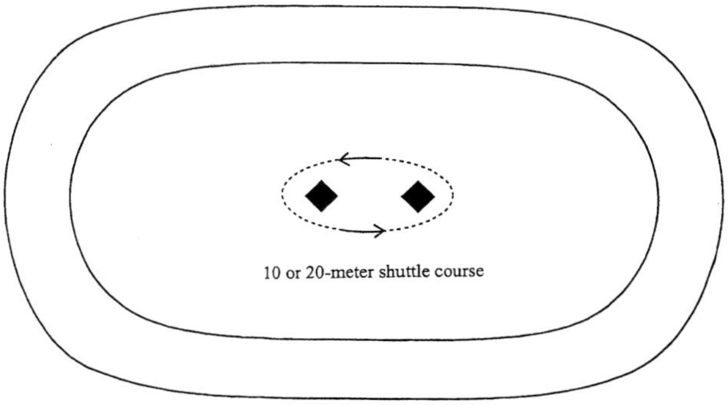


**Figure 2.4** Outdoor course layouts for timed walks, runs, and shuttle walks or runs. Any open space is appropriate for these purposes. A 400-m track, as shown, is ideal.

ant. Other laboratory instruments such as pedal cadence (r.p.m.) indicators and metronomes could be considered as timing devices.

### Chronometers

#### Description and principle of operation

Included in this category are laboratory clocks and stopwatches. Laboratory clocks typically are not used to time activities with great precision, but rather for gross estimates, signaling the timing of events such as taking blood pressure or administering psychometric scales during an exercise test. Thus, a laboratory clock should be visible throughout the exercise test.

Stopwatches are better suited for precise timing during data collection such as in collecting exhaled air in a Douglas bag for subsequent analysis, timed walking tests (see above), measurement of heart rate by palpation, or the precise duration of an exercise test. Additionally, accurate stopwatches are essential for calibrating treadmill speeds and cycle ergometer r.p.m. indicators.

#### Calibration, accuracy, and precision

Calibration of chronometers is usually performed against another chronometer that can be simultaneously started and stopped. Modern battery-powered digital stopwatches with tenth- or hundredth-second resolution possess sufficient accuracy and precision for laboratory use. Technician error may be of some concern if the chronometer is systematically actuated with the thumb instead of the index finger, the former resulting in poorer correspondence between the actual start of the event and the start of the watch due to a slower response time with the thumb. In the case of determining heart rate by palpation, starting the watch on a heart beat requires that the heart beat count corresponding with the start of the watch is zero. Errors may be magnified if the pulse count is for time intervals shorter than a minute.

### Maintenance

Chronometers should be handled carefully and not subjected to impact by dropping or coming in forcible contact with other objects. They should be kept dry and free from exposure to dirt or dust. Digital stopwatches are inexpensive and generally resistant to damage from all but gross mishandling.

## Counters

### Description and principle of operation

Counters may include pedal revolution counters and r.p.m. indicators. One or both of these are essential when exercise tests employ mechanically braked ergometers. For these ergometers, work rate calculations require knowledge of workload, distance traveled by the flywheel per revolution of the crank arms, and crank r.p.m. Since r.p.m. can be quite variable, especially at the end of a test or in subjects who have difficulty in maintaining a constant cadence, a counting device is indispensable. Pedal revolution counters are usually mechanical, incrementing numerically when a lever is tripped by the passing pedal crank. The r.p.m. indicator on mechanically braked ergometers (also known as a tachometer) is mechanically linked with a cable from the flywheel to an analog dial, providing visual feedback and thus enabling maintenance of a predetermined pedaling frequency.

### Calibration, accuracy, and precision

Calibration of the pedal revolution counter is simple, requiring only that a manual count of pedal revolutions is made simultaneously with the counter recording each revolution. For the r.p.m. indicator, calibration is obtained by turning the crank arms at a constant pedal frequency, e.g., 60 r.p.m., over a period of about a minute and noting the position of the tachometer needle on the analog dial. Although some variability in cadence is likely, an experienced human subject may be able to maintain a relatively constant r.p.m. allowing calibration. Alternatively, one feature of commercially available cycle ergometer dynamic torque meters (see below) is the ability to provide constant and known crank revolution rates.

### Maintenance

Counters typically require little maintenance other than occasional lubrication and alignment. As they are mechanical devices, they are subject to wear and may move from their original position.

## Metronomes

### Description and principle of operation

Metronomes are useful in helping subjects maintain pedaling cadence at fixed rates, e.g., 60 r.p.m. or, in the case of step tests, at a constant rate of stepping, such as 24 steps per minute. When possible, the metronome should provide both auditory and visual cues to assist the subject in maintaining the desired cadence. Metronomes may be either mechanical or electrical, emitting an audible tone precisely timed at the selected interval. In the case of electrical metronomes, a visual signal in the form of a flashing light may also be produced coincident with the audible signal. An alternative to the mechanical or electric metronome is a prerecorded audiotape with sounds recorded at precise intervals.

### Calibration, accuracy, and precision

Like pedal revolution counters and r.p.m. indicators, metronomes require calibration against an accurate chronometer. Correlating the audible signal with the digital display of a chronometer will provide a satisfactory approach to calibration. Counting a fixed number of tones from the metronome and dividing by the time elapsed over those tones will give the true rate. For example, if a metronome is set to deliver tones for 70 r.p.m. (140 tones in a minute, one for each pedal down stroke), the elapsed time for 35 tones should be 15 s (0.25 min). Metronomes, especially the electrical varieties, are usually precise. Accuracy of ±3 counts per minute is reasonable.

### Maintenance

Little maintenance is required other than careful handling and storage and protection against forcible contact with other objects as in dropping.

## Ergometers

### Introduction

Ergometers are used in the laboratory to provide an exercise stimulus in order to examine a subject's physiological response to that exercise. Different ergometers, e.g., leg cycles, arm cycles, and treadmills, provide different stimuli, abilities to quantify work rate, and physiological responses to the task-specific exercise. This section reviews typical laboratory ergometers, their characteristics, advantages and disadvantages, and appropriates uses. A typical selection of ergometers is shown in Figure 2.5. Of considerable importance is choosing the correct ergometer relative to the goals of the test. This is of particular importance in sports medicine applications in which training prescriptions and progress monitoring require attention to the law of task specificity, i.e., making assessments on apparatus as nearly identical to the training mode as possible.

The most common ergometers used in clinical exercise testing (CXT) are the cycle and treadmill ergometers. Each possesses distinct advantages and disadvantages that are summarized below. The choice of which apparatus to use should be based on the goals of the test and subject abilities. In view of these considerations, other ergometers, such as arm ergometers, rowing ergometers, or other work devices specific to the work task, may prove more appropriate. Recommendations for choice of work device are presented in Table 2.1. Figure 2.6 illustrates a comparison of physiological data collected with treadmills and cycle ergometers.

### Cycle ergometers

#### Description and principle of operation

*Mechanically braked ergometers*

With this type of cycle ergometer (which may be used for both leg work and arm work), resistance is typically applied by a heat-resistant friction apparatus (typically either a band surrounding a weighted metal flywheel of known circumference or caliper brakes). The resistance is increased or decreased by tightening or loosening the friction apparatus. It must be realized, however, that additional resistance arises from the ergometer drive train, which is comprised of the chain, sprockets, and bottom bracket. In a well-maintained ergometer, this added friction resistance is on the order of 5–10%. Only with dynamic calibration can this resistance be quantified. See the section on ergometer calibration in this chapter (below) for details.

The work rate on friction-braked ergometers is determined by the force in Newtons (N) or Kiloponds (kp) applied as resistance against the flywheel, pedal frequency (r.p.m.), and distance traveled by the flywheel per crank arm revolution. Although mechanically braked ergometers typically include an r.p.m. indicator, the work rate may be variable and unknown if pedal frequency is not known with a reasonable degree of accuracy. The

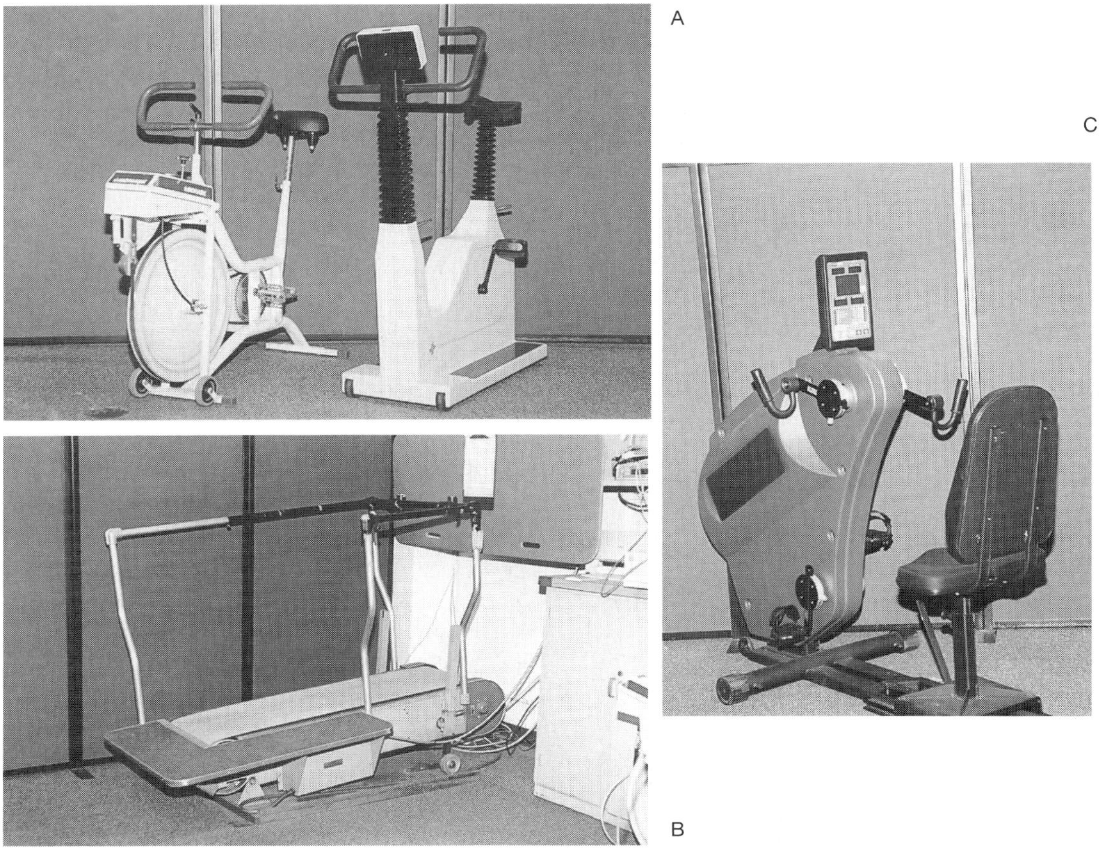


**Figure 2.5** Ergometers commonly used for exercise testing. (A) Cycle ergometers. Left: mechanically braked; right: electrically braked. (B) Treadmill ergometer. (C) Arm ergometer.

ergometer may be instrumented with revolution counters (see above) to verify pedal frequency and thus work rate. The actual work rates should always be used rather than making the assumption that work rate is a function of a constant pedal frequency, when this frequency is in fact variable. This is especially true at peak exercise where pedal rate may drop by more than 10 r.p.m.

*Effect of cadence errors on work rate and oxygen uptake* For every 1 r.p.m. above or below the expected value, $\dot{W}$ (in watts) will be in error by approximately 2%. Thus, a true work rate would be 10% lower than expected if the actual pedal frequency was 6 r.p.m. less than expected. The consequence on the expected $\dot{V}O_2$ at a given $\dot{W}$ would be slightly less, averaging about 1.3% higher or lower than expected for every one pedal revolution above or below expected. Hence, the 6 r.p.m. error noted above would result in a $\dot{V}O_2$ that was about 8% less than expected. Table C11 in Appendix C illustrates the effect of erroneous r.p.m. values on a range of $\dot{W}$ and predicted $\dot{V}O_2$ values.

One of the chief advantages of cycle ergometers is the capability of accurate presentation of work rate (also called power output). Work rate is expressed in watts or kilogram meters per minute ($kg \cdot m \cdot min^{-1}$), more correctly referred to as kilopond meters per

**Table 2.1.** Recommendations for choice of ergometer used in exercise testing

| Ergometer | Applications | Patient/subject | Comments |
|---|---|---|---|
| Leg cycle | Evaluate breathlessness, chest pain, claudication, baseline for exercise prescription or progress monitoring | Symptomatic<br>Apparently healthy, rehabilitation | Preferred ergometer for CXT due to increased control of work rate and ease of measurement |
| Treadmill | Evaluate functional capacity<br>Evaluate breathlessness, chest pain, claudication, baseline for exercise prescription or progress monitoring | Symptomatic<br>Apparently healthy, rehabilitation | Most common form of exercise; largest use of muscle mass; highest $\dot{V}O_{2max}$<br>Consider value of task-specificity between testing and training |
| Arm ergometry | Evaluate breathlessness, chest pain, claudication, baseline for exercise prescription or progress monitoring | Individuals using wheelchairs, spinal cord-injured, back pain, rehabilitation, pregnancy, task-specific sports | Back pain prohibits walking and/or sitting on cycle |

minute ($kpm \cdot min^{-1}$). The correct Système Internationale (SI) units are joules per second ($J \cdot s^{-1}$). Conversion constants for these different expressions of work rate are presented in Table B1 in Appendix B.

Estimation of the expected oxygen uptake at a given work rate may be more accurate in cycle ergometry since the power output of a subject at a given load and r.p.m. is similar for all subjects of similar body weight. This proves to be advantageous when performing biological calibrations.

Friction-braked ergometers have the additional advantage of being relatively inexpensive, rugged, easy to calibrate, and require no electrical supply. These characteristics make them ideally suited for safe transport and for field studies.

*Electrically braked ergometers*

As with the mechanically braked ergometers, electrically (or electromagnetically) braked ergometers may be used for either leg or arm work. Depending on the design of these ergometers, control of electrical current results in a braking action as the subject pedals. The load or braking force is inversely proportional to pedaling rate at any chosen work rate. If a subject pedals faster, the voltage, and thus the load, decreases. The converse is true for decreases in pedal frequency. Thus, electrically braked cycle ergometers have the distinct advantage over their mechanical counterparts in being able to maintain the desired work rate independent of any pedal frequency between about 40 and 80 r.p.m. Electrical braking and the negative feedback loop, which adjusts load inversely to pedal rate, is the most accurate method of determining external power output. Digital computer algorithms allowing small increments in work rate for ramp protocols (see Chapter 3) may control small voltage changes and thus enable very small increments in work rate, e.g., $0.25\,W \cdot s^{-1}$ for a $15\,W \cdot min^{-1}$ ramp.

Some electrically braked ergometers have the capability of regulating the ergometer work rate by a heart rate feedback circuit. The ergometer continuously monitors the heart rate and adjusts the braking voltage to allow maintenance of a preset heart rate. The work rates change in order to maintain the desired heart rate. Applications for this type of ergometer may be seen in the $PWC_{170}$ test in which the work rate at a heart rate of 170 beats $\cdot\, min^{-1}$ provides a measure of cardiovascular fitness, and also in training programs where strict maintenance of a target heart rate is required.

*Additional cycle ergometer concerns*

All cycle ergometers should provide visual feedback of the pedal frequency to the subject. An acoustical indicator, such as a metronome, is a valuable

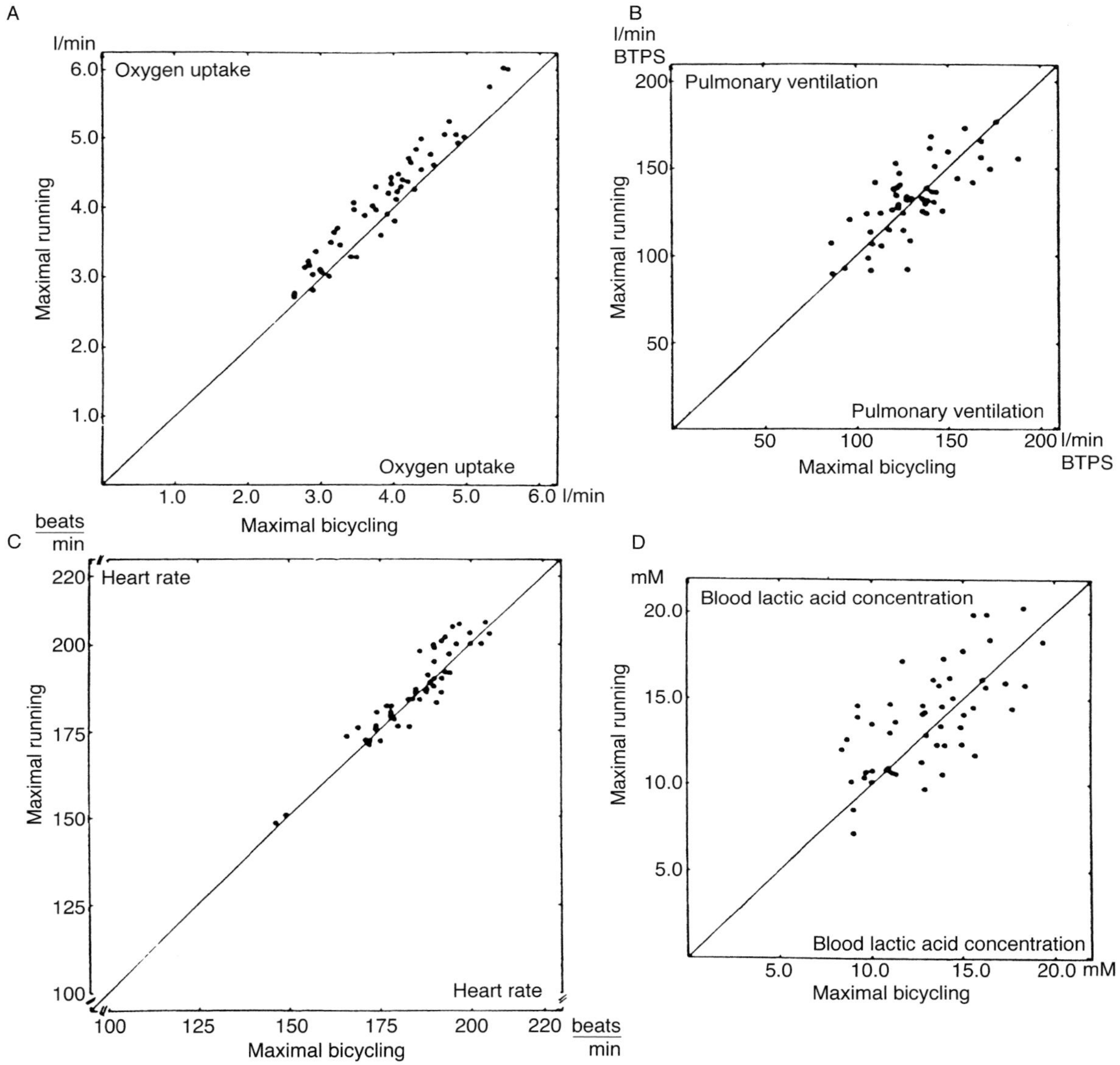


**Figure 2.6** Comparison of maximal responses to treadmill and cycle exercise. Reproduced with permission from Hermansen, L. & Saltin, B. (1969). Oxygen uptake during maximal treadmill and bicycle exercise. *J. Appl. Physiol.*, **26**, 31–7.

addition when using mechanically braked ergometers (see section on timing devices, above). Maintaining a constant pedal rate within 50–70 r.p.m. provides the most efficient range in which the lowest oxygen uptake is produced at a given load. Pedal frequencies above 80 r.p.m. increase the oxygen cost of the work, altering the expected relationship between work rate and oxygen uptake (Chapter 4).

Proper adjustment and recording of the saddle

height are also important for reproducible test results and subject comfort. Typically, the saddle height is adjusted so that when the ball of the foot is on the pedal with the crank arms vertical (pedal at its lowest position) the knee is just slightly bent (5–15° of knee flexion). This positioning may be facilitated if the subject first stands next to the ergometer and the saddle is adjusted so that the top of the seat is just opposite the greater trochanter of the femur. The subject then sits on the saddle and places the heel of the foot on the pedal when at its lowest position. If the knee is straight, the saddle height is about correct. This can be confirmed by placing the ball of the foot on the pedal, as described.

The length of the standard crank arm is 17.5 cm. This is good for most people, but attention should be given to changing the crank arm when testing very short or very tall individuals or children. Some commercially available ergometers allow an easy transition between leg and arm cycling. This convenience should be considered when making purchasing decisions if both leg and arm ergometry are used frequently.

Cycle ergometers afford the best instrumentation for assessing "anaerobic" power from tests such as the Wingate test. The cycle used for this test is usually a friction-braked ergometer modified to allow instant loading and specially instrumented to obtain precise measurements of power output over the 30-s data collection period. This ergometer may be used for either leg or arm exercise in ascertaining "anaerobic" power output.

The advantages and disadvantages of leg cycle ergometers are indicated in Table 2.2. These may be compared with a similar table for treadmills (Table 2.3).

**Table 2.2.** Advantages and disadvantages of leg cycle ergometers

| Advantages | Disadvantages |
|---|---|
| Quantification of external work | Less familiar mode of exercise in USA |
| Reduced motion artifact in ECG, ventilation, and gas exchange signals | Smaller total muscle mass, resulting in lower $\dot{V}o_{2max}$ |
| Reduced ambient noise improving detection of Korotkoff sounds | Unnatural form of exercise that may result in leg fatigue before cardiopulmonary limitation is reached |
| Ease in obtaining arterial blood samples | Intrinsic regulation of work rate |
| Safe; less subject apprehension | |
| Smaller space requirements | |
| Easily moved | |
| Less expensive | |
| May be applied to either arm or leg exercise | |

**Table 2.3.** Advantages and disadvantages of treadmill ergometers

| Advantages | Disadvantages |
|---|---|
| Familiar mode of exercise | Poor quantification of external work |
| Larger muscle mass involved, yielding larger $\dot{V}o_{2max}$ | Increased motion artifact in ECG, ventilation, and gas exchange signals |
| Intrinsic control over work rate | Increased ambient noise |
| Easy to calibrate | More difficult to obtain blood samples |
| | Occupies more space, less portable, expensive |
| | Greater safety risk |
| | Increased apprehension: may affect resting physiological measurements and/or limit attainment of maximal effort due to ensuing fear |
| | Difficult to use in kinetic studies |

## Calibration accuracy and precision

### *Mechanically braked ergometers*

Although some ergometer manufacturers suggest no need for recalibration following the initial factory calibration, experience as well as published reports indicate that regular, if not frequent,

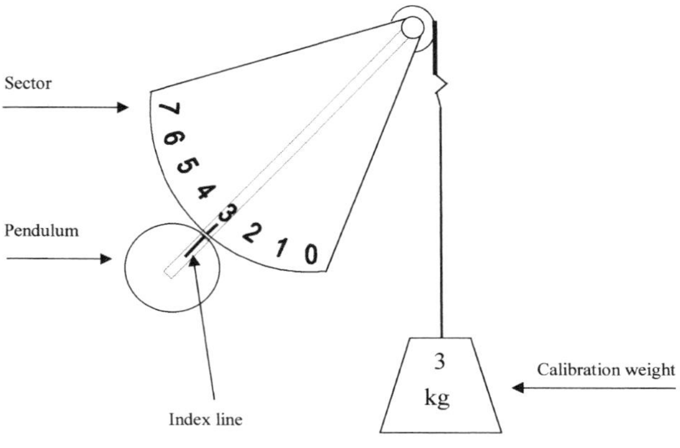


**Figure 2.7** Calibration of a mechanically braked cycle ergometer.

calibration is needed to ensure work rate accuracy during exercise testing. This is of significant importance when attempting to predict $\dot{V}O_{2max}$ from work rate and heart rate.

Calibration procedures will vary depending upon the type of mechanical braking and the design of the ergometer. Regardless of the type of ergometer used in the laboratory, attention to detailed and regular calibration is necessary for valid work rate measurements. Be sure to consult the owner's manual of your specific ergometer for calibration procedures. Calibration of mechanically braked cycles may be performed either statically or dynamically, with $\dot{W}$ as the key variable required of the cycle ergometer. The accuracy of each determinate of $\dot{W}$ should be ensured including load or braking force, distance traveled per revolution, and pedal cadence. When proper calibration procedures are performed as required, the work rates generated are reasonably accurate and precise. However, each laboratory must determine the required frequency for calibration with each type of ergometer. Older ergometers or those that have been poorly maintained may require more frequent calibration than others. It is clear from published reports that some ergometers require frequent calibration due to considerable and variable amounts of drift.

*Static calibration* This approach does not take into account the additional load due to friction of the drive train (chain, sprockets, bottom bracket, and bearings) which can be substantial. A well-maintained and lubricated drive train will still increase the frictional resistance of the ergometer by 5–10%.

1. Load: This requires application of a series of known loads (e.g., 0.5–7 kg) to the braking mechanism. Weights should be selected that bracket the expected range of measurement (e.g., 0.5 kg above and below the expected range). For some friction-braked ergometers, this requires hanging known weights from the friction band as shown in Figure 2.7 and described in Appendix D, Calibration of Monark cycle ergometer. Calibrating caliper-braked ergometers is difficult even using the dynamic calibration methods described below.
2. Distance traveled per revolution: This value is fixed as a function of the flywheel circumference and the number of times the flywheel passes a fixed spot on the cycle per complete revolution of the crank. The distance should be specified in the user's manual, but is also easily measured with a tape measure.
3. Pedal cadence: See section above on counters.

*Dynamic calibration* Dynamic calibration of mechanically braked (or electrically braked) cycle ergometers is the method of choice, since all sources of resistance may be accurately measured. The calibration devices attach to the crank arm with a coupler specific to each ergometer type. A precision motor turns the crank arm at known (but adjustable) rates and measures torque applied to the ergometer crankshaft at braking loads selected by the user. A load cell provides the torque measurement (kg.m) while a tachometer measures pedal cadence (r.p.m.). Power output from all frictional sources is then displayed, whether mechanical, electromagnetic, drive train, or other. These devices are commercially available and have been described in the literature.

*"Biological" calibration* In the absence of calibrating devices, human biological calibration may be performed. Laboratory personnel or subjects cycle at several constant work rates (such as 25, 50, 75, 100 W) below the metabolic threshold (see Chapter 4), while physiological variables such as $f_C$ and $\dot{V}O_2$ are monitored and recorded. Performing regularly, these "human calibrators" can indicate the reproducibility of physiological variables at standardized work rates, thus confirming a degree of ergometer calibration and at least reproducibility. Assuming accuracy of the system used to determine $\dot{V}O_2$, the oxygen cost of the work rate performed is predicable given the robust relationship between $\dot{V}O_2$ and $\dot{W}$ (see Chapter 4 and Equation 2.1). The following equation predicts $\dot{V}O_2$ at a given work rate as well as the increment in $\dot{V}O_2$ between work rates:

$$\dot{V}O_2 = (10.1 \cdot \dot{W}) + (5.8 \cdot BW) + 151 \qquad 2.1$$

where $\dot{V}O_2$ is expressed in $ml \cdot min^{-1}$, $\dot{W}$ is expressed in watts, and BW is body weight in kg.

While "biological" calibration is not good for detecting small changes in ergometer calibration, it can indicate larger errors that may then demand more rigorous calibration. It must be emphasized that biological calibration of ergometers assumes accuracy and reproducibility of the measured physiological variables, $f_C$ and $\dot{V}O_2$.

*Electrically braked ergometers*

*Static calibration* Most electrically braked ergometers provide a mechanism for static calibration where a known weight is suspended from a strain gauge built into the ergometer. This approach assumes strict linearity since the built-in calibration routine uses only one data point. Further, as with the mechanically braked ergometer, this static calibration does not take into account the friction introduced by the drive train. This is often considerable, amounting to as much as 12–20 W, and may obviate use of the ergometer in severely limited subjects.

*Dynamic calibration* Dynamic calibration of electrically braked ergometers employs the same methodology and need for dynamic torque meter described above for the mechanically braked cycle ergometers. It is the preferred method to ensure accurate work rates throughout the desired measurement range.

### Maintenance

Maintenance tends to be quite simple and straightforward for the mechanically braked ergometers. The chain should be lubricated as required and the tension adjusted so as to allow about 1 cm of play. The sprockets should be cleaned and oiled as needed. Bearings within the bottom bracket should be inspected annually and repacked or replaced as needed. The friction belt should be inspected for wear and accumulation of dirt or grease. If needed, the belt can be reversed before it is replaced. The flywheel should be cleaned and kept smooth and free of dirt and rust by cleaning with alcohol or emery cloth.

For electrically braked ergometers, maintenance needs include care in handling and movement, as even slight jars will adversely affect calibration. Otherwise, lubrication of moving parts inside the shrouding and regular clearing will suffice. The owner's manual for each type of ergometer should be consulted for complete details.

## Treadmill ergometers

### Description and principle of operation

Treadmill walking and running represents the most common form of laboratory exercise testing in the USA. This is undoubtedly due to the familiarity of the exercise among those subjects able to walk. In treadmill exercise, a continuous fabric belt is moved across a lubricated platform by an electric motor, powered by either alternating current (AC) or direct current (DC). Motor size is important, with 1 horsepower or more required for exercise testing. Greater power outputs up to 2 horsepower allow more demanding protocols with respect to higher speeds, steeper grades, and faster response times to speed and grade changes. Larger motors are also better suited for use with heavier subjects.

For clinical applications, treadmills should have variable speeds that begin at very low levels such as 0.1 m.p.h. (0.16 km $\cdot$ h$^{-1}$). Top end speeds of 5 m.p.h. (8.1 km $\cdot$ h$^{-1}$) are usually adequate for patient populations, whereas speeds up to if not exceeding 15 m.p.h. (24.1 km $\cdot$ h$^{-1}$) may be necessary in sports medicine applications. An adequate grade range for clinical purposes is 0–15%. Above about 15% grade, calf or back pain may be limiting. Some treadmill manufacturers provide negative slopes for downhill-running simulations that may be of interest in physical therapy, athletic, or research facilities.

A few manufacturers now make treadmills that have the capability of "ramping." That is, computer control of a special drive motor allows very small increments in either speed or grade each second. Such adjustments in speed or grade permit smooth work rate changes and the use of ramp protocols (see Chapter 3).

Similar to some electrically braked cycle ergometers, several treadmills are now equipped with mechanisms to regulate speed or grade from a predetermined heart rate. A heart rate, e.g. 140 beats $\cdot$ min$^{-1}$, is entered into the treadmill control panel along with the choice of either a constant speed or grade. Based upon the subject's heart rate response to the exercise, the nonconstant variable (speed or grade) changes to maintain the preset heart rate.

Additional considerations regarding treadmills include the size of the walking surface, side and front handrails, an emergency off switch or "panic button," height of the walking platform, and noise level. Electrical connections must also be planned, as some treadmills necessitate dedicated circuits with specific voltage and amperage requirements.

External work on the treadmill is difficult to quantify despite the simple equation used to calculate power output (in watts):

$$\dot{W} = 0.1634 \cdot \text{speed} \cdot (\text{grade}/100) \cdot \text{BW} \qquad 2.2$$

where $\dot{W}$ is expressed in watts, speed is expressed in m $\cdot$ min$^{-1}$ and grade is expressed as a percentage. BW is body weight in kg.

> **Example:** For an 80-kg subject walking at 53.6 m $\cdot$ min$^{-1}$ (2 m.p.h.) and 2% grade, the work rate would be 14 W. On a horizontal treadmill, the external work rate would be zero!

Compounding the problem of estimating work rates on the treadmill is handrail holding and inefficient walking gaits. Handrail holding may significantly reduce (15%) the oxygen cost of the work as the body weight is functionally reduced due to the handrail support. Running elicits a greater oxygen cost than walking at the same speed. While prediction equations for oxygen uptake utilizing speed and grade are available, the relationship between estimated work rate during treadmill exercise and oxygen uptake is often unpredictable.

Table 2.3 summarizes the advantages and disadvantages of motor-driven treadmills for XT.

### Calibration, accuracy, and precision

When a commercial-grade treadmill used for XT has been properly calibrated, it will tend to be both accurate and reproducible. This should be verified by regular calibration measurements.

*Grade*

At least upon installation, a treadmill should be set up so that the walking surface is absolutely level when set at 0% grade. This may be determined by placing a carpenter's level lengthwise on the walking surface of the treadmill. A 1–2-m level is best for this purpose. Shims may be added underneath one or more of the treadmill feet if after measurement the treadmill is found not to be level. Once the bubble in the carpenter's level is in the middle of the tube, the grade indicator on the treadmill control panel should read or be adjusted to read 0%. Calibration of grade may now be performed at several grade settings (e.g., 5% increments from 5% to 20% or higher if laboratory protocols call for steeper grades). A typical calibration routine is described below and can be followed with reference to Figure 2.8.

1. Place a carpenter's square with its long side along the long axis of the treadmill walking surface.

2. Place a carpenter's level on top of the square and ensure that the treadmill is level when the treadmill control panel reads 0%.
3. Use the treadmill grade control to elevate the treadmill to the desired grade, e.g., 5%.
4. While holding the long arm of the square and level, raise the short arm of the square until the bubble in the level is in the center of the window. Record the distance the short arm of the square was elevated to obtain the level position. This is known as the rise.
5. The length of the long arm from its end to where it joins the short arm is known as the run.
6. Calculate the grade by dividing the rise by the run and multiplying by 100%.
7. Repeat for additional grade settings.
8. If the grade indicator on the treadmill control panel does not correspond with the calculation, re-mark the dial using tape. Alternatively, construct a graph and regression equation as described earlier in this chapter, in the section on what to do with calibration data.

***Note:*** *If a carpenter's square is not available, a fixed distance can be measured on the floor (run) and the change in height from 0% grade to the new grade (rise) can be measured.*

> **Example:** The run on a standard carpenter's square is 22.5 in. If the short arm was raised by $1\frac{1}{8}$ in. (1.125 in.), the grade would be 1.125/22.5 or $0.05 \times 100\% = 5\%$.

This method of calibrating treadmill grade uses the tangent of $\angle\theta$ (rise/run) and is reasonably accurate for grades up to about 20%. For steeper grades, the same method can be used. However, the sine of that tangent should be calculated either by using a table of trigonometric functions or using a hand-held calculator. In this case, once the tangent is calculated, press ATAN (arc tangent), then press SIN. Multiply this value by 100% for the correct percent grade. Table 2.4 provides the relationship between percent grade and angle (°).

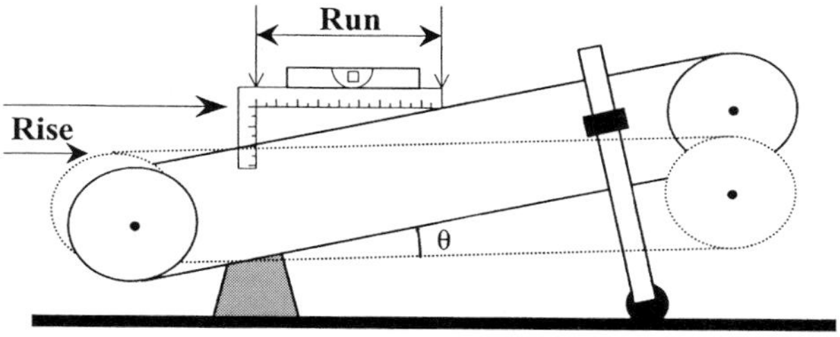


**Figure 2.8** Calibration of treadmill grade using carpenter's square and level.

*Speed*

Treadmill speed should be verified at several different speeds throughout the anticipated range of speeds to be used. Ideally, speed should be calibrated with someone walking on the treadmill. This is especially important with underpowered treadmills. Use the following procedures for speed calibration:

1. Consult the owner's manual (or the manufacturer) to determine the treadmill belt length (in meters).
2. Alternatively, measure the entire length of the treadmill belt in meters by marking two distant spots on the belt and then advancing the belt, marking and measuring back to the first mark.
3. Start the treadmill belt at the slowest speed anticipated.
4. Using a stopwatch, time and number complete revolutions of the belt by counting the number of times a mark on the belt passes a fixed place on the treadmill. Be sure to begin the count at zero when starting the watch. A convenient number of revolutions to count is 10.
5. Multiply the belt length (in meters) by the number of revolutions timed to obtain the number of meters the belt has moved in the time period. Divide that product by the time (converted to minutes) for the number of revolutions counted. The result will give speed in units of $m \cdot min^{-1}$ (see Equation 2.3).
6. The speed can be converted from $m \cdot min^{-1}$ to units of m.p.h. by dividing the value obtained using Equation 2.3 by 26.8 (see Equation 2.4).

**Table 2.4.** Relationship between percentage grade and angle for use in treadmill ergometry

| Grade | Angle (°) | Grade | Angle (°) | Grade | Angle(°) | Grade | Angle (°) |
|---|---|---|---|---|---|---|---|
| 0.0% | 0 | 5.0% | 2.86 | 10.0% | 5.71 | 15.0% | 8.53 |
| 0.5% | 0.29 | 5.5% | 3.15 | 10.5% | 5.99 | 15.5% | 8.81 |
| 1.0% | 0.57 | 6.0% | 3.43 | 11.0% | 6.28 | 16.0% | 9.09 |
| 1.5% | 0.86 | 6.5% | 3.72 | 11.5% | 6.56 | 16.5% | 9.37 |
| 2.0% | 1.15 | 7.0% | 4.00 | 12.0% | 6.84 | 17.0% | 9.65 |
| 2.5% | 1.43 | 7.5% | 4.29 | 12.5% | 7.13 | 17.5% | 9.93 |
| 3.0% | 1.72 | 8.0% | 4.57 | 13.0% | 7.41 | 18.0% | 10.20 |
| 3.5% | 2.00 | 8.5% | 4.86 | 13.5% | 7.69 | 18.5% | 10.48 |
| 4.0% | 2.29 | 9.0% | 5.14 | 14.0% | 7.97 | 19.0% | 10.76 |
| 4.5% | 2.58 | 9.5% | 5.43 | 14.5% | 8.25 | 19.5% | 11.04 |
| 5.0% | 2.86 | 10.0% | 5.71 | 15.0% | 8.53 | 20.0% | 11.31 |

7. Repeat for several speeds across the range of expected measurements in increments typically used in the XT protocol, e.g., 0.5 m.p.h.
8. Adjust the speed control on the treadmill control panel or develop a calibration curve (regression equation) as described earlier in this chapter, in the section on what to do with calibration data.

$$\text{Speed} = \frac{\text{Length} \cdot \text{Revolutions}}{\text{Time}} \qquad 2.3$$

where speed is expressed in $\text{m} \cdot \text{min}^{-1}$, belt length is expressed in meters, revolutions are counted, and time is expressed in min.

$$\text{m.p.h.} = \text{m} \cdot \text{min}^{-1}/26.8 \qquad 2.4$$

**Example:** A treadmill with a belt length of 6 m required 2 min 14 s (2.23 min) for 10 revolutions.

$$\text{Speed} = \frac{6 \cdot 10}{2.23} = 26.9\ \text{m} \cdot \text{min}^{-1} = 1.0\ \text{m.p.h.}$$

### Maintenance

Documentation accompanying the treadmill will generally include maintenance recommendations. This includes verifying speed and grade calibrations, lubricating the drive belt and elevation gear, alignment (tracking) and tensioning of the walking belt, and in some cases, waxing the platform below the walking belt. Newer treadmills have walking decks that are impregnated with a lubricant, essentially providing self-lubrication to the undersurface of the walking belt. The power cord and walking belt should be regularly inspected for wear. Handrails should be examined for tight connections to the treadmill. The treadmill should be cleaned daily to remove dust and debris. A complete service by qualified repair personnel should be performed according to manufacturer recommendations or after approximately every 1000 hours of use.

### Safety

Treadmills present increased safety risks as compared to other forms of ergometers. As such, care should be taken to minimize risks by attention to the following.

An emergency off switch should be installed and easily within the reach of both the subject and the test operator. Pressing this switch should result in the treadmill stopping within 2–3 s. It may also be wise to station lab personnel behind the subject if it appears that the risk of losing grip or balance and falling is great.

Handrails on the front and sides of the treadmill are important safety precautions, but should not be used for support during the test. Some patients are so frail and low-functioning that they cannot manage to walk without some handrail support. Although this practice should be discouraged as it interferes with accurate and reproducible measures of the exercise response, a technique that may be occasionally employed allows the use of one finger touching the top of the side rail. Alternatively, the back of the hand may be placed on the underside of a side rail. These techniques minimize handrail support and alterations in the physiologic response to the exercise while helping to ensure safety, increasing patient confidence and sense of security, and allowing a treadmill test to be taken to its normal completion.

An important safety precaution is to provide proper instruction for mounting, walking, and dismounting the treadmill. This should always be done with naïve subjects until they report a reasonable sense of security. Subjects should be instructed to grasp the handrails and begin walking normally as the treadmill belt starts underfoot. If the lowest speed on the treadmill is too fast for this approach, the subject may stand on the side platform while grasping the handrails and carefully step on to the treadmill with the inside foot, bringing the other foot forward as walking begins.

Treadmill walking should be done in an upright position without looking down at the feet. Bent-over walking, especially at increased elevations, may result in low back discomfort, leading to early test termination for reasons unrelated to the objectives of the assessment. Some subjects will attempt to march. This should be avoided, as it is less efficient than normal walking.

When the subject is walking normally and with confidence, the hands should be removed from the handrails and swung normally at the side.

## Arm ergometers

### Description and principles of operation

Arm ergometers are useful when leg cycling or treadmill exercise is inappropriate or contraindicated. Such cases might include testing those individuals using wheelchairs, people with back pain that is exacerbated by sitting or walking (particularly up a grade), pregnancy, or athletes for whom arm exercise is dominant. A potential limitation of arm ergometry is that $\dot{V}O_{2max}$ values are about 30% lower than in leg exercise due to the smaller total exercising muscle mass and increased static effort in arm exercise. Arm cycling ergometers are usually available in three forms: (1) a countertop arm-cranking device; (2) a modified mechanically or electrically braked cycle ergometer; or (3) a wheelchair ergometer. The countertop arm crank ergometers are smaller and can be effectively used by anyone, including people in wheelchairs. They are friction-braked with the tension controlled in a manner similar to that described above for friction-braked cycle ergometers. Alternatively, leg cycle ergometers (mechanically braked or electrically braked) can be elevated on to a table or suitable supports and used for arm work. Commercial arm ergometers typically have shorter crank arm lengths than leg ergometers. The shorter arm ergometer crank arm results in a shorter lever and therefore greater muscular effort at the same work rate setting. Recent evidence has suggested significantly higher $f_C$, $\dot{V}O_2$, $R$, rating of perceived exertion (RPE) responses, and lower gross efficiency to work rates above 25 W at the same power output in countertop arm crank ergometers compared with a leg ergometer from the same manufacturer used for arm cranking. It is important, therefore, to note the length of the crank arm, especially in serial testing. Wheelchair ergometers are also available or can be built, allowing task-specific assessment for those using wheelchairs. Additionally, other special ergometers for task-specific athletic populations may be available or specially constructed, e.g., kayaking, canoeing, or rowing ergometers.

### Calibration, accuracy, and precision

Methods used for calibrating arm ergometers are essentially identical to those used for leg ergometers whether performing static or dynamic calibration (see above). Since arm and leg ergometers utilize the same basic equipment configuration and mechanics, accuracy and precision are similar to those for leg ergometers.

### Maintenance

Maintenance of arm ergometers is essentially identical to that for friction-braked cycle ergometers. To ensure proper operation, all ergometers should undergo regular maintenance, including lubrication and checks for wear of the friction belt.

## Volume-measuring devices

### Introduction

Several devices are available for measuring exhaled or inhaled volumes of air for use in calculating pulmonary minute ventilation, oxygen uptake, carbon dioxide output, and other derived variables (see Chapter 4 for detailed discussion on these variables). Users should be aware of the need for careful and regular calibration of the volume-measuring instrument, its inherent limitations and recommended applications.

A number of volume- or flow-measuring devices are commercially available. These span a wide spectrum of applications from simple measurements of exhaled gas collected in bags as part of a teaching laboratory to sophisticated computer-controlled data acquisition systems for clinical exercise testing. Examples include Douglas bags and meteorological balloons, water-sealed spirometers (recommended as the "gold standard" for volume measurements), dry gasometers such as the Parkinson–Cowan gas meter, mass flow meters (hot-wire anemometers), pitot tubes, pneumotachographs, and turbine volume transducers. Each of these devices has its applications, advantages, and disadvantages. Desirable qualities of volume-measuring devices are listed in Table 2.5.

**Table 2.5.** Desirable qualities of volume-measuring devices

| |
|---|
| Demonstrated accuracy ( < 3% error) across the desired measurement range |
| Low resistance to inspired or expired airflow |
| Unaffected by pattern of airflow, gas viscosity, density, or gas concentration |
| Allows recording of each tidal breath |
| Comfortable patient interface: light-weight, portable, unobtrusive, no need for one-way valves or conducting tubing |
| Able to provide analog or digital output for computer signal processing |
| Easy to calibrate |
| Easy to clean and maintain |
| Cost-effective in case of need for replacement or multiple units |
| Leak-proof (including diffusion as with $CO_2$ in latex balloons) |
| Measurement unaffected by motion artifact |

### Gas collection bags

#### Description and principles of operation

Collection bags such as Douglas bags, Mylar® bags, aluminized polyester, or latex or neoprene meteorological balloons in the 100–300 l size range may be used to collect expired air for subsequent measurement. Figure 2.9 illustrates a typical bag–valve–tubing arrangement for the collection of expired air.

The collection bag is usually fitted with a large two-way stopcock used to direct the expired air either into the atmosphere or into the bag for collection over an appropriate time interval. The stopcock has a tap for gas sampling, allowing the analysis of the oxygen and carbon dioxide contents of the bag. Tubing leads from the stopcock to a one-way breathing valve and thence to the mouthpiece.

*Douglas bag technique*

The Douglas bag method remains the "gold standard" for measuring volume of exhaled air. Its usefulness is particularly apparent in validating other volume-measuring devices singularly or as part of an integrated metabolic measurement system. A true Douglas bag or alternatives such as Mylar® bags or latex or neoprene meteorological balloons serve

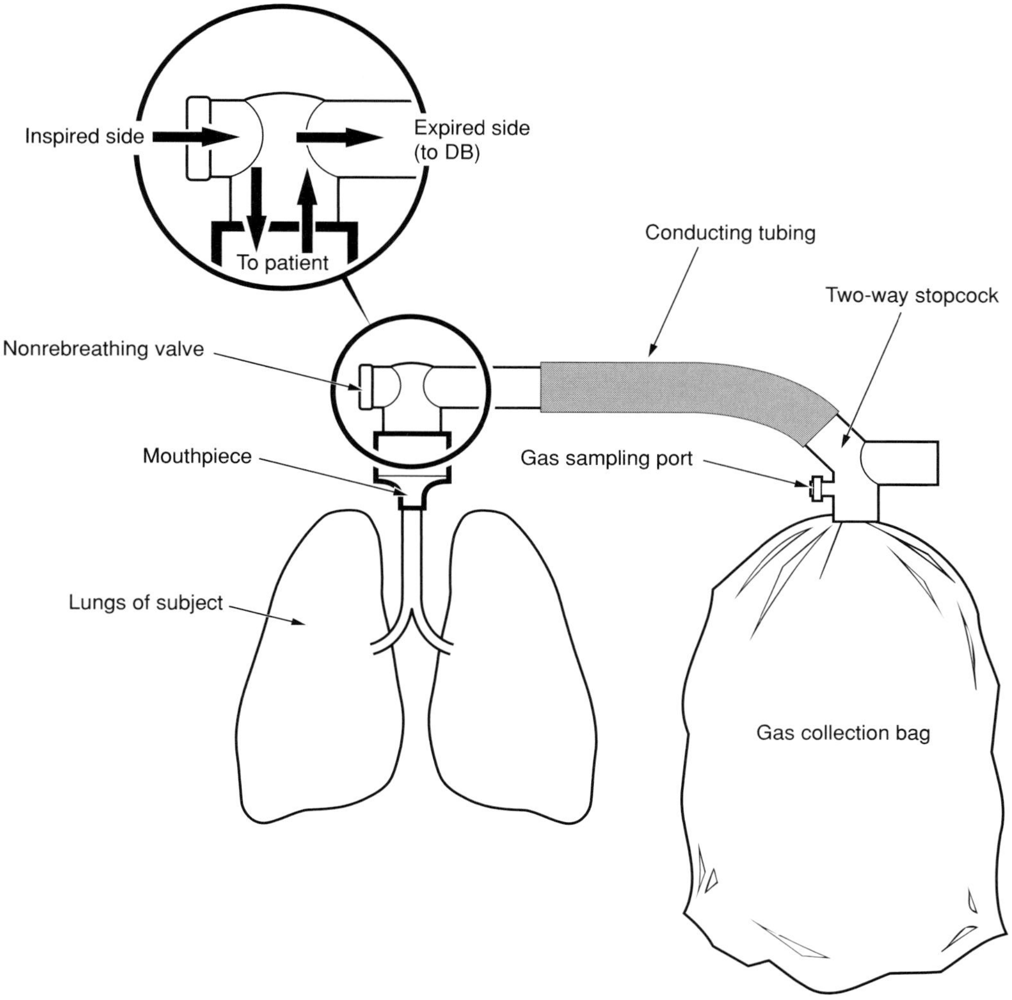


**Figure 2.9** Typical bag, tubing, and valve arrangement for collection of exhaled air. DB, Douglas bag.

to collect the exhaled air. Air acquired in the bag or balloon is carefully pushed into an appropriately sized spirometer such as a 120-l (or larger) Tissot water-sealed spirometer. The Tissot spirometer used alone is inappropriate for direct measurement of tidal breathing due to the large inertia of the bell and thus resistance to airflow. Furthermore, its limited capacity makes it unsuitable for direct use in exercise testing.

### Calibration, accuracy, and precision

The collection bags have no need for calibration, as they are simply reservoirs for the collection of exhaled air. However, care must be taken with latex meteorological balloons, as they are known to deteriorate when exposed to ozone and, even under the best conditions with a new bag, permit the diffusion of carbon dioxide. To avoid this potential problem, gas concentrations should be quickly measured with laboratory gas analyzers before the bag contents are pushed into the spirometer. Although manufacturers' specifications suggest up to 30 min before gas diffuses out of the latex- or neoprene-type bags, laboratory staff should verify this specification by completely evacuating bag contents then alternately filling and flushing the bag at least three times with a calibration gas. Gas concentrations within the bag are then measured immediately after the last fill and then at 1-min intervals until the gas concentrations change (typically carbon dioxide first).

***Note:*** *When performing the gas analysis, the gas removed from the bag for analysis must be accounted for and then mathematically "added back" to the volume measured by the spirometer. This is simply a process of timing the analysis period and multiplying by the analyzer sampling rate. For example, if the combined sample rate of discrete oxygen and carbon dioxide analyzers is 400 ml $\cdot$ min$^{-1}$ and the sample period is 30 s, 200 ml of gas was removed and must be added to the volume measured by the spirometer.*

The Tissot water-sealed spirometer typically needs no calibration; however, care must be taken to ensure a leak-free apparatus. This may be accomplished by avoiding pinhole leaks due to corrosion from tap water by using only distilled water in the spirometer and draining it when use is not anticipated for some time. Leak tests may also be performed as follows:

1. Draw the bell upwards several times at different levels (trials) throughout the expected range of measurements. Close all valves to "lock in" the air.
2. Then, for each trial, a reading is taken on the meter stick.
3. A 10-kg weight may then be placed on top of the bell and allowed to sit for approximately 1–2 min.
4. The weight is then removed and a reading once again taken on the meter stick.
5. There should be no difference between the two readings.

If changes in the bell spirometer volume are found, several sources of leaks may be possible. This includes the pinhole leaks indicated above, leaks from one or more of the valves, and leaks occurring at the mercury thermometer port.

Accuracy is also determined by careful attention to valving, timing, and collection of whole breaths in the collection bags. This requires use of a one-way valve between the patient and the collection bag, a two-way stopcock attached to the bag, and a small section of conducting tubing between the exhaust side of the one way valve and the inlet port of the two-way stopcock (Figure 2.9). The two-way stopcock is turned to direct the exhaled air into the bag when the subject starts to inhale. At this time a stopwatch is started in order to time the period of collection. The approximate length of the collection period will have been decided beforehand, e.g., as close as possible to 1 min. The stopcock is turned at the end of exhalation, directing the next exhaled breath to atmosphere. Timing is stopped when the stopcock is turned, e.g., at 58.5 s. Thus, only whole breaths are collected over a period that can be normalized to a minute value (58.5/60 = 0.975 min) for the calculation of minute ventilation ($\dot{V}_E$).

### Maintenance

Bags should be kept in airtight containers when not in use and checked frequently for deterioration and leaks. Collection bags should be handled with care, especially latex bags that tear easily. As indicated above, the Tissot spirometer should be checked for leaks, drained when not in use, and the valves regularly lubricated. Raising the bell out of the water and manually drying it at the end of the testing day is likely to retard any corrosive and thus leak-producing effect of prolonged exposure to the water. One-way valve leaflets should be replaced regularly as they wear and may leak. The two-way stopcock should be lubricated with stopcock grease.

## Spirometers and gasometers

### Description and principles of operation

*Water-sealed spirometers*

Examples of water-sealed spirometers include the Tissot, described above, as well as the small 9–13.5 l desktop spirometers that are used for pulmonary function testing. A description of these spirometers is included here for two purposes: firstly, to describe more fully the Tissot spirometer referred to above and secondly, to describe smaller spirometers that may be used for measurement of maximum voluntary ventilation (MVV) or forced expiratory volume in the first second ($FEV_1$) prior to conducting the XT. As discussed in Chapter 3, every diagnostic XT should be preceded by an MVV or $FEV_1$ measurement in order to estimate an individual's ventilatory capacity.

The general principle of water-sealed spirometers is the same, regardless of spirometer type or size. Figure 2.10 illustrates a typical configuration for water-sealed spirometers. An inner bell made of either metal or plastic is suspended from a pulley-and-chain mechanism. This bell is sleeved between an inner cylinder and an outer housing, usually made of metal. Water fills the space between the inner cylinder and outer housing, thus providing an airtight seal for the air contained within the bell. Rigid tubing supplies the inner cylinder with air from the patient or collection bags. Two-way valves direct airflow either into the inner cylinder or to the atmosphere. A canister containing a $CO_2$ absorbent may be present within the inner cylinder for studies requiring rebreathing of bell contents, such as in resting metabolic rate measurement. When used for MVV or other forced maneuvers such as $FEV_1$ and peak expiratory flow rate (PEFR), the $CO_2$ absorbent canister is removed to reduce resistance to airflow. As air moves in or out of the spirometer, the chain-suspended bell rises or falls with each breath or input of air. Also, these movements may be recorded on paper by means of pens moving in parallel with the movements of the bell or by linear transducers that send their signals to a computer for processing into volume measurements. To facilitate paper recording, a kymograph drum attached to a variable-speed motor turns at a preselected speed. In both cases, geometrically derived numerical "bell factors" are used to translate linear movements of the bell into volumes. In the case of the Tissot spirometer, movements of the bell cause movements of a meter stick. The difference in starting and ending positions of the meter stick can be used to calculate volume using the "bell factor." Knowledge of the time over which the volume changes

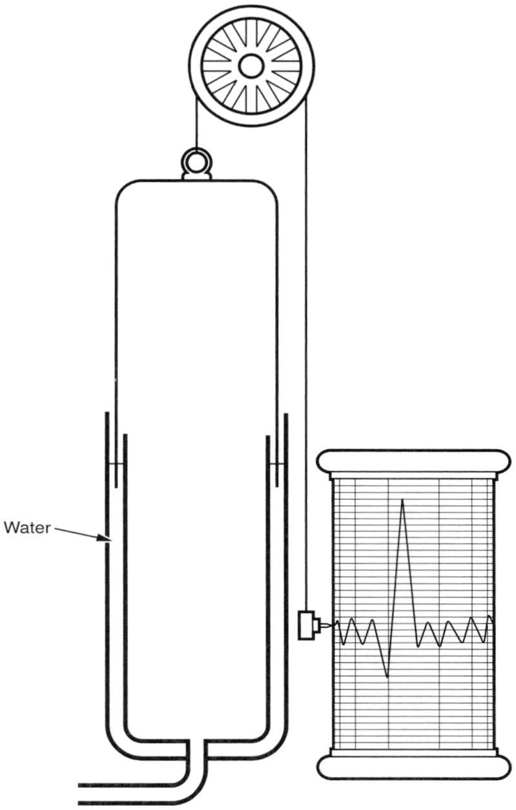


**Figure 2.10** Diagram of a water-sealed spirometer for the measurement of inhaled and exhaled lung volumes and flows.

were recorded, together with measurements of volume, allows measurements such as $\dot{V}_E$, $FEV_1$, and MVV.

*Dry rolling-seal spirometers*

Also known as the Ohio spirometer, this device consists of a horizontal cylinder to which is attached a flexible, cylindrical rolling seal. As air enters, the rolling seal allows the cylinder to move. Linear transducers are attached to the cylinder and interfaced with a computer allowing measurements of flow and volume.

*Dry gasometers*

An example of a dry gasometer is the Parkinson–Cowan dry gasometer. Two pairs of bellows are filled and emptied, the movements of which are transmitted to a pointer on a labeled circular dial. A potentiometer can be coupled to this dial to give an analog voltage signal proportional to the volume recorded. The dry gas meter is best used on the inspired side so as to avoid destruction of the bellows due to accumulation of moisture condensing from the exhaled airflow through the apparatus. Alternatively, if measurement of expired air is unavoidable, a portable hair dryer can be used to dry the inside of the gasometer, reducing potential damage.

### Calibration, accuracy, and precision

Calibration of spirometers and gasometers is essential. The American Thoracic Society has published standards on accuracy for pulmonary function and exercise testing (see Further Reading). According to these standards, volume-measuring devices must be accurate within ±3% of the true value. A 3-l syringe should be used to perform calibration checks for volume with syringe strokes applied at different speeds to simulate different flow rates. Care must be taken not to bottom out the syringe piston against the base of the cylinder as this may cause a rebound, producing an erroneous additional and unknown volume. Since the $FEV_1$ and MVV maneuvers are rate-dependent, exhaled volumes must be accurately measured over precisely known time periods. Calibration of the speed of the rotating kymograph drum on a water-sealed spirometer is performed at each of the speed settings as follows:

1. A stopwatch is used to time the movement of the spirometer paper attached to the revolving kymograph drum as it passes across the recording pen.
2. As the pen crosses a vertical line on the paper, the watch is started and then stopped several seconds later as the pen crosses a second vertical line.
3. The true paper speed is calculated by dividing the distance traveled by the pen by the corresponding time interval. For example, if the distance between two vertical lines on the recording paper is 192 mm and the time interval for the pen to travel between these lines is 6 s, then the drum speed is $32\,mm \cdot s^{-1}$ ($1920\,mm \cdot min^{-1}$).

### Maintenance

Water-sealed spirometers should contain only distilled water in order to avoid corrosion and possible leaks. This problem has been considerably reduced with the advent of plastic bells. Nevertheless, distilled water and frequent (if not daily) draining into a gravity-fed reservoir is advised. For all spirometers, rubber tubing and connectors should be inspected for cracks and replaced as needed. The bellows inside the dry gasometer should be inspected for leaks, especially if used to measure expired airflow.

## Flow and volume transducers

### Description and principles of operation

Mass flow tranducers measure instantaneous flow with a predetermined frequency (e.g., 100 Hz). The flow signals can be integrated with respect to time in order to obtain volume measurements. A significant advantage of these instruments is their capability of measuring individual breath volumes, both inspired and expired. The four commonest flow

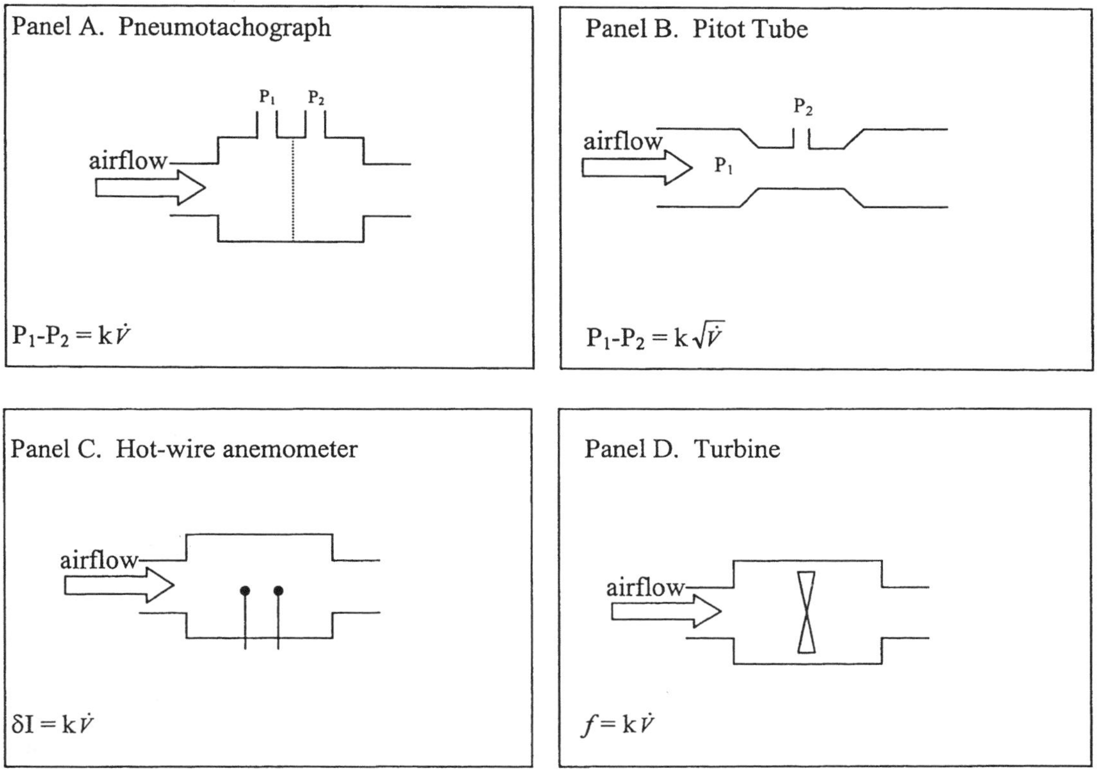


**Figure 2.11** Diagrammatic representation of four types of mass flow transducers. (In each example, $\dot{V}$ is flow. $P_1$–$P_2$ is the pressure difference in A and B. $\delta I$ is the difference in electrical current in C. $f$ is the frequency of rotation of the helical impeller in D.

transducers are described below and illustrated diagramatically in Figure 2.11.

*Pneumotachograph*

Pneumotachographs quantify airflow by measuring the pressure drop across obstructions placed within the tube. These obstructions may be bundles of parallel capillary tubes or low-resistance mesh screens of different gauges. Pneumotachographs are available in several different sizes, providing applications ranging from measurements in infants to maximal flow rates in large exercising subjects. Size of the pneumotachograph is important, as the change in pressure across the resistance is no longer proportional to airflow if the inappropriate size results in nonlaminar flow.

*Pitot tube*

The Pitot tube is a differential pressure sensor consisting of two tubes, one facing the air stream and the other perpendicular to it. The pressure gradient between the two tubes is measured with differential pressure transducers. Using an application of Bernoulli's law, airflow velocity is proportional to the density of the gas and to the square root of the pressure. Pitot tubes are advantageous in so far as they present low resistance to breathing, do not depend on laminar flow, are light-weight, and have minimal problems with heating and cooling of the gas. Some models are disposable, thus providing an additional precaution against communicable infections. However, corrections for the inherent nonlinearity of the quadratic relationship between airflow velocity and pressure as well as adjustments for gas density due to changes in gas composition throughout the respiratory cycle are necessary for accurate measurements of airflow and therefore volumes of exhaled air.

*Hot-wire anemometer*

This device measures mass flow – the number of molecules passing the point of measurement – by detecting the increase in the amount of electrical current needed to heat a wire placed in the air stream as air flows over the wire. A modification of this principle utilizes two wires heated to different temperatures in a bridge circuit. Flow is detected by the hotter wire losing heat faster than the colder wire. The amount of electrical current required to maintain the temperature ratio between the two wires is proportional to the airflow. Since the response to gas flow is nondirectional, an additional device, such as a pressure-sensing arrangement, must be added to detect phases of respiration. Digital computer algorithms are used to correct inherent nonlinearity.

*Turbine transducer*

This is an electromechanical device typically consisting of a low-mass helical impeller mounted upon jeweled bearings. The impeller is housed in a plastic support structure and inserted into an electronics cylinder consisting of pairs of light-emitting diodes. As the impeller blade spins with airflow, the light beams are broken and digital signals proportional to volume are sent to the processor. Bidirectional flow is easily sensed by the change in direction of rotation of the impeller. The turbine volume transducer may be used over a wide range of flow rates from rest to maximal exertion, although evidence exists for large errors at low (i.e., resting) flows attributable to impeller inertia at the onset and end of airflow.

### Calibration, accuracy, and precision

Calibration of flow and volume transducers is essential. Recommendations from the American Thoracic Society indicate that calibration should be performed with a 3-l calibration syringe with the transducer achieving an accuracy corresponding to no greater than a 3% error (see Further Reading). Flow and volume calibrations should be carried out prior to each test. Syringe strokes should be varied in speed so as to simulate the different flow rates that will be encountered during the XT. Care must be taken not to "bottom out" (slam the piston into the end of the cylinder) the piston as this will provide false volumes due to the potential for a rebound of the piston against the end of the cylinder adding an unknown quantity to the correct volume.

Considerations potentially affecting measurement accuracy include the temperature, viscosity, and density of the gas measured as well as flow characteristics (laminar or turbulent). Under optimal conditions where these variables are well controlled, the pneumotachograph, the Pitot tube, the hot-wire anemometer, and the turbine flow transducer have all been shown to provide measurements within the ±3% accuracy recommended by the American Thoracic Society.

### Maintenance

Cleaning and sterilization of mass flow meters presents the greatest maintenance requirement apart from the expected care in handling precision instruments. Cleaning with one of the many effective commercial sterilization solutions should be performed according to manufacturers' instructions after each use. Special care should be taken with pneumotachographs so as not to immerse the entire unit, which could damage the heater circuit or trap water inside the case. The screens or capillary tubes should be checked for obstructions. A portable hair dryer will facilitate drying of any of the mass flow sensors, although this practice should be used cautiously with turbines so as not to risk bending the impeller.

## Gas analyzers

### Introduction

Of primary interest in cardiopulmonary exercise testing is the measurement of oxygen uptake and carbon dioxide output. Requisite for these determinations is the measurement of the exhaled oxygen and carbon dioxide concentrations. Analyzers that use chemical, electronic, or spectroscopic methodologies perform these functions. Knowledge of the principle of operation among different analyzers will assist the user in understanding the inherent strengths and limitations underlying each. This is of particular importance when considering an integrated metabolic measurement system.

Chemical methods using the Scholander or Haldane apparatus and procedures provide "gold-standard" accuracy and are useful for validating calibration gases. Once so validated, these "grandfather" gas cylinders are used to validate subsequently purchased calibration gases. The methods are tedious and time-consuming, but in the hands of a practiced expert are invaluable for ensuring accuracy of calibration gases. The Scholander and Haldane methods are not practical for routine clinical use because of the time required per analysis (roughly 6–8 min for an experienced technician to perform duplicate measurements of a single aliquot sample). Discrete electronic analyzers for oxygen and carbon dioxide may exist either as stand-alone units or part of an integrated metabolic cart. When well calibrated, they perform remarkably well.

Alternatively, the mass spectrometer provides increased precision and the ability to measure multiple gas species in the same unit, albeit at a substantially increased cost.

### Oxygen analyzers

#### Description and principle of operation

Three types of discrete oxygen analyzers are in common use: paramagnetic, fuel cell, and zirconium oxide.

*Paramagnetic analyzers*

As first demonstrated by Faraday in 1851, oxygen possesses the property of paramagnetism, unlike other respiratory gases. The paramagnetic analyzers make use of this property, aligning oxygen molecules in a magnetic field located within a chamber, thus enhancing the field. Changes in the oxygen concentration change the magnetic field. The resulting signal is conditioned and linearized by electronic circuits within the analyzer or using digital computer algorithms. Typical applications of paramagnetic analyzers are in systems in which respiratory gases are measured from collection bags or mixing chambers. This is due to their slower response time (700–1000 ms) although pumps and signal processing may be used to enhance the response time to $<150$ ms, making them suitable for breath-by-breath measurements.

*Electrochemical or fuel cell analyzers*

With electrochemical or fuel cell analyzers, oxygen molecules diffuse through a sensing membrane and then through a thin layer of electrolyte. The molecules reach the cathode surface where they are reduced, gaining electrons. These electrons are furnished by the simultaneous oxidation of the anode. The flow of electrons from anode to sensing cathode results in a current proportional to the amount of oxygen in the sample gas. Over time, the fuel cell sensor becomes weaker and weaker, requiring replacement roughly every 2–3 years depending upon the frequency of use and the concentrations of oxygen typically measured. The fuel cell tends to be less sensitive to the effects of water vapor.

*Zirconium oxide analyzers*

In the zirconium oxide analyzer, the gas sensor (zirconium oxide ceramic), when heated, develops a voltage between its surfaces if they are exposed to different concentrations of oxygen. Porous electrodes deposited on the inside and outside surfaces of the cell serve as conductors for the cell output. The sample gas surrounds the exterior of the cell while the interior is exposed to ambient air. The output of the cell depends upon the differences in the partial pressure of oxygen on the inside and outside of the cell and also on temperature; the larger the difference, and the higher the temperature, the larger the output. The zirconium oxide analyzers operate at high (750 °C) temperatures, require an AC heater, heat shielding, and a large consumption of current. Analyzer response characteristics are quite fast, in the range of 50 ms, making them suitable for breath-by-breath applications.

*Laser diode absorption spectroscopy*
A recent development in oxygen analyzers makes use of laser diode absorption spectroscopy (LDAS). The absorption of oxygen is in the visible spectrum (760 nm) where there is no interference with other respiratory gases. The width of the laser beam and the absorption line width of oxygen are less than 0.01 nm, compared to 100 nm for the infrared measurement of carbon dioxide. As the oxygen concentration increases, light intensity is attenuated, with the photo detector varying linearly with the oxygen concentration. Analyzer response times are fast, i.e., in the 80 ms range. These analyzers are still in development and have limited application at present.

### Calibration, accuracy, and precision

When properly calibrated, a well-performing oxygen analyzer can be both accurate (±1% of full scale) and precise (0.01% $O_2$). Accurate calibration is critical for this performance. Oxygen analyzers are calibrated with gases of known concentration over the expected range of measurement, e.g., 12%–21% for XT without the use of supplemental oxygen. The accuracy of calibration gases is crucial since the accuracy of a gas analyzer can never be better than the accuracy with which the concentrations of calibration gases are known. Use of the Scholander apparatus and technique provides the best assurance of calibration gas accuracy. Alternatively, use of gases certified to be accurate within ±0.02% absolute is acceptable, although expensive (e.g., oxygen specified to 16% must be 15.98%–16.02%). To obviate the tedious Scholander procedure or the purchase of expensive certified gases, a practice used by many laboratories is "grandfathering" the Scholander tested or certified gases. These gases are then used only for the purpose of verifying the accuracy of subsequently purchased less expensive calibration gases along with electronic gas analyzers or a mass spectrometer.

With the exception of the mass spectrometer, most oxygen analyzers in current use are partial pressure-sensing devices. As such, care must be taken to ensure that the pressure of the gas reaching the sensing element is the same for calibration as it is for measurement during the XT. This is accomplished by maintaining the same tubing geometry and eliminating positive or negative pressures during the calibration routine or measurement of the expired gas. The need to maintain tubing geometry may be explained by Poiseuille's law which states that flow through a tube ($\dot{V}$) is proportional to the pressure gradient ($P_1$–$P_2$) and the fourth power of the tube's radius ($r^4$) and inversely proportional to length ($l$) and the viscosity ($\eta$) of the fluid (see Equation 2.5).

$$\dot{V} = (P_1 - P_2) \cdot r^4 \cdot \frac{\pi}{8l\eta} \qquad (2.5)$$

If the length or the radius of the tubing changes, the pressure difference changes at a given constant flow rate such as that maintained by the analyzer pump. As the pressure difference changes, so does the partial pressure of oxygen. Changes in pressure can be avoided by flowing the calibration gas from its source (usually a pressured gas cylinder) through an empty 10 ml syringe barrel. The sample line will not be pressurized since gas flow in excess of the vacuum pump flows to ambient air. However, the flow rate from the calibration gas tank must exceed the sensor pump flow rate so that ambient air is not drawn in to dilute the calibration gas. After calibration, no changes should be made to the sample flow rate or tubing that connects the subject's expired air to the gas analyzer. In summary, the following conditions must be met during gas analyzer calibrations.

1. Concentrations of the calibration gases must be precisely known.

2. The calibration gas pressure must not exceed or be lower than ambient pressure.
3. The flow rate of the calibration gas must be greater than the sample rate.
4. There must be no leaks in the sample circuit allowing dilution of the calibration gas by room air.
5. The configuration of the calibration circuit (including sample flow rate) must be identical to the measurement circuit so as not to alter the change in pressure from ambient to the sensing element.

*Water vapor*

A final important concern during calibration and measurement of gas analyzers is the effect of water vapor. Since water vapor pressure contributes to the total pressure in a mixture of gases, its presence decreases the concentration and therefore the partial pressure of all the other gases in the mix. The effect of water vapor may be eliminated with a tube of calcium sulfate placed in the sampling circuit between the distal end of the sample line and the gas analyzer sensor. Unfortunately, this slows the response and transit time and appreciably slower transit times are unacceptable for breath-by-breath applications. As an alternative, specialized sample lines composed of a perflourinated polymer that acts as a hygroscopic ion exchange membrane (Nafion®) may be used to cope with the water vapor problem. These sample lines selectively alter the water vapor content of the gas flowing through the line without changing the composition of the remaining gases. The water vapor content in saturated respiratory gases comes to equilibrium with the water vapor content in the atmosphere as the exhaled gas passes through the length of tubing. In this case the relative "drying" is determined by the amount of time the gas is in the tube (slower sample flow rates and longer tubes increase the "drying"). In the case of calibrating an oxygen analyzer through this special tubing using dry calibration gases, the dry gas is effectively made "wetter," achieving ambient water vapor pressure by the end of the sample line. Gases reaching the sensor of the gas analyzer are assumed to have water vapor content equal to ambient regardless of whether the gas was wet or dry at the inlet.

It is important to note that the gas reaching the gas analyzer through this tubing is never dry. It can only be as dry as the ambient air. This may present a problem in humid environments without air conditioning. Advantageously, this sample line may be used in breath-by-breath systems without appreciable compromise in transit times. In addition, removal of water vapor protects the analyzer from erroneous measurements or damage to the sensing element shortening its operating life. Experience with this special sample tubing suggests a finite time for effective use. The sampling tube should be changed after every three tests conducted in succession and allowed to dry. The sample line should be discarded after 3 months due to the degradation of its water vapor-handling properties.

***Remember the following:*** *Whenever analyzing a gas mixture, if the amount of water vapor in the mixture is underestimated, then the true gas concentrations (%) will be lower than those which you measure or calculate. Conversely, if the amount of water vapor in the mixture is overestimated, then the true gas concentrations (%) will be higher than those which you measure or calculate.*

## Maintenance

With regard to oxygen analyzers, little maintenance is required beyond normal calibration and adjustments recommended by the manufacturer. Care should be taken to maintain clear and clean sample lines. A daily log should be kept of calibration results, including response time and gain settings. With new sensors, the gain setting should be at the lower end of the adjustment range. As the sensor deteriorates with time and use, the analyzer may "run out of gain," meaning that there is little room left for adjustments to a calibration gas. When this happens, sensor replacement is imminently necessary. Some manufacturers recommend periodic service for cleaning and fine adjustments. It may be necessary to have this service performed by factory service personnel.

## Carbon dioxide analyzers

### Description and principles of operation

Most carbon dioxide analyzers in current use are of the nondispursive infrared type. The infrared beam is directed alternately through reference and measurement cells by means of a chopper wheel. A detector senses the alternating change in absorption of selected infrared wavelengths. The fractional concentration of carbon dioxide is proportional to the degree of infrared absorption. The resulting signal is processed and either displayed or output to digital computer algorithms. The response time of these analyzers can be $<100$ ms, making them acceptable for breath-by-breath measurements. The instruments are stable, although the sensing element is susceptible to vibration. Suspending the detector cell or placing it in foam significantly reduces this effect.

### Calibration, accuracy, and precision

The principles and procedures used for calibrating carbon dioxide analyzers are the same as those for oxygen analyzers noted above, with the exception of the selection of the calibration gas concentrations. For typical applications in XT, a "zero" gas containing no $CO_2$, (i.e., 100% nitrogen) and a "span" gas above the expected upper limit of physiological measurement (7–8% $CO_2$) is appropriate. All the concerns for partial pressures and water vapor-handling expressed above for oxygen analyzers are the same for $CO_2$ analyzers and may be dealt with in the same way (see above). Modern $CO_2$ analyzers are fast-responding, accurate (±1% full-scale), and precise.

### Maintenance

With regard to carbon dioxide analyzers, maintenance procedures are minimal. Depending on the model, adjustment of the optical balance and purging the sensor head may be required periodically. Otherwise, taking care not to jar the sensing element and maintaining daily records of the gain and zero settings together with calibration performance is adequate. Some manufacturers recommend periodic service for cleaning and fine adjustments. It may be necessary to have this service performed by factory service personnel.

## Mass spectrometry

### Description and principle of operation

Molecules of exhaled gas samples drawn through the sampling tube are first ionized then dispersed according to gas species on the basis of their mass-to-ionic-charge ratio. After separation, ions of a given species of gas reach an ion detector. The amplitude of the induced current is proportional to the partial pressure of the gas species. Mass spectrometers are linear, stable, and offer very fast response times. Despite these significant advantages, the high cost has limited the widespread use of mass spectrometers in performance and clinical exercise testing.

### Calibration, accuracy, and precision

Calibration of the mass spectrometer follows procedures identical to those described for oxygen and carbon dioxide analyzers above. Accurate calibration gases are required for accurate performance of the mass spectrometer. One of the advantages of the mass spectrometer is the ability to "dial out" water vapor in the gas measured, i.e., functionally eliminate its presence. This leaves only nitrogen, oxygen, carbon dioxide, argon, and other inert gases to comprise 100% of the sample. Consequently, algorithms for the calculation of $\dot{V}O_2$ and $\dot{V}CO_2$ must recognize the absence of water vapor when using a mass spectrometer (see Appendix B). Accuracy and precision of measurement with the mass spectrometer are excellent, varying only about ±0.1% of full-scale per day for $CO_2$ and ±1% of full-scale per day for $O_2$.

### Maintenance

Although an expensive investment and quite complicated in its principle of operation, the mass spectrometer is one of the most reliable gas analyzers available. Furthermore it requires relatively little maintenance. However, a mass spectrometer has two types of vacuum pump: one a priming pump and the other a deep vacuum pump. Both pumps are mechanical and require lubrication on a regular schedule. Occasionally the ionization chamber fails and needs replacement.

## Metabolic measurement systems

### Introduction

A major focus of this book is on the integrated exercise test in which measurement of pulmonary ventilation and gas exchange represent important objectives. The previous sections have outlined specific components for measuring the primary variables needed for this type of testing (i.e., minute ventilation and exhaled fractional concentrations of oxygen and carbon dioxide). Metabolic measurement systems enable the integration of these components using computer-controlled analog-to-digital signal processing. This additional capability allows for online and offline calculation and display of results, as well as storage of data. Several instrument configurations are available, ranging from very simple or semiautomated mixing chamber systems to highly sophisticated fully automated breath-by-breath measurement systems. Some systems provide options for both methods. Features, affordability, ease of use, product training, support, and service, in addition to the expected accuracy and reliability of the instrument, may differ among the commercially available systems. It is essential that users carefully evaluate the competing products and ask for validation data and current user lists, as well as having the opportunity to use the system in their own setting before purchase.

### Mixing chamber method

#### Description and principles of operation

Mixing chamber systems may be very simple manual systems, more complex semiautomated systems, or fully automated computer-controlled systems. Regardless of the degree of sophistication, all possess five basic components: (1) a one-way nonrebreathing valve to direct airflow; (2) conducting tubing; (3) an instrument to measure volume; (4) a device to mix the expired air for subsequent gas sampling; and (5) instruments to measure fractional concentrations of oxygen and carbon dioxide. Leak-free connections throughout the system are essential. The simplest approach is the Douglas bag method in which expired airflow is directed through the one-way valve into a collection bag (see above) over a precisely timed interval. The bag serves as a reservoir for the mixed expired air. Aliquot samples of the mixed air are analyzed with electronic gas analyzers or a Scholander method to give $O_2$ and $CO_2$ concentrations. Although the process is tedious and limited data are available with this approach, it is nevertheless extremely accurate when performed by well-practiced technicians. This method is the standard against which all other systems are validated for accuracy in the determination of $\dot{V}_E$, $\dot{V}O_2$, and $\dot{V}CO_2$.

Another approach replaces the collection bags with a dynamic configuration, directing the exhaled air through connecting tubing into a mixing chamber. At the same time, minute ventilation is determined by measuring either inhaled volume over time ($\dot{V}_I$) with a dry gasometer or exhaled volume over time ($\dot{V}_E$) with one of the mass flow meters, previously described. Mixing chambers may be cylindrical or rectangular-shaped containers in the range of 3–8 l containing baffles to encourage thorough mixing of the exhaled air (Figure 2.12). Some commercial systems use combinations of tubing and blenders as small "dynamic mixing chambers" to achieve this purpose. In any mixing chamber, the goal is to ensure thorough mixing of the dead space and alveolar air for subsequent sampling. Mixing occurs as a result of the turbulent flow-and-eddy

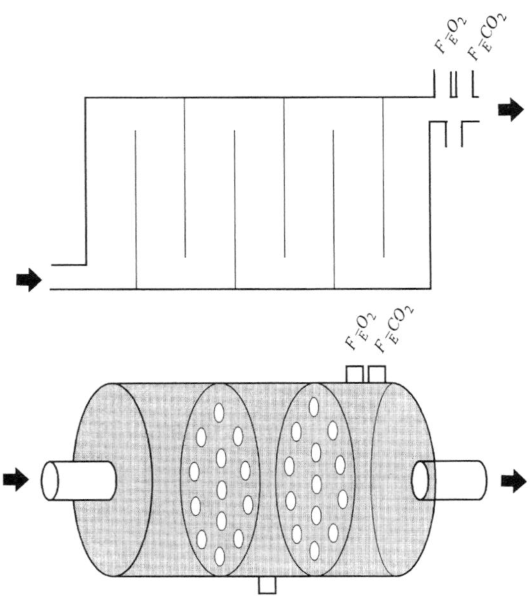


**Figure 2.12** A diagrammatic representation of two types of mixing chambers.

currents that develop when the entering airflow hits the baffles inside the mixing chamber. Properly mixed expired air is sampled near the exhaust port of the mixing chamber and should show no tidal variations in gas concentrations. The sample is drawn by a vacuum pump at known flow rate and passed through a drying tube to remove water vapor before entering the previously calibrated electronic gas analyzers.

In 1974, Wilmore and Costill described a semiautomated system in which a vacuum pump pulled samples of the air from the mixing chamber to small anesthesia bags. The vacuum pumps from the gas analyzers then pulled the mixed gas from the bags for determination of the fractional concentrations of oxygen and carbon dioxide. Three anesthesia bags were attached to a spinner valve at 120° intervals. The valve was manually turned so that, while one bag was filling with air from the mixing chamber, the gas analyzers were sampling from the second bag and the third bag was being evacuated. The interested reader should refer to the original publication for further details (see Further Reading).

Mixing chamber systems do not allow fast enough determinations of $\dot{V}O_2$ and $\dot{V}CO_2$ to be useful in studying gas exchange kinetics with exercise transitions. Typically, a mixing chamber method provides calculated values at best every 20 s.

### Calibration, accuracy, and precision

Of significant concern with mixing chamber systems, especially in non steady-state conditions, is the time alignment of the measurements of ventilation and the mixed expired gas concentrations. For proper calculation of $\dot{V}CO_2$ and $\dot{V}O_2$ the three primary variables, $\dot{V}_E$, fractional concentrations of mixed expired oxygen $F_{\bar{E}}O_2$, and carbon dioxide $F_{\bar{E}}CO_2$, must be measured at precisely the same time. Ventilation is measured without delay either before or after the expired gas is sampled from the mixing chamber. However, the measurement of gas concentrations is delayed since they must travel through conducting tubing, the mixing chamber, the drying tube, and thence to the gas analyzers for measurement. The introduction of Nafion® tubing has perhaps reduced this problem. The delay is not constant, but changes as a function of the flow rate. This is particularly important at low to moderate minute ventilation. During heavy exercise with high flow rates, the temporal misalignment is likely to be small with small errors in the calculated $\dot{V}O_{2max}$. Also, during constant-rate exercise in steady-state conditions, the mixed expired gas concentrations are not changing appreciably, thus eliminating the problem of temporal alignment. The accuracy of any mixing chamber method is dependent upon the accuracy of its component instruments as well as time alignment of the ventilation and gas concentration measurements. Whole breath cycles must be measured for the accurate calculation of ventilation and corrections made for any disparity between $\dot{V}_I$ and $\dot{V}_E$ when the respiratory exchange ratio ($R$) does not equal 1.0 (see Appendix B for computational formulae).

### Maintenance

It is important that the mixing chamber system is maintained in a leak-free condition. In addition to performing regular maintenance on each of the components of the system, the mixing chamber itself should be cleaned and kept free of water that condenses within the chamber. It should be inspected regularly for leaks, especially at the fittings for the gas sampling line(s).

## Breath-by-breath method

### Description and principles of operation

Whereas the mixing chamber method averages expired volumes and gas concentrations over a number of breaths, the breath-by-breath method takes each individual breath and computes its volume and gas composition. This is accomplished by sampling the inspired and expired flow signals at high frequency (e.g., 100 Hz) and integrating to give volume changes throughout the breath cycle. Inspired and expired gas concentrations must be sampled simultaneously with the same frequency and carefully time-aligned with the volumes. $\dot{V}O_2$ and $\dot{V}CO_2$ are then calculated by cross-multiplying the volumes and gas concentrations for the entire breath. In order to accomplish precision in the face of such complexity, precise flow transducers and rapidly responding gas analyzers are essential. Furthermore, processing of the signals would be impossible without the capability of digital computing. Current automated breath-by-breath systems include digital processing for data acquisition and real-time display for key response variables in both tabular and graphical format.

Skeptics of the breath-by-breath method question whether this approach conveys any advantage over a mixing chamber technique. Unquestionably, the breath-by-breath method provides a substantially higher density of data points yet it also exposes significant physiological variability in the data. Provided a carefully chosen method is used to smooth the data whilst at the same time preserving the data density then the display will lend itself more favorably to pattern recognition and detection of thresholds. This advantage can be likened to a television screen whereby the fidelity of the picture is dependent upon the number of lines of resolution. In this regard the rolling average approach to data smoothing is recommended (see Chapter 5).

### Calibration, accuracy, and precision

Automated breath-by-breath systems usually provide automated calibration routines for their flow transducers and gas analyzers. These routines are simple, quickly completed, and should be standard laboratory routine prior to every test (see Chapter 3). It is important to recognize that these calibration routines only check the accuracy of the component measuring devices and do not verify the integrated performance of the whole system.

Two methods are available for integrated system calibration. One approach, referred to as biological calibration, uses healthy human subjects with stable fitness levels. Each subject performs several constant work rates below the metabolic threshold on a well-calibrated cycle ergometer. $\dot{V}O_2$ is averaged across the subjects and compared to the expected $\dot{V}O_2$ calculated using Equation 3.9 (Chapter 3) for each work rate. Performed on a regular schedule (e.g., monthly), this approach assesses both accuracy and reproducibility. A second approach uses a device referred to as a metabolic simulator. This device produces a sinusoidal volume from a precision syringe pump and simulates gas exchange by displacement of room air with a gas mixture of known carbon dioxide and nitrogen concentrations.

### Maintenance

Maintenance of breath-by-breath measurement systems requires careful attention to the performance of their individual components, as previously described. The user should be particularly conscious of the deterioration of gas sampling tubes and slowing of gas analyzer response times. Cleaning and sterilization of nondisposable mass flow transducers is a routine part of system maintenance. To ensure optimal system performance, regular system calibration, as described above, should be included in the maintenance schedule.

## Peripheral measuring devices

### Introduction

Exercise testing can be significantly enhanced by the addition of peripheral measurements. This is particularly true in clinical exercise testing for diagnostic purposes. The peripheral measurements described here include electrocardiography, sphygmomanometry, pulse oximetry, and blood sampling. Once again, the purpose of this book is not to instruct on basic techniques but rather to draw attention to pitfalls commonly encountered in making such measurements and to suggest refinements that enhance the value of an exercise test.

### Electrocardiography

#### Description and principles of operation

The heart contracts as a result of the depolarization of myocardial cells initiated by an impulse from the sinoatrial node. Since the body is a large-volume conductor, this electrical signal may be monitored on the surface of the body with electrodes arranged in a particular configuration. Standard 12-lead electrocardiography (ECG) is the accepted standard for clinical exercise testing in which at least three leads can be simultaneously monitored (e.g., II, aVf, V5). Other lead configurations such as CM5 may be appropriate for performance exercise testing (see Chapter 3). ECG instruments should meet or exceed specifications published by the American Heart Association (see Further Reading). All ECG instruments consist of a recorder with properties of sensitivity, frequency response, and paper speed. Standard sensitivity is $10\,mm \cdot mV^{-1}$. Frequency response specifications should be from 0.5 to 100 Hz. This is important for accurate evaluation of ST segment changes. Standard paper speed is $25\,mm \cdot s^{-1}$. In some applications, sensitivity is increased to $20\,mm \cdot mV^{-1}$ in order to obtain improved detection of amplitudes. The sensitivity may be decreased to $5\,mm \cdot mV^{-1}$, especially when R or S waves are large, due to ventricular hypertrophy or in subjects with thin chest walls. Paper speed may be increased to $50\,mm \cdot s^{-1}$ for easier measurement of intervals and durations such as the QRS duration. The electrocardiograph should provide for continuous display of a minimum of three leads on an oscilloscope. Electrodes made of silver–silver chloride with aggressive adhesive are useful for decreasing motion artifact.

#### Calibration, accuracy, and precision

Modern electrocardiographs provide automatic calibration pulses that are recorded as part of every tracing. The $10\,mm \cdot mV^{-1}$ pulse should rise sharply with no overshoot to a height of 10 mm. Paper speed can be verified with marks and a stopwatch. While older electrocardiographs could be checked for frequency response by pressing and holding the calibration button and observing the subsequent decay of the calibration pulse, newer machines do not typically provide an option for manual calibration. Failure of the electrocardiograph to perform necessitates a service call.

#### Maintenance

Little maintenance is required other than preventing damage to the instrument due to impact. The patient cable should be kept clean, with lead wires hanging straight when not in use. Twisted or tangled lead wires may lead to breakage. Lead wire electrode attachments should be kept free of corrosion.

### Sphygmomanometry

#### Description and principles of operation

The indirect brachial artery auscultation technique using an inflatable cuff, mercury manometer, and good-quality stethoscope is the simplest and most reasonable method for blood pressure monitoring during exercise. Aneroid manometers are not recommended because they are less accurate, less precise, more difficult to calibrate, and require more frequent maintenance. Attention to proper technique (see Chapter 3), choice of correct cuff size, and stethoscope ear pieces that block out most ambient noise will facilitate accuracy, as will appropriate training in the detection of the Korotkoff sounds (see Chapter 4). Laboratories should have cuffs and bladders in multiple sizes from small adult to large adult (see Appendix D, Blood pressure measurement procedures, for correct cuff sizing). Audio and video training tapes are available for learning to distinguish between the distinct tonal qualities of these five sounds. Automated measurement systems have been developed that will inflate and deflate the cuff at preprogrammed intervals. A "physiological sounds" microphone placed over the brachial artery records the different sound frequencies of the Korotkoff phases. The American Heart Association and the British Hypertension Society have published recommendations for blood pressure measurement.

*Intraarterial blood pressure measurement*

Systemic arterial pressure can be measured by placement of an arterial catheter coupled to an electronic pressure transducer. This method is generally too invasive, complex, and time-consuming for performance or even clinical exercise testing. Invasive blood pressure monitoring may be preferred for research purposes.

### Calibration, accuracy, and precision

In sphygmomanometry, the mercury manometer is the calibration standard. When an arterial catheter is used for invasive blood pressure monitoring, the transducer should be calibrated against a mercury manometer. Furthermore, careful attention must be paid to the frequency response of the transducer as well as its accuracy.

### Maintenance

The mercury column should move quickly when pressure is applied through the cuff and tubing. A slow or sluggish-responding mercury column suggests the need for cleaning. The air filter at the top of the column should be regularly inspected and cleaned if necessary. All tubing (including stethoscope tubing), the bladder, and the bulb should be inspected regularly for cracks and leaks. Spares should be readily available, stored in plastic bags to prevent deterioration. Pressure control valves should operate smoothly. Cuffs may be washed in warm water and allowed to dry thoroughly before next use.

## Pulse oximetry

### Description and principles of operation

Pulse oximetry is used to estimate arterial oxygenation noninvasively using the differential absorption of light by reduced hemoglobin (Hb) and oxyhemoglobin ($HbO_2$). The resulting estimate of arterial oxygen saturation is denoted as $Spo_2$ to distinguish it from the saturation determined by blood gas analysis, which is normally denoted as $Sao_2$. The light source used in pulse oximetry is a light-emitting diode (LED) producing bright light in two wavelengths: 660 nm (red region of the spectrum) and 940 nm (near-infrared spectrum). A photo diode detects both wavelengths of transmitted light and produces electrical signals that each have two components: an AC component that varies with the pulsatile nature of arterial blood, and a much larger DC component that is relatively constant and represents light passing through tissue and venous blood without being absorbed. The AC component at each wavelength is corrected by dividing it by the corresponding DC component at each wavelength. The corrected AC component then represents only the differential absorption of light by Hb and $HbO_2$ at the two wavelengths. The absorption of 660-nm wavelength light is 10 times greater for Hb compared with $HbO_2$. At 940 nm, $HbO_2$ has 2–3 times greater absorption than Hb. The ratio of these different absorptions is determined by relating them to actual $Sao_2$ measurements, thus developing a calibration curve for the oximeter at all possible combinations of Hb and $HbO_2$ (from 0 to 100%). This calibration curve is stored in the memory of the microprocessor of the oximeter. Using the pulsatile nature of arterial blood flow, the pulse oximeter uses the AC component from either the 660 nm channel or the 940 nm channel to identify the peak of the waveform for counting. This count is displayed as the pulse rate.

### Calibration, accuracy, and precision

Validation of the pulse oximeter should be performed against simultaneous measurements of $Sao_2$. Most pulse oximeters are calibrated by simple electrical adjustment. Their accuracy is ±2% for $Spo_2$ above 90% and slightly less for $Spo_2$ between 85% and 90%. Accuracy and precision are affected by several factors (Table 2.6). Signal quality can in part be ascertained by examining the pulse rate. An inconsistent pulse rate that does not agree with palpation suggests poor perfusion. Changing between the finger and earlobe attachment site for the sensor may be helpful in some cases.

### Maintenance

Little maintenance is required apart from the normal care one would provide a delicate electronic instrument. Cables and sensors should be protected from damage.

## Arterial blood sampling

### Description and principles of operation

Accurate determinations about gas exchange during exercise necessitate arterial blood sampling at a minimum of two time-points: rest and maximum exercise. Assessment of muscle metabolism is aided by blood sampling for lactate and ammonia. Again, resting and end-exercise measurements are desirable. In addition to these two time-points, there might be indications for blood sampling at other times during testing, e.g., around the metabolic threshold or at a chosen intermediate work rate. Metabolites such as lactate and ammonia can be measured in venous blood; however, it is generally

**Table 2.6.** Factors affecting the accuracy of a pulse oximeter

| Factor | Comment |
|---|---|
| **Perfusion of the sensor site**<br>Poor vascularity<br>Low ambient temperature<br>Vasoconstrictive drugs<br>Hypotension | Poor perfusion causes the oximeter to underestimate $Spo_2$<br>Poor perfusion causes an inadequate pulse waveform and failure to detect accurately $f_C$<br>Perfusion can be improved by warming or rubbing the area |
| **Skin pigmentation** | Darker skin pigmentation causes the oximeter to underestimate $Spo_2$<br>Some oximeters adjust light intensity to compensate for denser pigmentation |
| **Movement of the probe** | Movement, especially during exercise, degrades the oximeter signal, usually resulting in underestimation of $Spo_2$ |
| **Carboxyhemoglobin** | When carboxyhemoglobin exceeds 3%, the oximeter overestimates $Spo_2$ |
| **Methemoglobin** | Low levels of methemoglobin cause the oximeter to overestimate $Spo_2$<br>Very high levels of methemoglobin result in a fixed $Spo_2$ of 84–86% |
| **Jaundice** | Increased bilirubin in the blood causes the oximeter to underestimate $Spo_2$ |
| **Nail polish or acrylic finger nails** | Artificial materials in the field of the oximeter probe cause the oximeter to underestimate $Spo_2$ |
| **Ambient light intensity** | Bright light can cause the oximeter to underestimate $Spo_2$<br>Opaque finger coverlets help |

accepted, at least for lactate, that arterial blood levels are more reliable. Therefore, depending on the type of test being performed, there could be a need for repetitive sampling, preferably of arterial blood. The exercise practitioner has the options of placing an arterial catheter or making multiple discrete arterial punctures.

*Arterial catheter*

Successfully inserted, an arterial catheter allows for rapid, easy, and repetitive sampling. Sterile polyethylene catheters of 18–22 gauge are suitable. Simple catheters can be threaded directly off the needle used for arterial puncture and probably offer the least expensive approach. An alternative approach is to use a guidewire method whereby a flexible wire is first threaded into the artery through the needle used for puncture. Either radial or brachial arteries are used. When a radial artery is chosen, a modified Allen test should be performed to ensure adequate collateral perfusion via the ulnar artery.

*Modified Allen test*

1. The exercise practitioner occludes both of the subject's radial and ulnar arteries using thumb pressure.
2. The subject clenches and releases the handgrip several times until the hand is blanched.
3. The practitioner releases the thumb compressing the ulnar artery and watches for reperfusion of the hand.
4. Lack of satisfactory reperfusion within 20 s indicates a failed Allen test and radial artery puncture on that side should be avoided.

An indwelling arterial catheter must be carefully secured and the arm supported to prevent the catheter from becoming bent or displaced during the study. A moulded plastic, padded splint with Velcro straps is ideal for this purpose. The catheter will require flushing with heparinized saline if not used for more than 2 min. Arterial catheters can readily remain in place for the whole duration of exercise testing. Indeed, in intensive care units patients have arterial catheters for several days with minimal complications. The incidence of thrombosis or occlusion is less than 1 in every 5000 catheterizations and surgical intervention is unlikely ever to be needed.

As well as allowing for repetitive blood sampling, an arterial catheter can be connected to a transducer to enable direct measurement of arterial blood pressure during exercise (see above). This set-up requires a three-way stopcock and heparinized normal saline flush, e.g., from a pressurized bag.

*Double arterial puncture*

A reasonable alternative to insertion of an arterial catheter, and an approach that might be preferred by the subject, is to obtain resting and end-exercise arterial blood samples by two separate arterial punctures. This technique can be useful when the exercise practitioner has a low degree of confidence about successful catheter insertion or when bilateral modified Allen tests are equivocal. Brachial puncture is preferred, since the artery is larger. One clear disadvantage of this technique is that difficulty might be encountered in obtaining the end-exercise sample at a precise time. Weighed against this is the advantage of having already located the artery during the resting puncture and therefore knowing of the site and depth of needle insertion required. Furthermore, the arterial pulse should be easily palpated at the time of maximum exercise. The ideal type of syringe for arterial puncture is preheparinized with a low-friction barrel that is self-filling up to 3 ml. The lactate assay can be performed on 2 ml of the heparinized sample, thus obviating the need for a third blood sample.

### Calibration, accuracy, and precision

Blood gas analyzers can be problematic if not used regularly and subjected to systematic quality control measures. Clinical laboratories performing blood gas analysis should participate in a recognized quality control program such as that offered by the American Thoracic Society. Quality assurance and reference ranges for other biochemical assays should be discussed with the laboratories performing the analyses.

### Maintenance

With regard to blood sampling, maintenance issues are straightforward. Every laboratory performing clinical exercise testing should have a supply of alcohol wipes, gauzes, syringes, needles, stopcocks, heparin, and tubing for blood sampling. Ice is required for transportation of the samples for arterial blood gases. Tubes containing 1 ml of perchlorate are required for lactate assay and need to be stored in a refrigerator until used. Some individuals experience a vasovagal reaction when arterial or venous puncture is performed. The symptoms are lightheadedness, and even fainting. The signs are pallor, sweating, bradycardia, and hypotension. When this happens the subject should be allowed to lie down comfortably for several minutes and the problems should resolve. With this in mind, initial blood sampling or catheter insertion is best performed with the subject seated in a secure reclining chair. The proximity of a gurney is helpful if problems develop.

After blood sampling or catheter removal there is no substitute for accurately applied and prolonged pressure at the puncture site to prevent a bruise or hematoma. This requires thumb or finger pressure by the exercise practitioner or an assistant. Two minutes is usually adequate following venepuncture. Five minutes is the minimum requirement following arterial puncture. A gauze pack, even tightly taped, in place is not a satisfactory substitute.

## FURTHER READING

American Heart Association Committee on Electrocardiography (1990). Recommendations for standardization and specifications in automated electrocardiography: bandwidth and digital processing. A report for health professionals by an ad hoc writing group of the Committee on Electrocardiography and Cardiac Electrophysiology of the Council on Clinical Cardiology, American Heart Association. *Circulation*, **81**, 730–9.

American Thoracic Society (ATS) (1995). Statement on standardization of spirometry – 1994 update. *Am. J. Crit. Care Med.*, **152**, 1107–36.

Consolozio, F. C., Johnson, R. E. & Pecora, L. J. (1963). *Physiological Measurements of Metabolic Functions in Man.* New York: McGraw-Hill.

Franklin, B. A. (1985). Exercise testing, training and arm ergometry. *Sports Med.*, **2**, 100–19.

Huszczuk, A., Whipp, B. J. & Wasserman, K. (1990). A respiratory gas exchange simulator for routine calibration in metabolic studies. *Eur. Respir. J.*, **3**, 465–8.

Laszlo, G. & Sudlow, M. F. (eds) (1983). *Measurement in Clinical Respiratory Physiology.* London: Academic Press.

Perloff, D., Grim, C., Flack, J. et al. (1993). Human blood pressure determination by sphygmomanometry. *Circulation*, **88**, 2460–70.

Ramsay, L. E., Williams, B., Johnston, G. D. et al. (1999). Guidelines for the management of hypertension; report of the third working party of the British Hypertension Society. *J. Hum. Hypertens.*, **13**, 569–92.

Ruhling, R. & Storer, T. (1980). A simple, accurate technique for determining work rate (WATTS) on the treadmill. *J. Sports Med. Phys. Fit.*, **24**, 387–9.

Serra, R. (1998). Improved simulation system for routine cardiopulmonary exercise test equipment. Part III: A new cycle ergometer check system. ECSC Working Group on Standardization of Stress Test Methods. *Monaldi Arch. Chest Dis.*, **53**, 100–4.

Wilmore, J. H. & Costill, D. L. (1974). Semiautomated systems approach to the assessment of oxygen uptake during exercise. *J. Appl. Physiol.*, **36**, 618–20.

Wilmore, J. H., Constable, S. H., Stanforth, P. R. et al. (1982). Mechanical and physiological calibration of four cycle ergometers. *Med. Sci. Sports Exerc.*, **14**, 322–5.

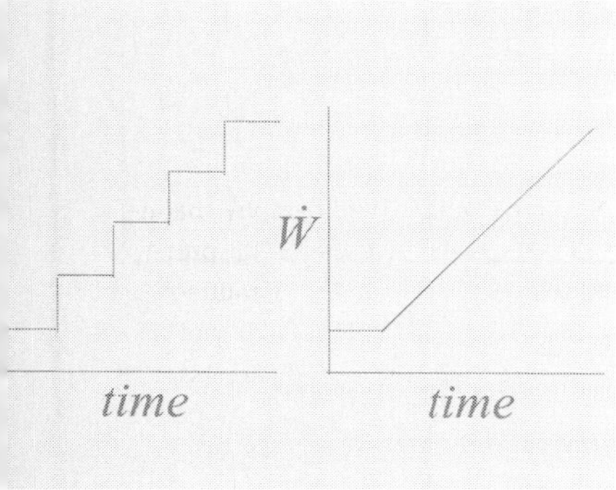


# 3

# Testing methods

## Introduction

A variety of methods is available for assessing the integrated response to exercise. This chapter presents detailed methodologies for conducting exercise tests where knowledge of this response is important for fitness or risk assessment, diagnostic, prescriptive, or monitoring purposes. As illustrated in Chapter 1, XT is conveniently partitioned into two general disciplines: performance exercise testing (PXT) and clinical exercise testing (CXT). The PXT is typically performed on the well population, often as part of preventive strategies, for health promotion, and to provide guidance for fitness improvement or as a basis for training athletes. The CXT is usually reserved for individuals presenting with signs or symptoms of illness or disease. In both PXT and CXT, the setting for the XT may be in the field or laboratory. The choice of a field or laboratory assessment depends upon the purpose of the test, the need for density, precision, and accuracy of the response variables, and the available instrumentation and personnel. Lastly, the protocol for field or laboratory tests describes how the test is conducted. Table 3.1 identifies several potential purposes within the two PXT and CXT disciplines along with possible settings and protocols. Clearly, some protocols will serve multiple purposes. For example, a maximal cycle ergometer test without arterial blood sampling may be appropriate for PXT fitness assessments, exercise prescription, progress monitoring, or CXT diagnostic exercise assessments, risk assessments, or in monitoring the progress of a patient undergoing rehabilitation.

The following two sections briefly introduce the two major types of protocols for exercise testing – submaximal and maximal – identifying their advantages, disadvantages, and assumptions.

### Submaximal testing

Submaximal tests are appropriate for both PXT and CXT. They may be conducted in the field or in the laboratory, may be incremental or constant work rate, but do not directly assess maximal exercise capacity. Many submaximal tests, particularly those used for PXT, attempt to predict aerobic capacity ($\dot{V}O_{2max}$), however, accuracy of the prediction is based on a number of assumptions, particularly the heart rate/work rate relationship. Generally, the predictions are made graphically (Figure 3.1) or through use of prediction equations specific to each test. The advantages, disadvantages, and assumptions underlying the use of the submaximal XT to predict aerobic capacity are presented in Table 3.2.

Submaximal constant rate tests may also be employed as a means to determine exercise endurance or the time constant for oxygen uptake ($\tau\dot{V}O_2$). These applications are described in the section on PXT below. See Chapter 4 for a discussion of $\tau\dot{V}O_2$.

### Maximal testing

Maximal or near maximal tests are also used as PXT and CXT, and may be conducted in the field or in the laboratory. Predictions of $\dot{V}O_{2max}$ may be improved since actual maximal data are obtained. If

**Table 3.1.** Potential purposes, settings, and protocols for performance and clinical exercise tests

| Discipline | Purpose | Setting | Protocol options |
|---|---|---|---|
| PXT | Fitness assessment<br>Exercise prescription<br>Progress monitoring | Field | Timed walk or run<br>Step test<br>Shuttle walk ro run |
| | | Laboratory | **Submaximal** (IWR or CWR)<br>Treadmill, cycle, or arm ergometer<br><br>**Maximal** (IWR or CWR)<br>Treadmill, cycle, or arm ergometer |
| CXT | Diagnostic<br>Integrative<br>Exercise-induced bronchospasm<br>Myopathy<br>Cardiac | Laboratory | **Symptom-limited maximal**<br>With or without arterial blood sampling<br>Treadmill, cycle, or arm ergometer |
| | Risk assessment<br>Cardiac<br>Preoperative<br>Return to work | Field | Timed walk<br>Step test<br>Shuttle walk<br>Stair climb |
| | | Laboratory | **Symptom-limited maximal**<br>With or without arterial blood sampling<br>Treadmill, cycle, or arm ergometer<br><br>**CWR**<br>With or without arterial blood sampling<br>Treadmill, cycle, or arm ergometer |
| | Progress monitoring | Field | Timed walk<br>Step test<br>Shuttle walk<br>Stair climb |
| | | Laboratory | **Symptom-limited maximal**<br>With or without arterial blood sampling<br>Treadmill, cycle, or arm ergometer<br><br>**CWR**<br>With or without arterial blood sampling<br>Treadmill, cycle, or arm ergometer |

IWR = incremental work rate; CWR = constant work rate.

instruments for the measurement of gas exchange are included, measurement of aerobic capacity ($\dot{V}O_{2max}$), as well as many other variables important for test interpretation, are also available. Because subjects are asked to exercise to the point of symptomatic or subjective limitation, the test is highly effort-dependent and can be influenced by a number of factors, including a desire for secondary gain. Table 3.3 indicates the advantages, disadvantages, and assumptions of the maximal XT.

## Performance exercise tests

### Introduction

In the apparently healthy population, performance tests are used for several purposes, including fitness assessments, developing exercise training prescriptions, and for progress monitoring. The key outcome variables for these purposes may be determined directly in the laboratory using maximal tests and metabolic measurement instrumentation. This approach usually provides the greatest accuracy and precision in acquiring the data needed to serve the purpose of the PXT. However, this is not always practical due to the risks, costs, equipment, and personnel required. Consequently, simpler tests have evolved in order to measure submaximal responses and to predict maximal variables such as $\dot{V}O_{2max}$ using nongas exchange data, including work rate, heart rate, or time. These simpler tests may be conducted in the field or in the laboratory and possess varying degrees of accuracy. The following sections review the purposes of PXT as well as field and laboratory tests that may be used to generate data needed for assessing subject performance.

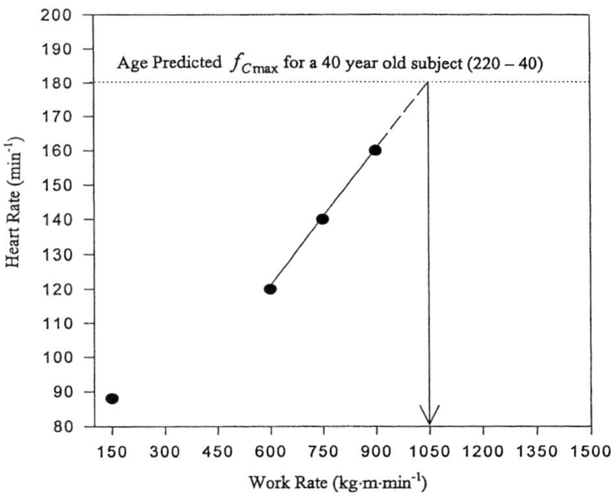


**Figure 3.1** Illustration of the extrapolation of maximal work rate from predicted maximal heart rate and the heart rate/work rate relationship obtained from a submaximal exercise test. In this example, the *x*-axis variable is work rate in kg · m · min$^{-1}$. However, the *x*-axis variable could contain other expressions of work intensity, such as $\dot{V}O_2$, calculated from treadmill speed and grade, or stepping. See Appendix B, Oxygen cost of exercise.

#### Fitness assessment

Fitness assessments are usually conducted to quantify aerobic capacity ($\dot{V}O_{2max}$) for subsequent comparison against reference values. These data may then be used to develop exercise prescriptions as well as to serve as a baseline for observing training status or progress. Testing may be conducted in the field or the laboratory and can be either submaximal or maximal. Field tests, submaximal tests, and some laboratory tests, even when maximal, only estimate $\dot{V}O_{2max}$ through use of prediction equations, thus decreasing accuracy when compared to direct measurements using gas exchange.

#### Exercise prescription

One purpose of PXT is acquisition of sufficient performance data to allow the development of an effective exercise training prescription. Accuracy of test data is of primary importance as its use now goes beyond simple profiling of a subject's aerobic fitness to creating an intervention for change. This suggests choosing the most accurate test available.

**Table 3.2.** Advantages, disadvantages, and assumptions of submaximal XT as compared to maximal XT

| Advantages | Disadvantages | Assumptions for predictive accuracy ($\dot{V}O_{2max}$) |
|---|---|---|
| Less exertion required | Estimates rather than measures aerobic capacity | Accurate ergometer work rates |
| Less time to complete | Misses potentially abnormal responses at work rates above termination point, e.g., ischemic or dyspneic thresholds, hypertension, signs of exercise intolerance | Accurate heart rate measurements |
| Safer, lower risk of complications | Limited data available for interpretation and use for guiding interventions | The $f_C$–$\dot{W}$ relationship is linear up to the predicted $f_{Cmax}$ |
| Fewer requirements for physician supervision (see section on level of supervision, later in this chapter) | Exercise prescriptions for intensity must not exceed the highest $\dot{W}$ achieved | Prediction of $f_{Cmax}$ (e.g., 220 – age) is accurate |
| Reproducible $f_C$–$\dot{W}$ relationship allowing a good method for progress monitoring | | The $\dot{V}O_2$–$\dot{W}$ is linear up to predicted $\dot{V}O_{2max}$ |
| Less dependent on motivation | | |

**Table 3.3.** Advantages, disadvantages, and assumptions of maximal XT as compared to submaximal XT

| Advantages | Disadvantages | Assumptions for predictive accuracy ($\dot{V}O_{2max}$)[a] |
|---|---|---|
| Can provide direct measurement of aerobic capacity | Highly effort-dependent | Ergometer work rates are accurate |
| Provides much additional data | Can require more time to complete | Prediction equations are appropriate to the population, have high correlations, and low SEE |
| Provides greater opportunity to observe an abnormal response if it exists | Increased safety concerns | The $\dot{V}O_2$–$\dot{W}$ is linear up to $\dot{W}_{max}$ |
| Reproducible $f_C$–$\dot{W}$ relationship allowing a good method for progress monitoring | Increased requirements for physician supervision | |
| | Can require more technical expertise to administer and interpret | |

[a]When $\dot{V}O_{2max}$ is not directly measured.
SEE = Standard error of estimate.

While it is beyond the scope of this book to discuss the intricacies of exercise prescription, Table 3.4 provides suggestions for PXT data that are required for this purpose. These data are used to develop the intensity portion of the exercise prescription. Type of exercise, duration, frequency, and rate of progression are other considerations.

**Table 3.4.** Data acquired from PXT for use in exercise prescription

| | Field tests | | Laboratory tests | |
|---|---|---|---|---|
| Variable | Submaximal | Maximal | Submaximal | Maximal |
| Resting heart rate ($f_{Crest}$) | ✓ | ✓ | ✓ | ✓ |
| Maximal heart rate ($f_{Cmax}$) | (✓) | ✓ | (✓) | ✓ |
| Maximal work rate ($\dot{W}_{max}$) | (✓) | ✓ | (✓) | ✓ |
| Resting oxygen uptake ($\dot{V}O_{2rest}$) | (✓) | (✓) | (✓)[✓] | (✓)[✓] |
| Maximal oxygen uptake ($\dot{V}O_{2max}$) | (✓) | (✓) | (✓) | (✓)[✓] |
| Metabolic threshold ($\dot{V}O_2\theta$) | | | [✓] | [✓] |
| Ventilatory threshold ($\dot{V}_E\theta$) | | | [✓] | [✓] |
| Rating of perceived exertion (RPE) | ✓ | ✓ | ✓ | ✓ |
| Walking or running speed | ✓ | ✓ | ✓ | ✓ |
| $f_C$–$\dot{W}$ relationship | ✓ | ✓ | ✓ | ✓ |

✓ Indicates data that may be collected in field or laboratory settings, (✓) indicates data that may be predicted, [✓] indicates data that may be measured if gas exchange measurements are included in the test.

### Progress monitoring

Performance exercise testing may also be used to document changes in aerobic performance due to exercise training. This allows the practitioner to evaluate the effectiveness of the training program and to modify the training elements based on subject responsiveness. Results from serial testing are often motivational, confirming the value of the training program through clear, objective measures of performance. In many cases, the greatest value in some of the field or submaximal tests is their reliability. As discussed in Chapter 2, a test may not exhibit great accuracy, but it may be quite reliable. The reliability of a test makes it ideally suited for progress monitoring when the change may be as or more important than knowledge of the true value.

## Field tests

### Introduction

Field tests for assessing fitness are often used when availability of more sophisticated instrumentation or practicality precludes the use of laboratory tests. Field tests are also appropriate when testing groups of people, providing quantitative and objective measures of exercise performance in a variety of settings. This section presents several field tests for the practitioner who desires a reliable, but simple method of quantifying exercise capacity. Table 3.5 summarizes these assessments.

### Timed walking tests

*Rockport walking test*

The Rockport walking test is a 1-mile (1.60 km) test developed and cross-validated ($r = 0.88$) in 1987 as a simple way to predict $\dot{V}O_{2max}$ in healthy people aged 30–69 years. The test protocol includes:

- Walking 1 mile as fast as possible without running.
- Measuring time for the mile walk to the nearest second.
- Recording a 15-s heart rate immediately upon completion of the mile walk.
- If a heart rate meter is available, record the average heart rate over the last 2 min of the walk.
- Recording body weight (kg) and age (years).
- A cool-down period.

Time and heart rate data are then used along with age, body weight, and a gender coefficient to predict $\dot{V}O_{2max}$:

$$\dot{V}O_{2max} = 132.85 - (0.169 \cdot BW) - (0.39 \cdot age) + (6.32 \cdot gender) - (3.26 \cdot t) - (0.16 \cdot f_C) \quad (3.1)$$

where $\dot{V}O_{2max}$ is expressed in $ml \cdot kg^{-1} \cdot min^{-1}$,

**Table 3.5.** Field tests for fitness assessment

| Test category | Test name and relative effort | Instruments required (optional) | Response variables | Predicted variables |
|---|---|---|---|---|
| Timed walks (submaximal) | Rockport 1-mile walk test<br>Cooper 3-mile walk test | Measured course<br>Stopwatch<br>Scale<br>($f_C$ monitor) | $f_C$<br>$\dot{W}$ (pace) | $\dot{V}O_{2max}$ |
| Timed runs (near maximal) | 12-min run or 1.5-mile run<br>20-meter shuttle run<br>Other distances | Measured course<br>Stopwatch | $f_C$<br>$d_w$<br>$\dot{W}$ (pace) | $\dot{V}O_{2max}$ |
| Step tests (submaximal) | Queens College step test<br>Siconolfi step test | Measured step<br>Metronome<br>Stopwatch or clock ($f_C$ monitor) | $f_C$<br>$\dot{W}$ (watts) | $\dot{V}O_{2max}$ |
| Other (near maximal) | 12-minute swim test<br>12-minute cycle test | Pool or traffic-free cycling area | Distance<br>Distance | Fitness category (quintile) |

BW = body weight in kg, age is in years, gender is 0 for females, 1 for males, $t$ is time to complete the mile walk (min), and $f_C$ is the heart rate (beats $\cdot$ min$^{-1}$). Alternatively, if a heart rate meter is used, the mean $f_C$ during the last 2 min of the test is used for the heart rate variable. The estimated $\dot{V}O_{2max}$ may be used with tables of reference values (see Tables C1 and C2, Appendix C) to obtain a fitness classification.

The standard error of the estimate for this test is 4.4 ml $\cdot$ kg$^{-1}$ $\cdot$ min$^{-1}$. The test has been further cross-validated on younger (20–29 years) and older (70–79 years) males and females and on overweight females with the correlation between estimated and measured $\dot{V}O_{2max}$ ranging from $r = 0.78$ to $r = 0.88$.

*The Cooper 3-mile walking test*

The 3-mile (4.80-km) walk test, developed by Dr Kenneth Cooper, is more challenging and effort-dependent than the Rockport 1-mile walk test. It is generally reserved for individuals who have been actively walking for at least 6 weeks and is applicable to healthy males and females aged 13–70 years. The walking course can be a measured indoor or outdoor track or any other suitable course that has been accurately measured. The procedures are as follows:

- Subject walks 3 miles as fast as possible without running.
- Time to completion is recorded to nearest second.
- Fitness category is determined using Table C8 in Appendix C.

Additional objective measures, such as $f_C$ and RPE, taken at regular intervals during the walk, add further documentation that can be used for progress monitoring.

### Timed run tests

In 1968, Cooper published the first description of his 12-minute run test for estimation of aerobic fitness. This was a modification of a 15-minute run test developed earlier by Balke on military personnel. Later, Cooper introduced the alternative 1.5-mile (2.40-km) run. These are very effort-dependent tests, requiring participants to give a near maximal effort. To be valid, the test requires previous exercise training (at least 6 weeks is recommended), presumably by running. Correlations between time for the 12-minute run or 1.5-mile run tests with measured $\dot{V}O_{2max}$ range from 0.30 to 0.90 depending on the population studied.

*Cooper 12-min running test*

The procedures are as follows:

- Subjects should be encouraged to warm up and stretch prior to the run.
- Subjects should be instructed to run as far as possible in 12 min; walking is permitted.
- Distance to the nearest yard is recorded. To facilitate greater precision in identifying the distance covered, the measured course should be marked every 55 yards (50 m). Distance is recorded by adding the number of complete laps to the distance represented by the last marked 55-yard interval passed.
- Convert distance (yards) to hundredths of a mile for use in Equation 3.2 below or Table B1 in Appendix B.

$$\text{miles} = \frac{\text{yards}}{1760} \tag{3.2}$$

- Subjects should cool down gradually upon completion of the test.
- Table C4 in Appendix C shows distance run in 12 min and the fitness category for that performance. The corresponding estimate for $\dot{V}O_{2max}$ is shown in Table C9.
- Instead of using Table C9, the following equation developed by Cooper provides an estimate of $\dot{V}O_{2max}$:

$$\dot{V}O_{2max} = (35.97 \times \text{miles}) - 11.29 \tag{3.3}$$

where $\dot{V}O_{2max}$ is expressed in $ml \cdot kg^{-1} \cdot min^{-1}$.

*Cooper 1.5-mile run test*

The protocol for the 1.5-mile (2.40 km) run test is identical to the 12-minute run except that the criterion is completion of a fixed distance rather than a fixed time. This is advantageous when testing larger groups of people, as it is easier to recognize and record a more precise endpoint for the test. For this reason and because people may be better able to pace themselves over a known distance rather than a known time (e.g., 12 min), the 1.5-mile run test is preferred. The procedures are as follows:

- Subjects should be encouraged to warm up and stretch prior to the run.
- Subjects should be instructed to complete the 1.5-mile distance as fast as possible; walking is permitted.
- Time is recorded to the nearest second.
- Subjects should cool down gradually upon completion of the test.
- Use of Tables C7 and C9 in Appendix C and the time to complete the 1.5-mile run will provide estimates of the fitness category and $\dot{V}O_{2max}$ for that performance.

*20-meter Shuttle running test*

The multistage 20-meter shuttle run test was originally developed by Léger & Lambert (1982) to assess $\dot{V}O_{2max}$ in healthy adults tested either individually or in groups. The protocol requires the following conditions:

- The 20-m course should be dry, firm, and flat and allow 5–10 m extra length for deceleration at each end (Figure 3.2).
- Subjects run back and forth on the 20-m course marked at each end with a line.
- Subjects must touch the line at the same time a sound cue is emitted from a prerecorded audiotape.
- The frequency of the cues is increased $0.5\ km \cdot h^{-1}$ ($8.33\ m \cdot min^{-1}$) every 2 min from a starting speed of $8.0\ km \cdot h^{-1}$ ($133.3\ m \cdot min^{-1}$ or 5.0 m.p.h.).
- Cues are provided so that an audible tone is sounded as a pacing mechanism. Table 3.6 indicates the pace time for each shuttle during each 2-min stage.
- When the subject is no longer able to reach the 20-m distance on cue (defined as more than 3 m away), the last fully completed stage number is recorded and used to predict maximal oxygen uptake corresponding to the final stage.

$$\dot{V}O_{2max} = (5.857 \cdot S) - 19.458 \tag{3.4}$$

where $\dot{V}O_{2max}$ is expressed in $ml \cdot kg^{-1} \cdot min^{-1}$, and $S$ is the speed corresponding to the last completed stage expressed in $km \cdot h^{-1}$. Speed can be obtained from Table 3.6 or calculated in $km \cdot h^{-1}$ using the formula $8 + [0.5(\text{completed stages} - 1)]$.

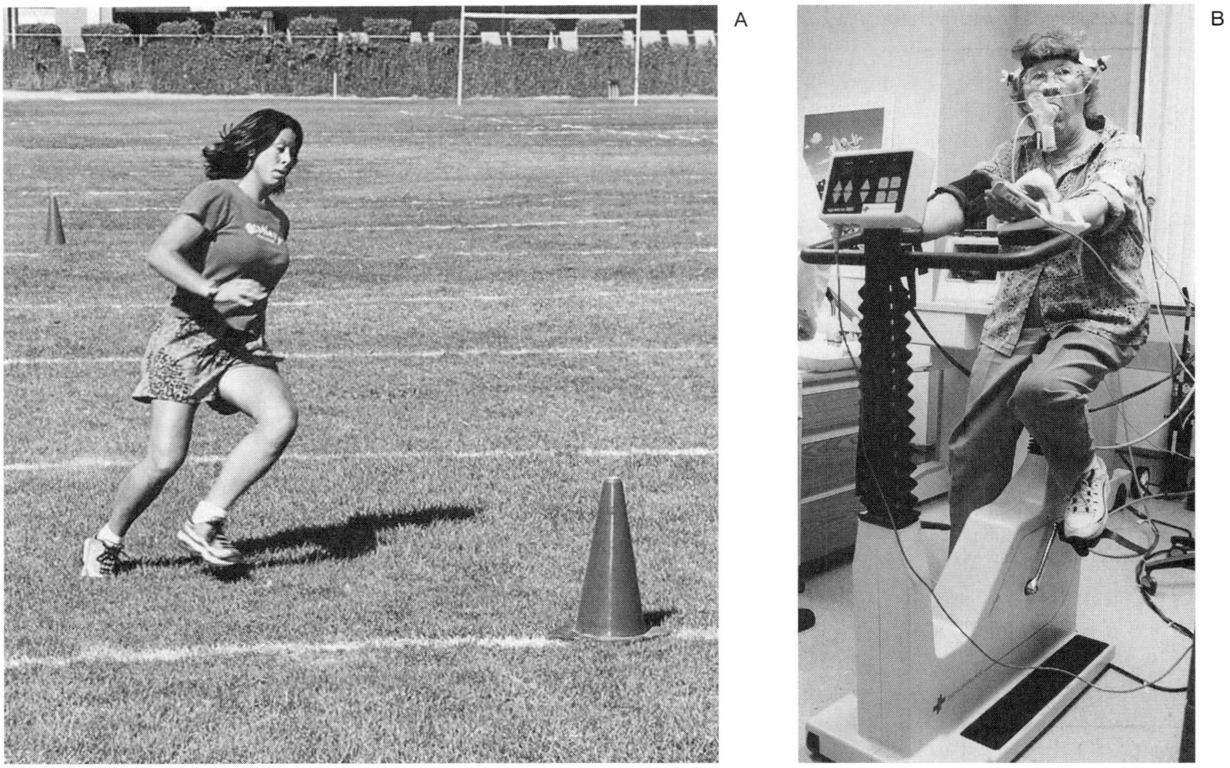


**Figure 3.2** Photographs of performance and clinical exercise tests in progress. (A) Healthy young adult performing a 20-m shuttle test. (B) Patient with chronic obstructive pulmonary disease performing a diagnostic exercise test on a cycle ergometer.

Table 3.6 indicates speed at each stage, the corresponding time per shuttle (for use in recording the audiotape), shuttles to be completed per minute, distance covered in each stage, and estimated $\dot{V}O_{2max}$.

> **Example:** If a subject completed nine stages and four shuttles, the speed would equal $8 + [0.5 \cdot (9-1)] = 12\ km \cdot h^{-1}$. Using Equation 3.4, or Table 3.6, $\dot{V}O_{2max} = 50.8\ ml \cdot kg^{-1} \cdot min^{-1}$ ($r = 0.84$, SEE $= 5.4\ ml \cdot kg^{-1} \cdot min^{-1}$).

### Step tests

*Queens College single-stage step test*

This step test is best suited for college-aged males and females and uses recovery heart rate to predict $\dot{V}O_{2max}$. The test is conducted in a single 3-min period and requires a 41.3-cm (16.25-in.) step or platform. In the USA, this height is standard for gymnasium bleacher seats. A metronome or prerecorded audiotape is used to set the stepping rate. Heart rate during recovery is recorded via palpation or a heart rate meter. The protocol requires that:

- Subjects have warmed up and stretched.
- The method of stepping is described and demonstrated as follows:
  - (a) On the first count (sound cue from the metronome or tape), step up on to the step with one foot.
  - (b) On the second count, subjects step up with the opposite foot, extending both legs and the back.

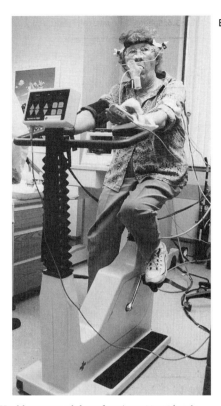

**Table 3.6.** Speeds, time intervals, and predicted $\dot{V}O_{2max}$ for each stage of the 20-m shuttle test

| Stage | Speed ($km \cdot h^{-1}$) | Speed ($m \cdot min^{-1}$) | Speed ($m \cdot s^{-1}$) | Speed (m.p.h.) | Shuttles per min | Time per shuttle (s) | Distance per stage (m) | Total distance (m) | Predicted $\dot{V}O_{2max}$ ($ml \cdot kg^{-1} \cdot min^{-1}$) |
|---|---|---|---|---|---|---|---|---|---|
| 1 | 8.0 | 133 | 2.22 | 4.98 | 6.7 | 9.00 | 267 | 267 | 27.40 |
| 2 | 8.5 | 142 | 2.36 | 5.29 | 7.1 | 8.47 | 283 | 550 | 30.33 |
| 3 | 9.0 | 150 | 2.50 | 5.60 | 7.5 | 8.00 | 300 | 850 | 33.26 |
| 4 | 9.5 | 158 | 2.64 | 5.91 | 7.9 | 7.58 | 317 | 1167 | 36.18 |
| 5 | 10.0 | 167 | 2.78 | 6.22 | 8.3 | 7.20 | 333 | 1500 | 39.11 |
| 6 | 10.5 | 175 | 2.92 | 6.53 | 8.8 | 6.86 | 350 | 1850 | 42.04 |
| 7 | 11.0 | 183 | 3.06 | 6.84 | 9.2 | 6.55 | 367 | 2217 | 44.97 |
| 8 | 11.5 | 192 | 3.19 | 7.15 | 9.6 | 6.26 | 383 | 2600 | 47.90 |
| 9 | 12.0 | 200 | 3.33 | 7.46 | 10.0 | 6.00 | 400 | 3000 | 50.83 |
| 10 | 12.5 | 208 | 3.47 | 7.77 | 10.4 | 5.76 | 417 | 3417 | 53.75 |
| 11 | 13.0 | 217 | 3.61 | 8.08 | 10.8 | 5.54 | 433 | 3850 | 56.68 |
| 12 | 13.5 | 225 | 3.75 | 8.40 | 11.3 | 5.33 | 450 | 4300 | 59.61 |
| 13 | 14.0 | 233 | 3.89 | 8.71 | 11.7 | 5.14 | 467 | 4767 | 62.54 |
| 14 | 14.5 | 242 | 4.03 | 9.02 | 12.1 | 4.97 | 483 | 5250 | 65.47 |
| 15 | 15.0 | 250 | 4.17 | 9.33 | 12.5 | 4.80 | 500 | 5750 | 68.40 |
| 16 | 15.5 | 258 | 4.31 | 9.64 | 12.9 | 4.65 | 517 | 6267 | 71.33 |
| 17 | 16.0 | 267 | 4.44 | 9.95 | 13.3 | 4.50 | 533 | 6800 | 74.25 |
| 18 | 16.5 | 275 | 4.58 | 10.26 | 13.8 | 4.36 | 550 | 7350 | 77.18 |
| 19 | 17.0 | 283 | 4.72 | 10.57 | 14.2 | 4.24 | 567 | 7917 | 80.11 |
| 20 | 17.5 | 292 | 4.86 | 10.88 | 14.6 | 4.11 | 583 | 8500 | 83.04 |

(c) On count 3, the first foot is returned to the floor.
(d) On count 4, the second foot returns to the floor. This four-step cycle is repeated in time with the counting device for the duration of the test.

- The subjects practice 15–30 s before the test is administered.
- Female subjects perform the test at 22 complete cycles per minute. Thus the metronome or audiotape emits 88 sounds per minute.
- Male subjects perform the test at 24 cycles (96 sounds) per minute.
- Heart rate is recorded for 15 s beginning precisely 5 s after the 3-min stepping period has ended. Thus, record $f_C$ between 5 and 20 s of recovery. Multiply by 4 to convert to beats $\cdot$ min$^{-1}$.
- For the test to be valid, both legs and the back must come to full extension at the top of each step, i.e., after count 2.

The following equations, also described in Appendix B, predict $\dot{V}O_{2max}$ in males and females respectively:

Males:

$$\dot{V}O_{2max} = 111.33 - (0.42 \cdot f_{Crec}) \tag{3.5}$$

Females:

$$\dot{V}O_{2max} = 65.81 - (0.1847 \cdot f_{Crec}) \tag{3.6}$$

where $\dot{V}O_{2max}$ is expressed in $ml \cdot kg^{-1} \cdot min^{-1}$ and $f_{Crec}$ is the recovery heart rate. The predicted $\dot{V}O_{2max}$ scores can be used to identify the fitness category using Tables C2 and C3 in Appendix C.

*Siconolfi multistage step test*

In contrast to the single-stage Queens College step test, the Siconolfi multistage step test predicts $\dot{V}O_{2max}$ from a test that consists of one, two, or three stages and is applicable to a wider range of age groups (males and females aged 19–70 years). The step height is lower (25.4 cm or 10 in.) and the stepping rate is varied with each 3-min stage. Recovery periods of 1 min are given between stages. A metronome or audiotape is used to set the cadence. Recovery $f_C$ is best obtained by a heart rate meter. Palpation in this test is difficult because of the need to measure $f_C$ during stepping. The protocol is as follows:

- Calculate and record the subject's age-predicted maximum heart rate (220 – age).
- Provide warm-up and stretching for the subject.
- Describe and demonstrate the stepping procedure as indicted for the Queens College step test (above).

*Stage 1*

- The subject steps at 68 steps (17 cycles) per minute for 3 min.
- Record $f_C$ during the last 30 s of the 3-min period.
- The subject sits for 1 min recovery.
- If the $f_C$ during stage 1 is less than 65% of the age-predicted maximum $f_C$, continue with stage 2 after the 1-min recovery period.
- If the $f_C$ during stage 1 is greater than 65% of the age-predicted maximum $f_C$, the test is ended.

*Stage 2*

- The subject steps at 104 steps (26 cycles) per minute for 3 min.
- Record $f_C$ during the last 30 s of the 3-min period.
- The subject sits for 1 min recovery.
- If the $f_C$ during stage 2 is less than 65% of the age-predicted maximum $f_C$, continue with stage 3 after the 1-min recovery period.
- If the $f_C$ during stage 2 is greater than 65% of the age-predicted maximum $f_C$, the test is ended.

*Stage 3*

- The subject steps at 136 steps (34 cycles) per minute for 3 min.
- Record $f_C$ during the last 30 s of the 3-min period.

$\dot{V}O_{2max}$ is predicted as follows:

1. First, the $\dot{V}O_2$ ($ml \cdot kg^{-1} \cdot min^{-1}$) for the stepping rate is determined from standard equations for stepping (Appendix B, Equations B11, B12, and B13). These $\dot{V}O_2$ values are 16.3, 24.9, and 33.5 ($ml \cdot kg^{-1} \cdot min^{-1}$), respectively, for stages 1, 2, and 3.
2. This $\dot{V}O_2$ is multiplied by the subject's weight (kg) and divided by 1000 to convert to $l \cdot min^{-1}$.
3. The $\dot{V}O_2$ in $l \cdot min^{-1}$ and the $f_C$ at the end of the last stage are used to predict $\dot{V}O_{2max}$ ($l \cdot min^{-1}$) from the Åstrand–Ryhming nomogram (Figure C5 in Appendix C). The estimated $\dot{V}O_{2max}$ so derived is corrected with the following equation, developed by Siconolfi et al. (see Further Reading):

$$\dot{V}O_{2max} = 0.302 \cdot (\text{nomogram}\dot{V}O_{2max}) - (0.019 \cdot \text{age}) + 1.593 \qquad (3.7)$$

where $\dot{V}O_{2max}$ is expressed in $l \cdot min^{-1}$ and age is expressed in years.

### Other field assessments

Additional assessments for fitness are available and include the Cooper 12-minute swim test and the Cooper 12-minute cycle test. Protocols for administering these tests are similar to the 12-minute run test described above. Fitness classifications based on distance completed for these tests are contained in Appendix C (Tables C5 and C6). Details on the conduct of these tests may be found by referring to Cooper's *The Aerobics Program for Total Well-being* (1982), listed in Further Reading.

## Laboratory tests

### Introduction

Laboratory tests offer greater control over the environment (temperature, humidity, surfaces, and distractions) and the subject. Use of more sophisticated instruments, including metabolic measurement equipment, within the laboratory allows greater accuracy and precision in the measurement of a greater number of response variables. Thus, more data of potentially higher quality are obtainable for interpretation. Whenever available and appropriate for the purpose, laboratory testing is preferred. This section presents several submaximal and maximal strategies that can be applied in the laboratory for assessing the integrated response to exercise. Table 3.7 summarizes these assessments.

### Submaximal incremental work rate tests

*Cycle ergometer tests*

Several tests are available in this category, most of which are modifications of the multistage test developed by Sjostrand in 1947. These tests are based on the same underlying principle: that the relationship between $f_C$, $\dot{W}$, and $\dot{V}O_2$ is linear and that estimates of $\dot{V}O_{2max}$ may be made from the extrapolation of the $f_C$–$\dot{W}$ relationship (Figure 3.1). Since estimates of $\dot{V}O_2$ are wholly dependent upon accurate ergometer work rates and accurate measurements of heart rate, extreme care must be exercised in ensuring this accuracy. Failure to do so increases error and decreases reproducibility. Error for these tests in predicting $\dot{V}O_{2max}$ is usually in the 10–15% range, but can be as high as 25%. The major source of error, assuming properly calibrated instruments and good procedures, is in the assumption that $f_{Cmax}$ is faithfully represented by the formula: 220 – age (or some other prediction equation). Other concerns include the potential for nonlinearity in the $\dot{V}O_2$–$\dot{W}$ response (see Chapter 4). Accuracy aside, submaximal cycle tests have potential for good reproducibility and thus for tracking changes.

The multistage YMCA cycle ergometer test is one of the most commonly used submaximal cycle tests for fitness assessment. The test consists of four 3-min stages, incrementing in a heart rate-dependent branching protocol, as illustrated in Figure 3.3. After an initial 3 min of cycling at 150 kg · m · min$^{-1}$ (~25 W), work rate is increased in the next 3-min stage based on the $f_C$ response to the first work rate (Figure 3.3). For subsequent stages, work rate is further increased following the initial branch until a fourth stage is completed (12 min) or until the subject reaches 85% of age-predicted $f_{Cmax}$ or 70% of the heart rate reserve (age-predicted $f_{Cmax} - f_{Crest}$).

$$f_{Creserve} = f_{Cmax} - f_{Crest} \qquad (3.8)$$

The following protocol should be undertaken to perform the YMCA multistage cycle test:

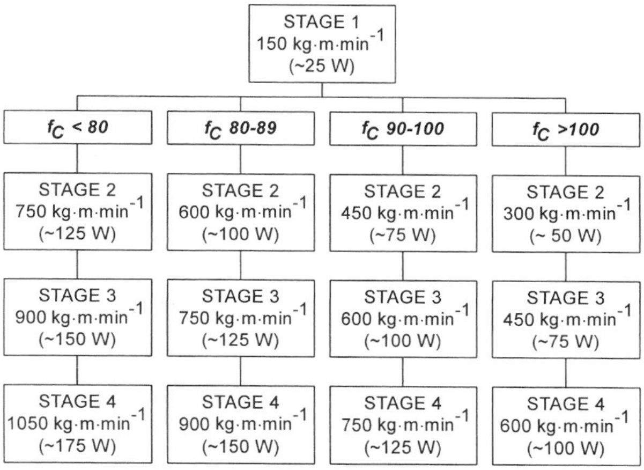


**Figure 3.3** Branching protocol for submaximal cycle ergometer exercise testing. Adapted with permission of the YMCA from Golding, L., Myers, C. & Sinning, W. E. (eds) (1989). *Y's Way to Physical Fitness: The Complete Guide to Fitness Testing and Instruction*, 3rd edn. Chicago, IL: Human Kinetics Publishers.

- Verify calibration of the ergometer.
- Adjust the saddle height so that the knee angle is between 5 and 15° of flexion when the foot presses the pedal to the bottom of its stroke. The seat height should be recorded for future tests. Failure to do so and the use of a different seat height in subsequent tests may result in biomechanical changes and differences in $\dot{V}O_2$ at every work rate.
- Attach a heart rate meter (a pulse oximeter can be used for this purpose) or find and mark a peripheral artery such as the radial or carotid artery to be used with palpation. If the carotid artery is used, care should be taken to press lightly on one side only and not to massage the area so as to avoid provoking the baroreceptor reflex. Obtain $f_C$.
- Attach a sphygmomanometer cuff and measure the resting blood pressure.
- Explain the protocol and allow familiarization with pedal cadence during stage 1. A pedal cadence of 50–60 r.p.m. is recommended.
- Record $f_C$ near the end of minutes 2 and 3 of each of the 3-min stages.
- Record blood pressure and rating of perceived exertion (RPE) near the end of each stage.

**Table 3.7.** Laboratory tests for fitness assessment

| Test category | Test name | Instruments[a] required and optional[b] | Variables that can be measured[c] | Predicted variables |
|---|---|---|---|---|
| Submaximal, incremental work rate | YMCA cycle[d] test<br>Modified Bruce or Balke treadmill test | Cycle ergometer<br>Treadmill ergometer<br>Arm ergometer<br>Sphygmomanometer<br>Stethoscope<br>Timing device<br>($f_C$ monitor)<br>(ECG)<br>(Pulse oximeter)<br>(Metabolic measurement system)[a]<br>(Arterial blood sampling)<br>(Psychometric scales) | $f_C$<br>$\dot{W}$ (watts) or BP<br>$t$<br>(ECG)<br>($Spo_2$)<br>($\dot{V}o_2$, $\dot{V}co_2$, $\dot{V}_E$ plus derived variables)[e]<br>($Pao_2$, $Paco_2$, $Spo_2$, $HCO_3^-$, La, BP)<br>(RPE, VAS) | $\dot{W}_{max}$<br>$\dot{V}o_{2max}$ |
| Submaximal, constant work rate | Åstrand–Ryhming cycle test<br>Constant work rate cycle[c] test<br>Single-stage treadmill test | Cycle ergometer<br>Treadmill ergometer<br>Sphygmomanometer<br>Stethoscope<br>Timing device<br>($f_C$ monitor)<br>(ECG)<br>(Pulse oximeter)<br>(Metabolic measurement system)[a]<br>(Arterial blood sampling)<br>(Psychometric scales) | $f_C$<br>$\dot{W}$ (watts) or BP<br>$t$<br>(ECG)<br>($Spo_2$)<br>($\dot{V}o_2$, $\dot{V}co_2$, $\dot{V}_E$ plus derived variables)[e]<br>($Pao_2$, $Paco_2$, $HCO_3^-$, La, BP)<br>(RPE, VAS) | $\dot{V}o_{2max}$<br>$\dot{W}_{max}$ |
| Maximal, incremental work rate | Stair step or ramp cycle[d] test<br>Stair step or ramp treadmill test | Cycle ergometer<br>Treadmill ergometer<br>Arm ergometer<br>Sphygmomanometer<br>Stethoscope<br>Timing device<br>($f_C$ monitor)<br>(ECG)<br>(Pulse oximeter)<br>(Metabolic measurement system)[a]<br>(Arterial blood sampling)<br>(Psychometric scales) | $f_C$<br>$\dot{W}$ (watts) or BP<br>$t$<br>(ECG)<br>($Spo_2$)<br>($\dot{V}o_2$, $\dot{V}co_2$, $\dot{V}_E$ plus derived variables)[e]<br>($Pao_2$, $Paco_2$, $HCO_3^-$, La, BP)<br>(RPE, VAS) | $\dot{V}o_{2max}$ |

[a]See Chapter 2.
[b]Instruments in parentheses are optional.
[c]Variables in parentheses are optional depending on equipment used.
[d]May also be used with arm ergometry. See below.
[e]See Chapter 4.
See Appendix A for definition of variables.

**Table 3.8.** Suggested timing for measurement of $f_C$, blood pressure, and RPE during each 3-min stage of a submaximal exercise test

| Time of each stage | $f_C$ | Blood pressure | RPE |
|---|---|---|---|
| 0:00–1:40 | | | |
| 1:40–1:55 | X | | |
| 2:00–2:30 | | X | |
| 2:40–2:55 | X | | |
| 2:55–3:00 | | | X |

Although there are no specific times that are necessarily better than others, the schedule shown in Table 3.8 works well, allowing all necessary data to be collected.

- The $f_C$ at the end of minutes 2 and 3 must agree within ±6 $min^{-1}$ before the work rate is increased to the next stage.
- Monitor signs and symptoms of exercise intolerance throughout test.
- Verify that the pedal cadence is maintained at the desired rate. This is of utmost importance in mechanically braked ergometers since changes in r.p.m. directly affect the work rate (see Chapter 2).
- Terminate the test when the subject reaches 85% of age-predicted $f_{Cmax}$ or 70% of the heart rate reserve (see Equation 3.8).
- Provide a recovery period during which the subject cycles at a work rate equivalent to or lower than stage 1 of the test.
- In an emergency or if the subject develops adverse symptoms such as angina, dyspnea, or claudication, remove the subject from the cycle and elevate the feet. Monitor $f_C$, blood pressure, and symptoms for at least 4 min of recovery. Extend the recovery period if untoward signs persist.

Upon completion of the test, $f_C$ and $\dot{W}$ are tabulated as shown in Table 3.9. The $\dot{W}_{max}$ may be estimated by graphical analysis from the linear portion of the $f_C$–$\dot{W}$ relationship, extrapolating the curve upwards to the predicted $f_{Cmax}$ (Figure 3.1). Alternatively, the slope and intercept of the linear portion of the $\dot{W}$–$f_C$ relationship along with the predicted $f_{Cmax}$ can be used to estimate $\dot{W}_{max}$. Following estimation of $\dot{W}_{max}$ by either method, $\dot{V}O_{2max}$ is predicted from the estimated $\dot{W}_{max}$ (either W or kg · m · $min^{-1}$) and the subject's body weight (kg) using either Equation 3.9 or 3.10 below.

**Table 3.9.** Data table for $\dot{W}$–$f_C$ regression and prediction of $\dot{V}O_{2max}$ from $f_C$–$\dot{W}$ responses from the YMCA submaximal branching protocol

| Stage | $f_C$ ($min^{-1}$) | $\dot{W}$ (kg · m · $min^{-1}$) |
|---|---|---|
| 1 | 88 | 150 |
| 2 | 120 | 600 |
| 3 | 140 | 750 |
| 4 | 160 | 900 |

Either, using the equation of Whipp and Wasserman (see Further Reading):

$$\dot{V}O_{2max} = (10.3 \cdot \dot{W}_{max}) + (5.8 \cdot BW) + 151 \quad (3.9)$$

where $\dot{V}O_{2max}$ is expressed in ml · $min^{-1}$, $\dot{W}_{max}$ is in watts, and BW is in kg.

Or, using the equation of the American College of Sports Medicine (see Further Reading):

$$\dot{V}O_{2max} = (2 \cdot \dot{W}_{max}) + (3.5 \cdot BW) \quad (3.10)$$

where $\dot{V}O_{2max}$ is expressed in ml · $min^{-1}$, $\dot{W}_{max}$ is in kg · m · $min^{-1}$, and BW is body weight in kg.

**Example:** Calculating the slope and intercept ($\dot{W}$ as the dependent, e.g., *y*-axis variable) from the sample data in Table 3.9 for a 40-year-old male yields a slope of 7.5 and *y*-intercept of –300. Since a 40-year-old male has a predicted $f_{Cmax}$ of 180 min, predicted $\dot{W}_{max} = 7.5 \cdot 180 - 300 =$ 1050 kg · m · $min^{-1}$ (172 W). Using the graphical approach for this 40-year-old subject as shown in Figure 3.1, $\dot{W}_{max}$ is predicted as 1050 kg · m · $min^{-1}$ (172 W). Using the subject's body weight of 75 kg and predicted $\dot{W}$ with Equation 3.9, the predicted $\dot{V}O_{2max}$ is 2319 ml · $min^{-1}$. Using Equation 3.10, $\dot{V}O_{2max}$ is 2363 ml · $min^{-1}$.

**Table 3.10.** Data for $\dot{V}O_2$–$f_C$ regression and prediction of $\dot{V}O_{max}$ from a submaximal Bruce protocol

| Stage | Speed m.p.h. $(m \cdot min^{-1})$ | % Grade | $f_C$ $(min^{-1})$ | $\dot{V}O_2$ $(ml \cdot kg^{-1} \cdot min^{-1})$ |
|---|---|---|---|---|
| 1 | 1.7 | 10 | 100 | 16.3 |
| 2 | 2.5 | 12 | 130 | 24.7 |
| 3 | 3.4 | 14 | 160 | 35.6 |

*Treadmill tests*

While submaximal fitness testing is often performed on the cycle ergometer, submaximal treadmill tests may be advantageous from the point of view of task specificity. If a subject is planning to walk or run as the primary mode of training, use of a similar exercise mode for assessment will optimize the chance of documenting real change. The advantages and disadvantages of the various ergometers were presented in Chapter 2.

The Bruce or Balke protocols (see Tables D1 and D2 in Appendix D) are often used, although these tests are generally terminated at 85% of the $f_{Creserve}$ (see Equation 3.8). An estimation of $\dot{V}O_{2max}$ may be obtained using either regression analysis or the extrapolation method, described in Figure 3.1. Unlike the method described for cycle ergometry, values of $\dot{V}O_2$ are used instead of $\dot{W}$ for the $x$-axis variable. Table 3.10 gives an example of this approach for a submaximal Bruce protocol.

Appendix B explains how to derive the required values for $\dot{V}O_2$. Equation B21 predicts $\dot{V}O_2$ for the Balke treadmill protocol and Equations B22a–c predict $\dot{V}O_2$ for the Bruce treadmill protocol. Alternatively, $\dot{V}O_2$ can be calculated from any treadmill speed and grade, using Equation 3.11 below in conjunction with Equations B4–6 in Appendix B.

$$\dot{V}O_2(ml \cdot kg^{-1} \cdot min^{-1}) = \dot{V}O_2H + \dot{V}O_2V + \dot{V}O_2R \qquad (3.11)$$

where $H$ is the horizontal component in $m \cdot min^{-1}$, $V$ is the vertical component expressed as percentage grade/100, and $R$ is the resting component (generally assumed to be $3.5\,ml \cdot kg^{-1} \cdot min^{-1}$).

**Example:** Calculating the slope and intercept ($\dot{V}O_2$ as the dependent, e.g., $y$-axis variable) from these data for a 40-year-old male yields a slope of 0.322, and a $y$-intercept of –16.3. Hence this 40-year-old male with a predicted $f_{Cmax}$ of $180\,min^{-1}$ has a predicted $\dot{V}O_{2max}$ of $41.6\,ml \cdot kg^{-1} \cdot min^{-1}$.

This same approach may be adopted for any protocol developed by the user. The Balke protocol can be favorably modified, maintaining a constant speed while incrementing the grade each minute. Choice of speed is based on subject history and clinical judgment. The grade is chosen so as to terminate the test in 8–12 min at a level corresponding to about 85% of the $f_{Creserve}$. A simple spreadsheet can be used to calculate the optimal percentage grade (see Figure D4 in Appendix D, Calculating a treadmill protocol).

*Arm ergometry*

The smaller muscle mass employed in arm ergometry, in addition to lack of regular training stimulus (except in upper-extremity athletes such as swimmers, rowers, kayakers), results in early fatigue and lower $\dot{V}O_{2max}$ (60–80% of leg cycling). This suggests a selection of protocols that utilize smaller $\dot{W}$ increments than typically used in leg ergometry. The $\dot{W}$ increment is selected individually on the basis of subject history and test purpose (see section below on selecting the optimal exercise test protocol). Maximal arm ergometer protocols generally use work rate increments of 10–25 W and may be continuous or discontinuous, applied in stages of 1–6 min. Continuous protocols save time whilst discontinuous protocols facilitate easier measurement of blood pressure, $f_C$, and the ECG if included. Cranking frequency is 40–60 r.p.m. Application of the $f_C$–$\dot{W}$ relationship provides an appropriate basis for designing a submaximal arm ergometer protocol. Prediction of $\dot{V}O_{2max}$ is accomplished through the same regression procedures described above for leg cycling, although the equation for predicting $\dot{V}O_{2max}$ from predicted $\dot{W}_{max}$ is different, as shown in Equation 3.12.

A submaximal arm ergometer protocol for

younger, healthy subjects might consist of:

- 3-min warm-up at 0 W.
- Increasing the $\dot{W}$ by 15–25 W every 3 min while measuring and recording $f_C$ at the end of each minute. $f_C$ should be in steady state (±6 min$^{-1}$) during the last 2 min of each stage.
- If $f_C$ is >6 min$^{-1}$ different, the $\dot{W}$ is held for another minute until the steady-state $f_C$ criterion is achieved.
- Blood pressure may be measured by momentarily stopping the test every 3 min.
- RPE should be obtained at the end of each 3-min stage.
- The test is terminated when the subject reaches 85% $f_{Cmax}$ or 70% of the $f_{Creserve}$ ($f_{Cmax} - f_{Crest}$) or if the subject cannot maintain the cranking frequency, or exhibits signs of intolerance to the exercise.
- A recovery period is provided at a low $\dot{W}$ (e.g., 0–10 W) with continued $f_C$ and blood pressure monitoring.
- Regression is obtained for $f_C$ and $\dot{W}$ as described above for leg cycling.
- $\dot{W}_{max}$ is estimated from the age-predicted $f_{Cmax}$ and the $f_C$ – $\dot{W}$ relationship.
- The estimated $\dot{W}_{max}$ is used with Equation 3.12 to estimate $\dot{V}O_{2max}$.

$$\dot{V}O_{2max} = (18.36 \cdot \dot{W}_{max}) + (3.5 \cdot BW) \qquad (3.12)$$

where $\dot{V}O_{2max}$ is expressed in ml · min$^{-1}$, $\dot{W}_{max}$ is in watts, and BW is body weight in kg.

### Submaximal constant work rate tests

Single-stage tests to predict fitness level have been developed for use on both the cycle ergometer and the treadmill. As with the multistage tests, these tests rely on the relationship between $\dot{V}O_2$ and $f_C$ to predict $\dot{V}O_{2max}$.

*Åstrand–Ryhming cycling test*

The Åstrand–Ryhming test requires setting a cycle ergometer load using a pedal frequency of 50 r.p.m. so that the work rate is 75 W, 100 W, or 150 W for untrained, moderately trained, or well-trained subjects, respectively. This work rate is then maintained for 6 min. If values for $f_C$ recorded during minutes 5 and 6 are not different by more than 5 min$^{-1}$, and if $f_C$ is between 130 and 170 min$^{-1}$, the test is terminated. If $f_C$ is less than 130 min$^{-1}$, the work rate is increased by 50–100 W and the test continued for another 6 min. Again, if $f_C$ is different by more than 5 min$^{-1}$ between minutes 5 and 6, the test is continued until the $f_C$ between two consecutive minutes does not differ by more than 5 min$^{-1}$. The final $f_C$ and $\dot{W}$ are then used with the Åstrand–Ryhming nomogram (see Figure C5 in Appendix C), to determine $\dot{V}O_{2max}$. This value is then corrected for age with the table included on the nomogram.

*Submaximal treadmill tests*

Submaximal constant work rate treadmill exercise tests for prediction of $\dot{V}O_{2max}$ are uncommon. While it is conceivable that a modification of the Åstrand–Ryhming nomogram could be applied to treadmill exercise, unknown and variable work rates obtained from a single $f_C$–$\dot{W}$ relationship would undoubtedly result in decreased accuracy and precision in prediction. A nomogram to predict $\dot{V}O_{2max}$ from a single submaximal treadmill stage remains to be developed.

*Constant work rate tests for endurance*

Constant work rate (CWR) tests have applications in fitness assessment other than predicting $\dot{V}O_{2max}$. One such use is in assessing exercise endurance. Although reference values are not available to evaluate performance in this way, the CWR test provides an excellent baseline for further comparisons of change in fitness. For this purpose, a predetermined work rate is selected, usually as a percentage of the previously performed maximal exercise test. After warm-up (see section below on data acquisition), the load is abruptly increased to provide the preselected CWR. Appropriate CWR settings are in the range of 60–100% of the peak work rate achieved in the maximal XT.

The CWR test is highly reproducible and is somewhat less effort-dependent, especially at lower percentages of the peak $\dot{W}$. Measurement variables include endurance time ($t$), $f_C$, and systemic arterial pressures, as well as the other variables indicated in Table 3.7. See Chapter 4 for detailed descriptions of these variables.

*Constant work rate tests to determine the time constant for oxygen uptake*

The time constant for oxygen uptake ($\tau\dot{V}O_2$) is a parameter of aerobic fitness, representing the approximate time (in seconds) for $\dot{V}O_2$ to reach 63% of its steady-state value. Measurement of $\tau\dot{V}O_2$ typically requires application of a series of CWR tests at a preselected work rate below the metabolic threshold. Suprathreshold work rates disallow the observation of a $\dot{V}O_2$ steady state and are thus not used for this purpose.

The CWR protocol to determine $\tau\dot{V}O_2$ requires a baseline of low-intensity work followed by an abrupt increase ("square wave") in work rate to the desired level. This is known as the on-transient. Since more breath-by-breath variability is observed during unloaded cycling, a 10–20-W baseline with a two- to fourfold increase in work rate appears optimal (provided the steady-state $\dot{V}O_2$ remains below $\dot{V}O_2\theta$). Since $\tau\dot{V}O_2$ is typically 35–45 s in healthy subjects, breath-by-breath data acquisition provides the only appropriate measurement of $\dot{V}O_2$ for the determination of $\tau\dot{V}O_2$.

The high signal-to-noise ratio in breath-by-breath measurements suggests that a single CWR test is generally inappropriate for measurement of $\tau\dot{V}O_2$. Thus, multiple CWR tests at the same CWR are required to improve the fidelity with which $\tau\dot{V}O_2$ is reported. Interestingly, the off-transient for $\tau\dot{V}O_2$, measured immediately upon the return of a CWR to the baseline work rate, appears to be equivalent to $\tau\dot{V}O_2$ measured from the on-transient. Hence, two CWR XTs will yield four estimates of $\tau\dot{V}O_2$. Since the work rates utilized for these tests must be below the metabolic threshold, duplicate tests can be administered after only about 15 min of recovery. Responses from the multiple transitions are then averaged to obtain $\tau\dot{V}O_2$. See Chapter 4 for a discussion of the normal and abnormal response of this parameter.

The CWR test offers additional value in helping to verify $\dot{V}O_2\theta$. Examination of values for $\dot{V}O_2$ after 3 and 6 min of a CWR protocol (the so-called $\dot{V}O_{2(6-3)}$) indicates whether or not a true steady state exists. Identical values over this time interval confirm that the work rate was below $\dot{V}O_2\theta$. Alternatively, the identification of an upward "drift" in $\dot{V}O_2$ confirms that the work rate was above $\dot{V}O_2\theta$. For the purposes of confirming that a work rate is below $\dot{V}O_2\theta$, $\dot{V}O_{2(6-3)}$ should be less than 100 ml · min$^{-1}$.

The protocol for constant work rate tests used to determine $\tau\dot{V}O_2$ should be as follows:

- Selection of an appropriate constant work rate protocol (depending on the purpose of the test).
- A work rate near but below the metabolic threshold is desirable for measurement of $\tau\dot{V}O_2$ or for confirming $\dot{V}O_2\theta$.
- A work rate at 75–80% of the previously measured maximum work rate is desirable for tests of endurance or progress monitoring.
- 3–4 min of baseline exercise at a low work rate, e.g., 20–25 W.
- 6–8 min of constant work rate exercise at the chosen work rate.
- 6–8 min of recovery if gas exchange measurements are required to define the off-transient.
- Averaging of a minimum of two CWR tests in order to reduce the signal-to-noise ratio.

### Maximal incremental work rate tests

Maximal XTs provide the greatest amount of data with which to evaluate exercise performance and aerobic capacity. Data collected from a maximal XT also allow more precise interpretations of exercise performance, especially when ventilation is measured and gas exchange data are acquired. Response variables may be observed, recorded, and plotted throughout the range of rest to maximal exertion. These data allow observations of the pattern of response as well as discrete individual responses at particular work rates, including $\dot{W}_{max}$ or $\dot{V}O_{2max}$. If oxygen uptake is not directly measured, prediction of $\dot{V}O_{2max}$ is possible from $\dot{W}_{max}$ (e.g., Bruce and Balke treadmill protocols, American College of

Sports Medicine (ACSM) and Storer cycle protocols, and various arm ergometer protocols). Actual measurement of $\dot{W}_{max}$ is expected to improve prediction of $\dot{V}O_{2max}$.

Maximal XTs require the greatest dependence on subject effort and the subject's ability to withstand the discomfort of high-intensity exercise. Endpoints for maximal XT include fatigue (exhaustion) as well as a variety of symptoms. The term symptom-limited usually refers to patient populations in which test termination criteria may be based on the observance of specific symptoms. Typical limiting symptoms include muscle discomfort, breathlessness, chest pain, claudication, muscle strain or cramps (common in steep-grade walking on a treadmill), inability to maintain adequate cycle cadence, or inability to keep pace with the treadmill belt.

Incremental exercise protocols are the most commonly used laboratory tests for integrated assessment of ventilatory, cardiovascular, and musculoskeletal function. These tests possess the attributes of being graded (increasing in work intensity over time) and continuous up to maximal exercise or the occurrence of symptoms suggesting termination of the test (see the section on safety considerations, below). The various incremental protocols differ with respect to their metabolic cost at each stage, duration of the stages, and total duration of the test. Two common types of incremental tests are used; stair-step and ramp.

*Stair-step test*

The stair-step protocols use the common feature of discrete increases in work rate, typically occurring in stages of 1, 2, or 3 min duration. Using the cycle or arm ergometer, work rates are increased with each stage, by increments typically in the range of 5–50 W. The most commonly used treadmill protocol, the Bruce protocol, requires increases in both speed and grade every 3 min in stair-step fashion. The increment in the oxygen cost of each stage is variable, ranging from 4.1 to 11.6 ml $\cdot$ kg$^{-1}$ $\cdot$ min$^{-1}$.

The original Balke protocol uses a constant speed of 3.3 m.p.h. (88.4 m $\cdot$ min$^{-1}$) with 1% increases in grade each minute, thus yielding equal increases in the oxygen cost of each stage. Use of incremental protocols with the work rate increased each minute rather than every 2 or 3 min as with some protocols increases the fidelity of the key response variables enabling easier pattern recognition. This is particularly important in identifying the metabolic threshold ($\dot{V}O_2\theta$), as discussed in Chapter 4. With protocols that increment work rate every 2–3 min, the key response variables for identifying $\dot{V}O_2\theta$ are slurred, making detection more difficult. Additionally, clinicians should not ruthlessly apply a single protocol, e.g., a Bruce protocol, to every subject. Rather, total test duration must be considered and constrained ideally to 8–12 min, as described in the section on selecting the incremental exercise test protocol, below. Examples of incremental exercise test protocols for treadmill, leg, and arm cycling exercise are provided in Appendices B and D.

*Ramp test*

The ramp protocol is one in which the work rate continuously increases in small increments throughout the test. Such fine control over the work rate is generally attained through use of a programmable microprocessor that controls the voltage signal to the ergometer. Small increments in work rate can be achieved each second, allowing for smooth work rate transitions throughout the test. This form of work rate increase facilitates pattern recognition of the physiological variables used to interpret the exercise test. While ramp protocols are more common in cycle ergometer testing, some treadmill manufacturers provide for this function as well. Typical cycle ergometer ramp protocols offer a range of ramp rates of 5–50 W $\cdot$ min$^{-1}$. Treadmill ramp protocols should be designed so that the work rate increases smoothly, resulting in a steady rate of increase in oxygen cost throughout the test, terminating in 8–12 min at $\dot{V}O_{2max}$ or at the limit of subject tolerance.

## Clinical exercise tests

### Introduction

In the clinical population, that is to say individuals with recognized illness or disease, clinical exercise tests are used for specific purposes, such as assistance with diagnosis, definition of specific pathophysiological limitations to exercise, and preoperative risk assessment. Also, in the clinical discipline, CXT can be used for progress monitoring in response to physical rehabilitation or various therapeutic interventions. The following sections review the purposes of CXT as well as field and laboratory tests that may be used to generate data useful in clinical management.

#### Diagnostic tests

Impaired exercise capacity, fatigue and exertional breathlessness are remarkably common symptoms in clinical practice. Frequently they lead to exhaustive investigation without definite conclusions. The role of diagnostic exercise testing is to reproduce these symptoms while obtaining precise physiological measurements with which to evaluate the exercise response. This approach usually necessitates a maximal exercise test, which is limited by the symptoms in question. A cycle ergometer is often chosen for its precision in controlling external work rate. Sometimes the test gives definitive diagnostic information, pointing to a particular disease entity, but more often than not the test indicates specific physiological or pathophysiological limitations to exercise. These limitations are usually explained by one or more disease processes and, most importantly, give guidance as to what therapeutic interventions are necessary to relieve the symptoms and improve exercise capacity.

#### Risk assessment

A second category of CXT is used for risk assessment. Again, tests for risk assessment demand precision. They will usually be maximal exercise tests, performed on a cycle or treadmill ergometer. Many of these tests are focused on clinical risks and lead to therapies aimed at risk modification. However, task-specific exercise testing can be used in a rehabilitative sense to assess potential risks associated with return to work.

Perhaps the best known type of risk assessment is the evaluation of cardiac risk from myocardial ischemia or dysrhythmia. This type of risk assessment carries important prognostic and therapeutic implications. Secondly, exercise testing is used to assess suitability for surgery and can predict postoperative mortality and morbidity, e.g., after thoracotomy. A less well-recognized type of risk assessment is the detection of exercise-induced hypertension. This finding, even in the presence of normal resting blood pressures, indicates compromised vascular conductance and predicts the development of hypertension later in life. Finally, exercise testing can detect significant hypoxemia, even in the presence of normal resting oxygenation. This problem, which reflects gas exchange failure, if chronic and uncorrected can lead to permanent vascular damage to the pulmonary circulation. Thus, exercise testing can identify those patients at risk and aid in the prescription of supplemental oxygen which ameliorates the problem.

#### Progress monitoring

Progress monitoring assessments in the clinical setting are often performed to evaluate responses to rehabilitation, pharmacotherapy, surgery, and other interventions. Progress monitoring tests may include field or laboratory, submaximal or maximal tests. Any of the protocols listed below may be used to monitor progress, although the laboratory tests typically offer greater precision and thus increased ability to detect changes. Regardless of the test chosen, care must be taken to perform the test precisely since the important concern is change in one or more variables previously measured. Failure to do so increases error and may obscure the ability to detect any real change.

## Field tests

### Introduction

Field tests used in the clinical setting are essentially modifications of those used in PXT. Their value is best seen in providing a means to monitor progress in rehabilitation rather than in assessing fitness. Prediction of $\dot{V}O_{2max}$ is generally not the primary goal of these tests. Observation and recording of symptoms or subject responses to these tests (e.g., $f_C$, $t$, $SpO_2$, RPE, $\beta$–) can also be used to adjust the elements of the exercise program. See Chapter 4 for descriptions of these variables as well as normal and abnormal responses.

### 6- and 12-minute walk

These tests are modifications of the Cooper 12-minute run test, as described in PXT above. The 6- and 12-minute walk tests are field tests appropriate for use with certain patient groups. They have gained considerable popularity in patients with chronic pulmonary disease. These tests are submaximal and may have a variable rate depending upon the pacing characteristics of the patient. Equipment requirements are modest, requiring only an accurately measured course and a stopwatch (see Chapter 2). The addition of RPE and visual analog or angina rating scales, along with $f_C$ and $SpO_2$ monitoring (portable pulse oximeter) add substantially to the data available to assess performance. While these tests possess certain advantages, including an estimate of the ability to perform everyday activities, they should not be considered for diagnostic purposes. Reproducibility is enhanced when the protocol is standardized with respect to encouragement offered to the patient during the test, whether or not the patient carries supplemental oxygen, or how tests conducted indoors might vary from tests conducted outdoors. Additionally, a learning effect is common, yielding significantly increased walking distances with repeat trials.

Correlations between 6-min or 12-min walking distance and $\dot{V}O_{2max}$ are in the range of $r = 0.4$–$0.6$, thus accounting for only 16%–36% of the common variance. Correlations between the 6-min and the 12-min walk are higher ($r > 0.9$), suggesting improved time efficiency with the 6-min test. An effective timed walk test protocol requires standardized procedures, including:

- Clear instructions to the subject regarding the test procedures, including expected level of effort (see Appendix D, Standard instructions for the 6-minute walk test).
- Standardized statements of encouragement to the subject during the test.
- A requirement for the test administrator to walk behind the patient so as not to provide pacing.
- Standardized feedback with respect to time remaining in the test.
- At least 2–3 practice trials for familiarization.

### 10-meter shuttle

As with the 20-meter shuttle test described above in PXT, the 10-meter shuttle is an incremental maximal test. The endpoint of this test is either fatigue or observation of symptoms. The protocol for this clinical application reduces the distance to 10 m per shuttle and the starting speed to $30\ m \cdot min^{-1}$. Speed is incremented by $10\ m \cdot min^{-1}$ every minute for each of the 12 stages. Like the 20-meter shuttle, the 10-meter shuttle depends on keeping pace with audio signals emitted from a prerecorded tape. The intervals of these tones may be seen in Table 3.11 under the heading Time per shuttle (s). Table 3.11 also shows speeds for each stage, distance walked per stage, total distance, and an estimation of $\dot{V}O_{2max}$ derived from a regression of shuttle performance against $\dot{V}O_{2max}$ determined by treadmill testing (see Further Reading). The regression equation was:

$$\dot{V}O_{2max} = 0.025 \cdot \text{distance} + 4.19 \qquad (3.13)$$

where $\dot{V}O_{2max}$ is expressed in $ml \cdot kg^{-1} \cdot min^{-1}$ and distance is expressed in m. The correlation coefficient was 0.88. A separate study showed reliability to be high: $r = 0.98$.

The protocol includes:

- Explanation of test procedures:

**Table 3.11.** Speeds, time intervals, and predicted $\dot{V}O_{2max}$ for each stage of the 10-meter shuttle test

| Stage | Speed ($km \cdot h^{-1}$) | Speed ($m \cdot min^{-1}$) | Speed ($m \cdot s^{-1}$) | Speed (m.p.h.) | Shuttles per min | Time per shuttle (s) | Distance per stage (m) | Total distance (m) | Predicted $\dot{V}O_{2max}$ ($ml \cdot kg^{-1} \cdot min^{-1}$) |
|---|---|---|---|---|---|---|---|---|---|
| 1 | 1.8 | 30 | 0.50 | 1.12 | 3 | 20.00 | 30 | 30 | 4.94 |
| 2 | 2.4 | 40 | 0.67 | 1.49 | 4 | 15.00 | 40 | 70 | 5.94 |
| 3 | 3.0 | 50 | 0.84 | 1.87 | 5 | 12.00 | 50 | 120 | 7.19 |
| 4 | 3.6 | 60 | 1.01 | 2.24 | 6 | 10.00 | 60 | 180 | 8.69 |
| 5 | 4.2 | 70 | 1.18 | 2.61 | 7 | 8.57 | 70 | 250 | 10.44 |
| 6 | 4.8 | 80 | 1.35 | 2.99 | 8 | 7.50 | 80 | 330 | 12.44 |
| 7 | 5.4 | 90 | 1.52 | 3.36 | 9 | 6.67 | 90 | 420 | 14.69 |
| 8 | 6.0 | 100 | 1.69 | 3.73 | 10 | 6.00 | 100 | 520 | 17.19 |
| 9 | 6.6 | 110 | 1.86 | 4.10 | 11 | 5.46 | 110 | 630 | 19.94 |
| 10 | 7.2 | 120 | 2.03 | 4.48 | 12 | 5.00 | 120 | 750 | 22.94 |
| 11 | 7.8 | 130 | 2.20 | 4.85 | 13 | 4.62 | 130 | 880 | 26.19 |
| 12 | 8.4 | 140 | 2.37 | 5.22 | 14 | 4.29 | 140 | 1020 | 29.69 |

(a) "Walk at a steady pace with a goal of turning around each marker cone when you hear the signal."
(b) "You will increase speed at the end of each minute. This will be signaled by a distinctly different tone. Try to keep pace with the signals as long as you can."
(c) To facilitate pacing, the examiner may walk alongside the subject for the first minute.

- Monitoring the subject so that pace is maintained and signs and symptoms are observed.
- The test is terminated when the subject is more than 0.5 m away from a marker. If the subject is less than 0.5 m from the marker, another 10 m is allowed to come back on pace. If the subject cannot make up the distance, the test is terminated.
- The number of completed levels and shuttles is recorded in order to calculate total distance in meters.

**Example:** If the subject completes level 5 plus two additional shuttles (each shuttle equals 10 m) the total distance is 250 + 20 = 270 m.

### Symptom-limited maximal stair-climb

This simple test is used to estimate $\dot{V}O_{2max}$ and minute ventilation in patients with chronic obstructive pulmonary disease. Subjects are instructed to climb stairs (or flights of stairs) until they stop at their symptom-limited maximum.

## Laboratory tests

### Introduction

As with PXT, laboratory tests offer greater control over the environment (temperature, humidity, surfaces, and distractions) and the subject. Use of more sophisticated instruments, including metabolic measurement equipment, within the laboratory allows greater accuracy and precision in the measurement of a greater number of response variables. Thus, more data of potentially higher quality are obtainable for interpretation. Whenever available and appropriate for the purpose, laboratory testing is preferred. This section presents several submaximal and maximal strategies that can be applied in the laboratory for assessing the integrated response to exercise. The reader is referred again to Table 3.7 for a summary of laboratory tests.

### Without arterial blood sampling

Many clinical laboratories will perform a majority of their exercise tests without arterial blood sampling (Figure 3.2). This approach offers a simpler protocol but information regarding gas exchange is limited. Regardless of whether or not arterial blood samples are obtained, certain elements are necessary for this type of CXT. The resting phase should continue long enough to obtain stable data within acceptable limits (see section on data acquisition, below). A warm-up phase of 3 min is recommended as a standard. This enables a new steady-state baseline to be established prior to the systematic increase in external work rate. The work rate increment should be carefully selected with a view to obtaining 8–12 min of exercise data. Peripheral measurements can include ECG monitoring, blood pressure measurements, and pulse oximetry. A convenient frequency for recording these measurements is once towards the end of each of the resting and warm-up phases, every 2 min during the exercise phase, at maximum exercise, and after 2 min of recovery. Further recovery measurements might be indicated to ensure that the subject returns appropriately towards baseline.

Use of psychometric scales for rating of perceived exertion (RPE) and breathlessness (*β*–) is strongly encouraged. Examples of these scales are given in Appendix D. These scales can be administered multiple times during the test but the most valuable assessment is as soon as possible after termination of exercise. A meaningful test can certainly be performed without any blood sampling. However, depending on subject acceptance and laboratory expertise, any test can be enhanced by the addition of certain blood measurements. One sample that can be considered is a single venous blood sample after 2 min of recovery for lactate. Notwithstanding the fact that arterial blood gives more reliable lactate measurements, a venous sample usually tells whether a significant increase in lactate has occurred and gives some indication of subject motivation. Lastly, it must be acknowledged that if a pulse oximeter is to be relied upon to evaluate oxygenation, the instrument should be calibrated by a simultaneous arterial blood gas. Again, if acceptable to the subject and laboratory staff, a single arterial sample obtained during the resting phase enables calibration of the oximeter and also calculation of gas exchange indices at rest. Subsequent indirect measures of gas exchange such as end-tidal gas tensions and ventilatory equivalents can be judged accordingly.

### With arterial blood sampling

Among the most difficult decisions facing an exercise laboratory is the choice of when to perform exercise testing with serial arterial blood gas sampling. Essentially this question is about whether precise determination of gas exchange is necessary at maximum exercise. Calculation of physiological dead space and alveolar–arterial partial pressure gradient for oxygen necessitate arterial blood sampling and the moment of exercise limitation is the most valuable time at which to evaluate these indices. Given these considerations, it is clear that whenever a gas exchange abnormality might be suspected, then serial arterial sampling is required. This consideration might apply to many diagnostic exercise tests. Also, it applies when testing a patient with known pulmonary disease who might be at risk of exercise-induced hypoxemia. The availability of narrow-gauge plastic or Teflon catheters renders the decision about arterial blood sampling easier since these catheters are relatively easy to insert and well tolerated by the subjects (see Chapter 2). Alternatively, the double arterial puncture technique can be used (see Chapter 2).

Once an arterial catheter is inserted, blood samples become readily available. The most important samples are those obtained at rest and at maximum exercise. In both instances timing is important. The resting sample must be obtained whilst breathing through the mouthpiece in order to allow precise calculation of gas exchange indices. The end-exercise sample should be obtained as close to maximum exercise as possible. Since the exercise practitioner can usually anticipate the end of an exercise test, it is preferable to obtain this arterial blood sample during the last 30 s of exercise rather than during recovery when rapid hemodynamic changes are occurring. An indwelling arterial catheter enables other samples to be obtained. A convenient sampling frequency might be to include samples towards the end of the warm-up phase and every 2 min during the exercise phase. In practical terms these additional samples add limited value to the exercise test interpretation.

### Exercise-induced bronchospasm test

Exercise-induced bronchospasm (EIB) or, as some prefer, exercise-induced asthma (EIA), is caused by bronchiolar smooth muscle contraction that is stimulated by the increased ventilation associated with exercise. The increased ventilation results in loss of heat and water, and changes in mucosal osmolarity, which then appear to trigger bronchoconstriction. Alternatively, airways cooling during exercise may provoke a reduction in bronchial blood flow. When exercise ceases, a reactive hyperemia ensues, resulting in mucosal edema, thus inducing airflow obstruction. Higher intensities and longer duration of the exercise as well as breathing cool, dry air seem to increase the occurrence of EIB. Following exercise, symptoms include wheezing, shortness of breath, chest discomfort, coughing, and decreased performance. This is usually not a life-threatening condition and tends to abate spontaneously within 30–40 min.

Confirmation of EIB is a two-step process, first requiring 6–8 min of exercise at an intensity that increases ventilation to about 20 times the predicted forced expiratory volume in the first second ($FEV_1$). Following this exercise, the subject performs repeated $FEV_1$ maneuvers at 1, 3, 5, 7, 10, 15, and 20 min. The forced expiratory flow between 75% and 25% of vital capacity ($FEF_{25-75}$) may also be measured, particularly in athletes. The lowest $FEV_1$ measured after exercise is compared with the preexercise $FEV_1$ and expressed a percentage fall. A change of $\geqslant$10% is abnormal and $\geqslant$15% is diagnostic for EIB. Salient features of the EIB protocol are as follows:

- Subjects should not have had an occurrence of EIB within the past 3 h, should be at least 6 weeks free from infection, and have bronchodilator medication withheld 6–24 h before the test depending upon their duration of action. Caffeine, antihistamines, and steroids should also be withheld on the day of the test.
- Patient risk factors should be assessed and oxyhemoglobin saturation monitored during the test using a pulse oximeter. Supplemental oxygen and rapidly acting inhaled bronchodilators (e.g., salbutamol) should be available.
- $FEV_1$ is measured before the exercise test at least in duplicate with <10% variability between the best two tests.
- Cycle ergometry or treadmill exercise is performed such that minute ventilation ($\dot{V}_E$) is increased to about 20 times the $FEV_1$ measurement and held at this level for at least 4 min. Some believe that cycle exercise does not provoke EIB symptoms as well as treadmill exercise, as lower $\dot{V}_E$ is observed in cycle exercise.
- The target $\dot{W}$ should be approached with an initial $\dot{W}$ of 60% of the target value in minute 1. The $\dot{W}$ is increased to 70% of the target value in minute 2, 90% of the target value in minute 3, then achieving and maintaining the target work rate for an additional 4–5 min.
- The inspired air should be <25 °C and <50% relative humidity. If laboratory conditions do not favor these requirements, breathing compressed air through a respiratory valve is an ideal alternative.
- $\dot{V}_E$, $\dot{V}O_2$, and $\dot{W}$ should be recorded in order to identify the level of ventilation and work at which symptoms occur.
- In some circumstances, it may be necessary to conduct the exercise portion of the test in field conditions specific to the activity causing the EIB if laboratory methods fail to duplicate symptoms.

The target work rate for the cycle ergometer may be calculated as follows:

$$\dot{V}O_2 = (\dot{V}_E - 0.27)/28 \tag{3.14}$$

where $\dot{V}_E$ and $\dot{V}O_2$ are both expressed in $l \cdot min^{-1}$ and $\dot{V}_E$ is estimated from $FEV_1 \times 20$.

$$\dot{W} = \frac{\dot{V}O_2 - 500}{10.3} \tag{3.15}$$

where $\dot{W}$ is expressed in W and $\dot{V}O_2$ is expressed in $ml \cdot min^{-1}$.

**Example:** If $FEV_1 = 4.2$ l
Desired $\dot{V}_E \cong 20 \times 4.2 = 84$ l · min$^{-1}$
Estimated $\dot{V}O_2$ (l · min$^{-1}$) = 84 − 0.27)/28
= 2.99 l · min$^{-1}$
Estimated $\dot{W}$ (W) = (2990 − 500)/10.3 = 241 W

For treadmill exercise, calculation of the correct speed and grade combination is more tedious, although possible:

1. Estimate $\dot{V}O_2$ using Equation 3.14.
2. Convert to ml · kg · min$^{-1}$ by dividing this $\dot{V}O_2$ by the subject's body weight.
3. Use Equations B3–6 in Appendix B to calculate a grade at any desired treadmill speed.
4. Alternatively, use Figure D4 in Appendix D to provide an automated approach for this calculation.

### Myopathy evaluation

Various myopathies limit exercise capacity and are associated with specific patterns of cardiovascular and ventilatory abnormality (see Chapters 4 and 5). However, more specific myopathy evaluation requires blood sampling to assess changes in lactate, ammonia, and perhaps other metabolites. These samples could be obtained from an indwelling venous catheter, although an arterial catheter is more reliable for rapid and complete sampling and allows simultaneous determinations about gas exchange. Practicality and economy govern when to obtain samples. A resting sample is clearly necessary as a baseline and a sample at maximum exercise is also necessary for obvious reasons. A third sample might be considered after 4 min of the exercise phase. The rationale for this sample is as follows. An intermediate sample between rest and maximum exercise helps characterize the pattern of increase in lactate or ammonia. Furthermore, in normal subjects substantial increases in these metabolites would not be expected below 40% of predicted $\dot{V}O_{2max}$ (see Chapter 4). Assuming that the exercise protocol was carefully selected with the goal of obtaining 10 min of data, then the subject would be expected to achieve predicted $\dot{V}O_{2max}$ after 10 min of exercise. Thus, after 4 min of steadily incrementing exercise the subject will have an oxygen uptake approximately 40% of predicted $\dot{V}O_{2max}$ and, if blood is sampled at this time, premature increases in lactate or ammonia can be detected. Adoption of a standard protocol for myopathy testing, such as the one described here, eventually leads to improved pattern recognition and better ability to identify abnormalities.

### Cardiac exercise testing

Although it is preferable not to distinguish a cardiac exercise test from an integrative exercise test, historically the former clinical evaluations have been performed specifically to detect myocardial ischemia and as a test to identify symptoms such as angina. These purposes were generally served with incremental treadmill exercise, terminating at 85–90% of predicted $f_{Cmax}$. Respired gases were rarely measured as part of the so-called cardiac stress test. Rather, exercise tolerance was assessed on the basis of treadmill time at termination along with ECG changes and symptoms. Several protocols exist for this purpose, the most popular of which is the aforementioned Bruce treadmill protocol (Appendix D). Other protocols exist, such as the Naughton protocol and the Ellestad protocol. No matter which of these protocols is used, much potentially valuable diagnostic information is lost when the integrated XT is not performed.

### Preoperative assessment

The literature regarding preoperative risk assessment, at least for thoracotomy, relies upon determination of $\dot{V}O_{2max}$ and $\dot{V}O_2\theta$. With this in mind, a laboratory CXT that aims to assess preoperative risk should be designed to facilitate reliable determination of these parameters. Clearly, a symptom-limited maximal test is required with all of the considerations that improve threshold detection, such as a ramp increase in work rate and careful selection of the work rate increment. The cycle ergometer is preferred for its precision in controlling external work rate and for enabling peripheral measurements that might also impact risk stratification.

Table C10 in Appendix C summarizes five studies of operative risk assessment using maximal exercise testing. Low risk, with mortality of 0% and complications less than 10%, is characterized by $\dot{V}O_{2max}$ $> 1.5 l \cdot min^{-1}$ or $20 ml \cdot kg^{-1} \cdot min^{-1}$ and $\dot{V}O_2\theta$ $> 15 ml \cdot kg^{-1} \cdot min^{-1}$. High risk, with mortality up to 18% and complications up to 100%, is characterized by $\dot{V}O_{2max} < 1.0 l \cdot min^{-1}$ or $10–15 ml \cdot kg^{-1} \cdot min^{-1}$ and $\dot{V}O_2\theta < 10 ml \cdot kg^{-1} \cdot min^{-1}$.

### Constant work rate tests

CWR tests were described above, in the section on PXT laboratory tests. Use of CWR tests in clinical exercise testing allows quantification of the kinetic responses of $\dot{V}_E$, $\dot{V}CO_2$, and $\dot{V}O_2$. These responses are known to be significantly slower in both pulmonary and cardiac disease. While theoretically sound, the clinical utility of documenting these responses remains to be established.

CWR tests are useful, however, in confirming the identification of $\dot{V}O_2\theta$, or in assessing endurance performance at a percentage of maximum work rate or at a fixed percentage of a metabolic marker such as $\dot{V}O_2\theta$ or $\dot{V}O_{2max}$. The CWR test is also beneficial in establishing parameters for exercise prescription such as target heart rates, ratings of perceived exertion, minimal oxygen saturation, and appearance of symptoms such as dyspnea, angina, claudication, and serious dysrhythmias. Serial CWR tests at the same work rate are useful in documenting the effectiveness or ineffectiveness of a therapeutic intervention. CWR tests can be modified to determine requirements for supplemental oxygen.

## Subject preparation

### Before the test

A successful exercise test necessitates careful subject preparation. The following sections describe approaches that enhance the professionalism of the exercise practitioner and improve the efficiency of the laboratory or other setting for exercise testing.

1. A date and time for the test should be mutually agreed upon at least 48 h before the test appointment. A 24-h reminder telephone call might prove valuable in confirming the appointment, potentially saving time, as well as demonstrating professionalism.
2. The subject should be given written instructions prior to the test date providing information about how to prepare for the tests, what to wear, when to eat, and what to do about medications. A sample of such instructions is contained in Appendix D.
3. Prepare a file folder for the subject with the appropriate data collection forms needed for the tests, the medical history questionnaire or Physical Activity Readiness Questionnaire (PAR-Q), the informed consent (see Appendix D). Other documentation needed should include the purpose of the test and physician approval when indicated. Additional information can be gathered from subjects with respect to their goals, medications, habits, and exercise history.

### Subject arrival

The subject should arrive at the designated location at a scheduled time. Greet the subject in a professional and friendly manner. Ask the subject to be seated so that a short rest period may begin, after which resting heart rate and arterial blood pressure will be taken. Ensure that the medical history questionnaire and informed consent have been completed (see Appendix D). Explain the events of the day. That is, explain the nature of the assessment planned for that appointment. Ask the subject, if relevant, for a goal statement with respect to exercise training, weight management, fitness, and health. Perhaps offer several examples to stimulate the appropriate responses.

### Completion of medical history questionnaire

If the client has not already done so, a medical history questionnaire and informed consent should be given to the client. These important documents should be completed and available for your review at the start of the test appointment. Samples of a medical history questionnaire and the PAR-Q, as well as basic elements of the informed consent are contained in Appendix D.

### Informed consent

The informed consent is an important part of the preparation for XT. The consent form is designed to advise the client fully of: (1) the purpose and characteristics of the test; (2) the benefits and risks inherent with the test; (3) alternatives to not testing; (4) responsibilities of the client; (5) confidentiality of results and potential use of information; and (6) freedom to make inquiries about the test as well as to remove consent. It is recommended that all clients read, understand, agree to, and sign the informed consent before testing. Since laws vary from state to state, individualized legal advice should be sought before adopting a consent form. Basic elements of the informed consent are contained in Appendix D.

### Resting 12-lead electrocardiogram

#### Skin preparation for electrodes

Skin preparation is important to ensure that a high-fidelity signal, free from motion artifact or electrical interference, is sent to the electrocardiograph and the metabolic measurement system where $f_C$ will be recorded. Proper skin preparation involves removing hair with a disposable safety razor, cleansing the skin with alcohol or acetone to remove skin oils, followed by light abrasion to remove the stratum corneum. Scratching the next layer of skin, the stratum granulosum, will further reduce motion potentials. Ideally, for exercise testing, skin abrasion should reduce impedance to less than 5000 Ω. This may be verified once the electrode is in place with a hand-held multimeter. A small amount of electrode gel on the pregelled electrode will facilitate signal conduction. Care must be taken to prevent gel from seeping out under the electrode adhesive.

#### Lead placement

The standard 12-lead ECG with the limb lead electrodes placed on the wrists and ankles cannot be used during exercise. Placement of these electrodes is modified for exercise testing by moving them to the trunk in the Mason–Likar configuration, shown in Figure 3.4. In this arrangement, limb lead electrodes are moved from the wrists and ankles to the anterior trunk as follows:

- The right-arm electrode is positioned just below the distal end of the right clavicle.
- The left-arm electrode is placed just below the distal end of the left clavicle.
- The right-leg electrode is positioned just above the right iliac crest in a right mid clavicular line.
- The left-leg electrode is positioned just above the left iliac crest in a left mid clavicular line.

***Note:*** *Movement of the limb electrodes in this manner changes the ECG waveforms from those obtained in the standard 12-lead ECG. It is important to indicate the lead configuration for comparison to past or future tracings.*

The chest (precordial) leads remain in their standard configuration as follows:

- V1: fourth intercostal space just to the right of the sternum.
- V2: fourth intercostal space just to the left of the sternum.
- V3: on a diagonal line halfway between V2 and V4.
- V4: fifth intercostal space in the left mid clavicular line.
- V5: on the same level as V4, on the left anterior axillary line.
- V6: on the same level as V4 and V5 in the left mid axillary line.

On some occasions such as PXT, the standard 12-lead ECG is not employed except for recording a resting 12-lead ECG. The exercise ECG may be acquired using a simpler, bipolar lead configuration such as $CM_5$ in which the positive electrode is in the V5-left position and the negative electrode is on the manubrium sterni. This configuration is considered to be the most sensitive for ST segment changes.

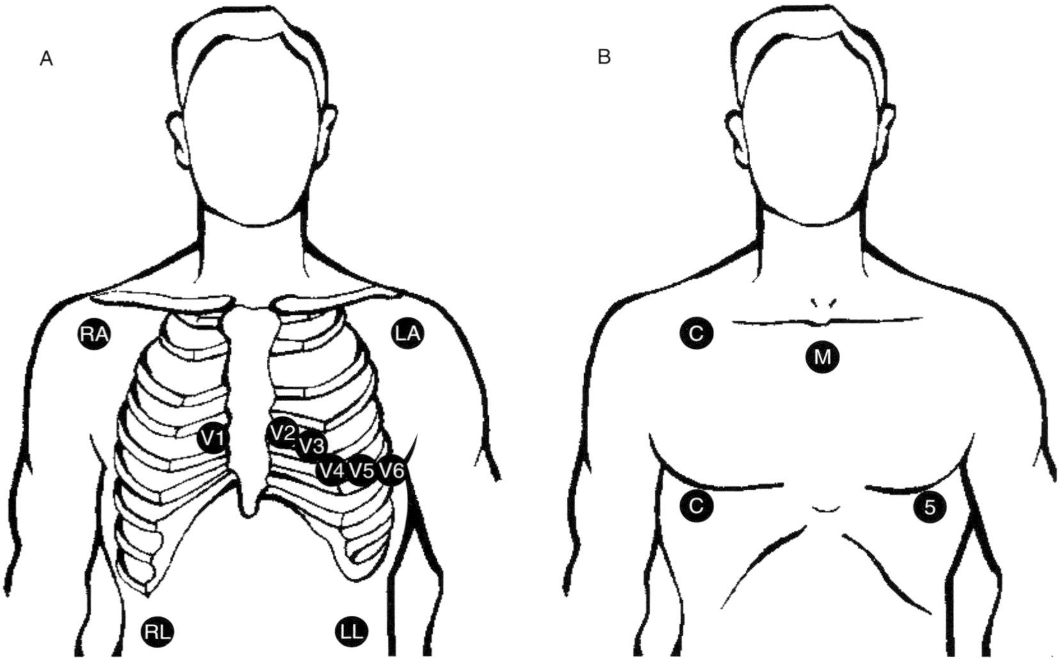


**Figure 3.4** Placement of electrodes for the exercise ECG. (A) Mason–Likar configuration. (B) Simple bipolar $CC_5$ and $CM_5$ configurations. See text for description of anatomical locations.

Another alternative is the $CC_5$ configuration in which the positive electrode is placed in the V5-left position and the negative electrode is located at the level of the fifth intercostal space on the anterior axillary line. The $CC_5$ configuration decreases the influence of the atrial repolorization (Ta wave) and is thus thought to reduce the incidence of false-positive tests (ST segment depression reaching the criteria for a positive test when in fact ischemia is not present).

## Measurement of resting blood pressure

After the subject has been resting quietly during the ECG preparation and measurement, blood pressure should be measured by auscultation or with a reliable and valid automated device. If laboratory or field tests are conducted in which ECG measurements are not included, blood pressure measurements should be taken only after the subject has rested for at least 5 min after arrival. Ideally, arterial systolic pressure K1 (first Korotkoff sound) and diastolic pressure K4 and K5 (fourth and fifth Korotkoff sounds) will be recorded. See Table 4.5 in Chapter 4 for a description of the Korotkoff sounds. The recording of both K4 and K5 is of particular importance during exercise since blood flow may remain turbulent without disappearance of K5 at manometer readings of 0 mmHg. See Chapter 2 and Appendix B for additional equipment and procedural information.

## Determination of ventilatory capacity

Especially before CXT, if not already performed, ventilatory capacity ($\dot{V}_{Ecap}$) should be determined by maximal voluntary ventilation (MVV) or predicted from $FEV_1$ (see Chapter 4). Ventilatory capacity, like the estimated $f_{C\max}$, provides a physiological boundary with which to interpret the exercise response. For example, ventilatory capacity can be compared with the measured $\dot{V}_{E\max}$ to determine if a true ventilatory limitation occurred during exercise (see Chapter 5).

### Explanation of test procedures

The subject should be given a complete explanation of what is expected during the course of the test. This includes instructions on how to use psychometric scales such as the Borg RPE scale, the visual analog scale for breathlessness, and other angina or dyspnea scales that may be employed. General testing procedures should also be explained. The following example is appropriate for maximal PXT or CXT. This example is given for an electrically braked cycle ergometer, but a treadmill or other ergometer may be substituted.

1. "You will be exercising on this special exercise bike beginning with a 1–2-minute rest. This will be followed by 3 minutes of warm-up exercise at a very light level of work. After the warm-up, the intensity of the exercise will increase very gradually until you are no longer able to continue. We anticipate that you will be exercising for about 10 minutes after the warm-up."
2. "At no time during the test should you rise out of the seat. We will ask that you maintain a constant pedaling cadence of 60."

   ***Note:*** *The cadence may be higher when testing trained cyclists for the purpose of exercise prescription. Cadences of 90–110 may be appropriate, although this will cause an increase in the oxygen cost of the work, displacing the* $\dot{V}O_2$–$\dot{W}$ *curve upward along the y-axis.*

3. "Since you will not be able to speak, nor should you try to do so, you should use hand signals for communication: Thumbs-up means yes or that everything is OK. Thumbs-down means no. Hold up your index finger if you think you can continue one more minute. Hold up a half-finger if you can only last 30 seconds longer."
4. "If you develop any untoward symptom such as pain, point to the part of your body affected (e.g., head, chest, a joint, or legs). Then use one, two, or three fingers to indicate mild, moderate, or severe, respectively."

   ***Note:*** *This method enables early detection of potentially concerning or limiting symptoms and also enables the subject to indicate if the symptom is worsening.*

5. "At certain times during the test we will be presenting you with the RPE scale. Please point to the appropriate number when asked to do so. We will take your blood pressure periodically throughout the test. At the end of the test we will show you the visual analog scale (VAS) and ask you to mark the scale somewhere between not all at breathless and extremely breathless, depending upon your feelings at the time. We will also ask you to tell us why you stopped exercise."
6. "We may decide to stop the test before you feel ready to stop. This will be for your safety or for technical reasons."
7. "Do you have any questions about the test?"

### Familiarization with ergometer

Whenever possible, subjects should be allowed practice on the ergometer selected for the XT and its specific requirements and movement patterns. This is especially true with the treadmill since it is the only work device that has extrinsic control over the work rate. The fact that subjects must mount and then keep up with a moving belt may be anxiety-provoking. Initial balance and gait patterns are unsure, leading to further apprehension. Although holding the handrails may reduce this, such action should be discouraged since it decreases the work rate by a variable and unknown amount. Handrail holding thus affects test interpretation by affecting the $\dot{V}O_2$–$\dot{W}$ relationship and makes comparison with previous or future tests difficult. At near maximal levels, subjects unfamiliar with treadmill exercise often stop prematurely because of their unease and fear of falling. These concerns can largely be alleviated with good pretest familiarization.

## Equipment preparation

### Ergometer settings

If the cycle ergometer is chosen, the seat height must be correctly set, allowing for a knee bend of 5–15° when the pedal is at the bottom of its stroke. The seat height should be recorded for future tests. Failure to do so and the use of a different seat height may result in biomechanical changes and differences in $\dot{V}O_2$ at every work rate. Cycling cadence should be maintained at between 50 and 80 r.p.m. with 60 r.p.m. an optimal target. It is important to maintain a constant pedaling rate, even with electrically braked ergometers. Variable pedaling rates affect oxygen uptake, changing their expected relationship with work rate. As mentioned previously, when testing cyclists for the purpose of exercise prescription, cadence should be increased to that commonly used during training. This may mean 90–110 r.p.m. In addition, consideration for modification of the ergometer to include clipless pedals, drop bars, and a racing saddle will make the test more task-specific.

No additional treadmill settings are required to accommodate most subjects. Although atypical in most laboratory settings, treadmills with very short walking surfaces may present a safety hazard when used with subjects having very long legs or stride lengths. It is good practice to keep all subjects walking or running near the front of the treadmill.

With arm ergometry, care must be taken to position the ergometer so that subjects can maintain an upright position with feet on the floor. The height of the arm ergometer should allow crank arms when horizontal to be at or slightly below shoulder level. The seat position should allow full extension of the arms during cranking.

### Calibration

The work device (cycle or treadmill) should have been previously calibrated. Just prior to the exercise test, the volume-measuring device and gas analyzers should be calibrated. While many mass flow meters and gas analyzers are quite stable, it is of primary importance that they be calibrated with known values prior to the administration of each exercise test.

### Patient interface

The patient interface consists of the mouthpiece and nose clip or the respiratory mask. These should be sterile before use and carefully applied to ensure leak-free connections. Facemasks tend to leak when $\dot{V}_E$ exceeds about $90\,\text{l}\cdot\text{min}^{-1}$. If the laboratory staff prefer the use of facemasks, they should perform their own independent leak check. This can be accomplished by having two or three of the staff perform duplicate bouts of exercise using the same protocol, once with a standard mouthpiece and nose clip arrangement and once with the facemask. Work rates should slightly exceed the highest expected work rate anticipated when facemasks are to be used.

Nose clips may become loose due to perspiration during the test. Some nose clips have foam pads that are less susceptible to this problem. As an added precaution, a small strip of gauze between the nose and nose clip will avert this concern.

### Preset data displays

Many of the commercially available metabolic measurement systems allow real-time graphical and tabular data display, including the ECG signal. The tabular and graphical configurations shown in Table 3.12 are recommended, when possible, to optimize patient data monitoring and safety during exercise testing.

## Selecting the optimal exercise test protocol

Selection of the optimal protocol is crucial for subject comfort and safety, as well as to obtain the most interpretable data for addressing the purpose of the test. This is equally true for treadmill ergometer, cycle ergometer, and arm ergometer testing.

**Table 3.12.** Recommended tabular and graphical real-time data displays for integrative XT

(a) Tabular display

| Time (min: s) | $\dot{W}$ (W) | $f_C$ ($min^{-1}$) | $\dot{V}O_2$ ($ml \cdot min^{-1}$) | $\dot{V}CO_2$ ($ml \cdot min^{-1}$) | $R$ | $\dot{V}_E$ ($l \cdot min^{-1}$) | $\dot{V}_E/\dot{V}O_2$ | $\dot{V}_E/\dot{V}CO_2$ | $P_{ET}O_2$ (mmHg) | $P_{ET}CO_2$ (mmHg) |
|---|---|---|---|---|---|---|---|---|---|---|

(b) Graphical display

| *y* axis | | *x* axis |
|---|---|---|
| $f_C$ | vs | time |
| $\dot{V}O_2$ | vs | time |
| $\dot{V}CO_2$ | vs | $\dot{V}O_2$ |
| $\dot{V}_E$ | vs | time |
| $\dot{V}_E/\dot{V}O_2$ and $\dot{V}_E/\dot{V}CO_2$ | vs | time (dual criterion plot) |
| $P_{ET}O_2$ and $P_{ET}CO_2$ | vs | time (secondary dual criterion plot) |

The Bruce and Balke treadmill protocols are perhaps the most widely used examples of stair-step incremental work rate tests. Tables D1 and D2 in Appendix D show the speed and grade as well as the oxygen cost at each stage. Table D2 indicates the standard Bruce protocol (stages Ic through IV), and modified stages (denoted Ia and Ib) for patients with low functional aerobic capacity. A potential concern with the standard protocol (beginning at 1.7 m.p.h. and 10% grade) is the large increase in work rate and thus oxygen cost between each stage. Using the equation for estimating work rate in treadmill exercise (Chapter 2, Equation 2.2) with a 70-kg subject, the increase in work rate between stages is about 50 W – a formidable undertaking for patients with cardiovascular or pulmonary disease who might have a maximal work capacity of 50 W. Advantageously, the large increase in work rate from stage to stage may be an important stimulus for detecting ischemic ECG changes.

The Balke protocol is less troublesome in regard to the work rate increments as they are smaller, with an average increase of about 10 W between stages. However, the constant speed of 3.3 m.p.h. is likely to be too fast for patient groups. An oxygen uptake of over 20 $ml \cdot kg^{-1} \cdot min^{-1}$ is required after only 5 min of exercise. This value may represent maximal oxygen uptake in many patient groups. As indicated in the next section, 5 min is not optimal for protocol duration.

Other standard incremental protocols exist for both cycle (arm and leg) as well as treadmill exercise. However, use of a previously developed protocol may not provide the appropriate work stimulus nor the opportunity for high-fidelity test interpretation based on pattern recognition. The next section suggests optimal protocol design for achieving these purposes.

It is now well established that the optimal duration of the CXT and PXT used for fitness assessment is between 8 and 12 min. Shorter or longer tests tend to underestimate $\dot{V}O_{2max}$. Decisions should be made a priori as to the work rate increment to be applied to the stair-step or ramp protocol. This section provides step-by-step instructions for determining the work rate increment for maximal cycle and treadmill exercise tests.

## Maximal cycle exercise tests

1. Determine the expected $\dot{V}O_{2max}$ for the patient in $ml \cdot min^{-1}$. This is facilitated by using appropriate reference standards based on age and gender as well as clinical experience (see Appendix C).
2. Calculate and subtract the unloaded oxygen requirement:

$$\dot{V}O_{2unloaded} = (5.8 \cdot BW) + 151 \qquad (3.16)$$

where $\dot{V}O_2$ is expressed in $ml \cdot min^{-1}$ and BW is body weight in kg.

3. Divide the remainder by 103. This divisor represents the product of the expected oxygen cost of leg cycling (10.3 ml · min$^{-1}$ · W$^{-1}$) and the optimal test duration (10 min).
4. The resulting quotient represents the desired work rate increment per minute.

$$\ddot{W} = \frac{(\text{Predicted } \dot{V}o_{2max} - \dot{V}o_{2unloaded})}{103} \quad (3.17)$$

where $\ddot{W}$ is the rate of work rate increment in W · min$^{-1}$.

**Example:** Using the reference values from Hansen et al. (see Further Reading), a 55-year-old 65 kg sedentary female would have a predicted $\dot{V}o_{2max}$ of 1450 ml · min$^{-1}$. The following steps would be used to calculate the optimal rate of work rate increment:

(a) The unloaded cycling $\dot{V}o_2$ would be:

$(5.8 \times 65 + 151) = 528$ ml · min$^{-1}$

(b) The expected increase in $\dot{V}o_2$ for a maximal test would be:

$1450 - 528 = 922$ ml · min$^{-1}$

(c) The expected rate of work rate increment would be:

$922/103 = 9.2$ W · min$^{-1}$

This result suggests a 9 W · min$^{-1}$ (or, nominally, 10 W · min$^{-1}$) protocol. This estimate would be either increased or decreased, usually in 5 W · min$^{-1}$ increments based on the nature of the subject. For example, this same 55-year-old female weighing 65 kg, with clinical evidence of ventilatory abnormalities, e.g., asthma, might require a 5 W · min$^{-1}$ work rate increment. Conversely, a healthy, regularly exercising 55-year-old female weighing 65 kg might require a protocol of 20 W · min$^{-1}$. In most cases, it is better to overestimate the work rate increment slightly, as this will result in a shorter test. If necessary, after recovery, the test can be repeated with an adjusted work rate increment.

**Table 3.13.** Guide for setting the work rate increment for leg cycling in a variety of subject groups

| Work rate increment (W · min$^{-1}$) | Patient characteristics |
|---|---|
| 5 | Severely impaired (e.g., subject who is confined to home or walks only short distances) |
| 10 | Moderately impaired (e.g., subject who walks one or two city blocks before developing symptoms) |
| 15 | Mild impairment or sedentary older adult |
| 20 | Sedentary younger subject (no physical activity beyond activities of daily living) |
| 25 | Active younger subject (regular physical activity) |
| 30 | Athletic and fit (competitive) |
| 40 | Extremely fit (highly competitive, particularly as a cyclist) |

Table 3.13 presents a guide for setting work rate increments for leg cycle ergometer testing in a variety of subject groups. This table has been developed from experience and use of the above equations. Selection of the increment should be modified based on clinical assessment of the person's exercise capacity. Smaller subjects, even though more fit, might require smaller increments.

## Maximal treadmill exercise tests

Designing the optimal treadmill protocol for ramp or stair-step incremental exercise testing requires knowledge of the expected $\dot{V}o_{2max}$ in units of ml · kg$^{-1}$ · min$^{-1}$. Reference standards appropriate to the subject's age, gender, and weight along with clinical experience will aid in this determination (see Appendix C). Use of standard equations will allow the algebraic calculation of a speed or grade increment. Importantly, during treadmill exercise the total $\dot{V}o_2$ equals the sum of a horizontal component related to treadmill speed ($\dot{V}o_2H$), a vertical component related to treadmill speed and grade ($\dot{V}o_2V$), and a resting component ($\dot{V}o_2R$).

$$\dot{V}o_2 = \dot{V}o_2H + \dot{V}o_2V + \dot{V}o_2R \quad (3.18)$$

where all measures of $\dot{V}O_2$ are expressed in $ml \cdot kg^{-1} \cdot min^{-1}$.

The following example is used with walking speeds ($50–100\ m \cdot min^{-1}$):

1. Estimate $\dot{V}O_{2max}$ for the patient being tested using subject characteristics and clinical experience.
2. Substitute the estimated $\dot{V}O_{2max}$ for $\dot{V}O_2$ in Equation 3.18.
3. Subtract the $\dot{V}O_2R$ component ($3.5\ ml \cdot kg^{-1} \cdot min^{-1}$) from both sides of Equation 3.18.
4. Choose a constant treadmill speed (Speed) for the calculation of $\dot{V}O_2H$ and $\dot{V}O_2V$.
5. Calculate $\dot{V}O_2H$ using Equation 3.19 or Equation 3.20.

$$\dot{V}O_2H = Speed \cdot 0.1 \qquad (3.19)$$

where $\dot{V}O_2H$ is the horizontal component of oxygen uptake expressed in $ml \cdot kg^{-1} \cdot min^{-1}$ and Speed is the treadmill speed expressed in $m \cdot min^{-1}$. Alternatively:

$$\dot{V}O_2H = Speed \cdot 2.68 \qquad (3.20)$$

where $\dot{V}O_2H$ is the horizontal component of oxygen uptake expressed in $ml \cdot kg^{-1} \cdot min^{-1}$ and Speed is the treadmill speed expressed in m.p.h. ($1\ m.p.h. = 26.8\ m \cdot min^{-1}$).

6. Subtract $\dot{V}O_2H$ from both sides of Equation 3.18. The remainder represents $\dot{V}O_2V$.
7. Calculate the maximum treadmill grade using Equation 3.21 or Equation 3.22.

$$\dot{V}O_2V = Speed \cdot Grade \cdot 0.018 \qquad (3.21)$$

where $\dot{V}O_2V$ is the vertical component of oxygen uptake expressed in $ml \cdot kg^{-1} \cdot min^{-1}$, Speed is the treadmill speed in $m \cdot min^{-1}$ and Grade is the treadmill grade expressed as a percentage. Alternatively:

$$\dot{V}O_2V = Speed \cdot Grade \cdot 0.482 \qquad (3.22)$$

where $\dot{V}O_2V$ is the vertical component of oxygen uptake expressed in $ml \cdot kg^{-1} \cdot min^{-1}$, Speed is the treadmill speed in m.p.h. and Grade is the treadmill grade expressed as a percentage ($1\ m.p.h. = 26.8\ m \cdot min^{-1}$).

8. Divide the maximum percent grade by 10 min (optimal test duration) to obtain the percentage grade increment for each minute.

**Example:** If the estimated $\dot{V}O_{2max}$ is $20\ ml \cdot kg^{-1} \cdot min^{-1}$ and the chosen treadmill speed is 1.5 m.p.h., assuming an optimal test duration of 10 min:

$$\dot{V}O_2 = \dot{V}O_2H + \dot{V}O_2V + \dot{V}O_2R$$
$$20 = \dot{V}O_2H + \dot{V}O_2V + 3.5$$
$$16.5 = \dot{V}O_2H + \dot{V}O_2V$$

since:

$$\dot{V}O_2H = (1.5 \cdot 26.8 \cdot 0.1)$$

then:

$$\dot{V}O_2H = 4.02$$
$$16.5 = 4.02 + \dot{V}O_2V$$
$$12.48 = \dot{V}O_2V$$

since:

$$\dot{V}O_2V = (1.5 \cdot 26.8 \cdot 0.018) \cdot \text{Maximum grade}$$

therefore:

$$\text{Maximum grade} = 12.28/(1.5 \cdot 26.8 \cdot 0.018)$$
$$\text{Maximum grade} = 17.2(\%)$$
$$\text{Grade increment} = 1.7\ (\% \cdot min^{-1})$$

The calculations detailed above can be condensed into a single equation to estimate the minute-by-minute grade increment (Equation 3.23 or Equation 3.24). Again, these equations assume an optimal test duration of 10 min and require knowledge of the expected $\dot{V}O_{2max}$ and the desired treadmill speed.

$$\text{Grade increment} = \frac{\dot{V}O_{2max(expected)} - 3.5 - (Speed \cdot 0.1)}{Speed \cdot 0.18} \qquad (3.23)$$

where Grade increment is expressed in $\% \cdot min^{-1}$, $\dot{V}O_{2max}$ is expressed in $ml \cdot kg^{-1} \cdot min^{-1}$ and Speed is the treadmill speed in $m \cdot min^{-1}$. Alternatively:

$$\text{Grade increment} = \frac{\dot{V}O_{2max(expected)} - 3.5 - (Speed \cdot 2.68)}{Speed \cdot 4.82} \qquad (3.24)$$

where Grade increment is expressed in $\% \cdot min^{-1}$,

$\dot{V}O_{2max}$ is expressed in $ml \cdot kg^{-1} \cdot min^{-1}$ and Speed is the treadmill speed in m.p.h. (1 m.p.h. = $26.8\ m \cdot min^{-1}$).

> **Example:** Using the same example as above; where the estimated $\dot{V}O_{2max}$ is $20\ ml \cdot kg^{-1} \cdot min^{-1}$ and the chosen treadmill speed is 1.5 m.p.h.:
>
> $$\text{Grade increment} = \frac{20 - 3.5 - (1.5 \cdot 26.8 \cdot 0.1)}{(1.5 \cdot 26.8 \cdot 0.18)}$$
>
> $$= 1.7\ (\% \cdot min^{-1})$$

A spreadsheet that allows calculation of the optimal percentage grade increment by inputting the expected $\dot{V}O_{2max}$ and chosen constant treadmill speed is shown as Figure D4 in Appendix D.

## Maximal arm ergometer exercise tests

For young, healthy subjects, typical work rate increments range between 10 and $25\ W \cdot min^{-1}$ and may be continuous or discontinuous. Stage durations range between 1 and 6 min. Discontinuous protocols facilitate measurement of blood pressure and acquisition of artifact-free ECG tracings during the interposed 1-min rest period. Many investigators have reported comparable $\dot{V}O_{2max}$ values between the continuous and discontinuous protocols, although the continuous protocols are more time-efficient. Cranking frequency usually ranges between 40 and 60 r.p.m. For patients with cervical spinal cord injuries resulting in quadriparesis, choice of the work rate increment is important, with increments of $2\text{–}6\ W \cdot min^{-1}$ yielding higher $\dot{V}O_{2max}$ values than $8\ W \cdot min^{-1}$ or greater protocols. For persons with paraplegia, the work rate increment may be increased to $10\ W \cdot min^{-1}$ or greater. Elderly persons and patients with cardiac or pulmonary disease may terminate at low work rates (e.g., 25–50 W), thus suggesting low initial work rates and small ($2\text{–}5\ W \cdot min^{-1}$) work rate increments. Unlike leg cycling and treadmill ergometry, there is no direct evidence that the optimal duration for maximal arm exercise XT is 8–12 min. However, it may be reasonable to apply this approach to arm ergometry as well. In doing so, one would:

- Identify the expected $\dot{V}O_{2max}$ according to subject history, physical training history, and clinical experience. Alternatively, since arm $\dot{V}O_{2max}$ is approximately 25–35% lower than leg cycling, reducing the predicted $\dot{V}O_{2max}$ for leg ergometry by an appropriate value within that range for a given subject would provide good initial guidance in setting the work rate increment.
- Use the expected $\dot{V}O_{2max}$ along with Equation 3.25, below, to estimate the appropriate work rate increment:

$$\text{Arm}\dot{V}O_{2max} = (\dot{W}_{max} \cdot 18.36) + (BW \cdot 3.5) \qquad (3.25)$$

where Arm $\dot{V}O_{2max}$ is expressed in $ml \cdot min^{-1}$, $\dot{W}_{max}$ is expressed in W, and BW is body weight in kg.

> **Example:** If the expected leg cycling $\dot{V}O_{2max}$ for a 70-kg subject is $2700\ ml \cdot min^{-1}$, using Equation 3.25 and assuming arm ergometry $\dot{V}O_{2max}$ to be 70% of leg cycling $\dot{V}O_{2max}$:
>
> $$2700 \cdot 0.7 = (\dot{W}_{max} \cdot 18.36) + (70 \cdot 3.5)$$
> $$\dot{W}_{max} = (1890 - 245)/18.36$$
> $$= 90\ W$$
>
> Hence, for a 10-min protocol, a work rate increment of $9\ W \cdot min^{-1}$ would be recommended. For most ergometers, the nominal value of $10\ W \cdot min^{-1}$ would be used.

## Exercise testing in pregnancy

Formal guidelines for XT during pregnancy are not readily available. Whilst the American College of Obstetrics and Gynecology as well as the ACSM have position statements on exercise training during pregnancy, guidelines for specific XT protocols are lacking, apart from the ACSM's recommendation that maximal exercise testing is not recommended in nonclinical settings. Occasions might exist when CXT would be useful. However, the benefits of XT must clearly outweigh the risks to warrant testing during pregnancy rather than waiting and test-

**Table 3.14.** American College of Sports Medicine recommendations for physician supervision during exercise tests

| Type of test | Apparently healthy: Male aged $\leqslant 40$ Female aged $\leqslant 50$ | Apparently healthy: Male aged $>40$ Female aged $>50$ | Increased risk: No symptoms | Increased risk: Symptoms | Known disease |
|---|---|---|---|---|---|
| Submaximal testing | No | No | No | Yes | Yes |
| Maximal testing | No | Yes | Yes | Yes | Yes |

ing postpartum. Treadmill exercise testing may present greater risk than necessary because of the potential of falling. Cycle ergometry offers a desirable alternative because it provides a nonweight-bearing form of work with increased stability due to the seated position and handlebar holding. However, in later stages of pregnancy, the cycle seat may prove uncomfortable and the leg action may be affected by the encumbrance of the fetus. Arm ergometry is also a reasonable alternative. The woman is seated on a more comfortable chair or bench seat and the increased size of the abdomen presents a smaller hindrance. Care should be taken to optimize heat dissipation, especially during the first trimester, by advising rehydration prior to the test, appropriate close-fitting clothing, and cool (e.g., 66°), dry testing environments. Morning appointments might be avoided because of the nausea experienced in early pregnancy by some women.

## Personnel recommendations

### Level of supervision

Every cardiopulmonary exercise test should be properly supervised. Depending upon the setting, purpose of the test, and characteristics of the subject, this may require a physician experienced with exercise testing to be in attendance, directly supervising the test. The ACSM has provided recommendations for physician supervision, as shown in Table 3.14. *Apparently healthy,* according to the ACSM, refers to those individuals with less than two risk factors and no signs or symptoms of cardiac, pulmonary, or metabolic disease. *Increased risk* is defined by the ACSM as persons with two or more risk factors or one or more signs or symptoms. *Known disease* refers to people with known cardiovascular, pulmonary, or metabolic disease. *Yes* in the table indicates that physician supervision is recommended or that a physician is in close proximity and readily available if needed. *No* in the table response means physician supervision is not necessary and does not mean that the test should not be performed.

### Experience and qualifications

Generally for CXT, a physician's presence will be appropriate during the test. The ACSM recommendations are moot in a clinical setting where the physician is in charge of the exercise test. When this is not the case, for example in university, corporate, health club, or fitness center settings, care should be taken that test personnel are appropriately trained and experienced. The ACSM provides certification for this purpose and, when tests are to be conducted with patient groups, the ACSM Exercise Specialist™ certification is ideal. In an apparently healthy population, particularly when submaximal tests are administered, the ACSM Health and Fitness Instructor™ certification is appropriate. While ACSM certifications are not absolutely necessary, they do suggest that the certified individual has achieved a particular level of competency and proficiency in conducting the integrated exercise test. Such competency and proficiency may be acquired through alternative means such as formal courses of study, internships, or job experience. Nevertheless, it behooves those planning to conduct and interpret cardiopulmonary exercise tests to become knowledgeable and practiced.

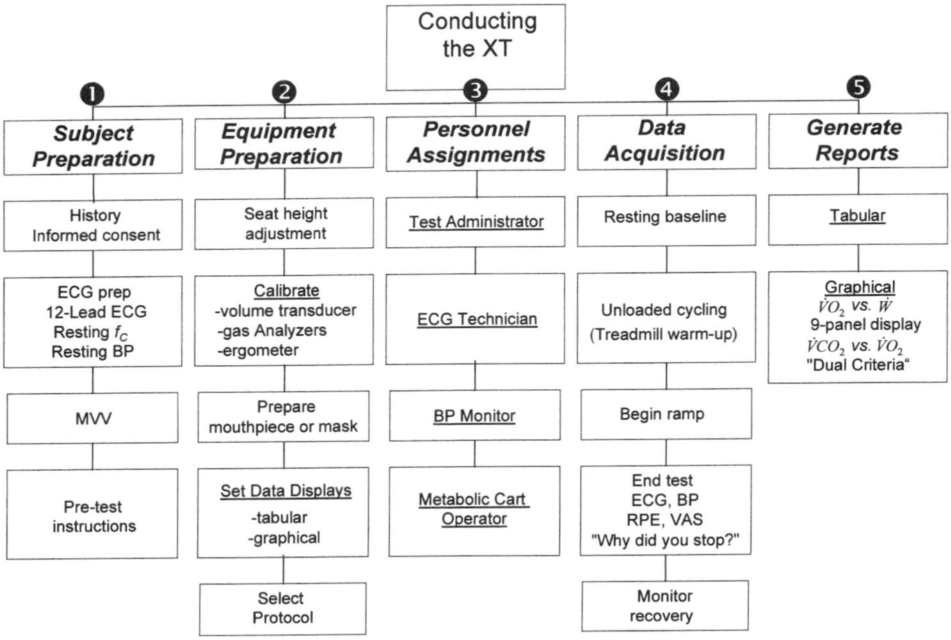


**Figure 3.5** Flow chart indicating the sequence for conducting an exercise test (XT).

## Assignments

The XT should be conducted with a minimum of key personnel, each assigned to specific roles. Excess personnel are potentially distracting to both subject and test administrators and should be kept away from the test environment. Typically, a good XT can be conducted with the personnel listed below and shown in Figure 3.5. While this list is somewhat luxurious, it serves to identify key roles. Two experienced persons can easily perform all the functions listed below.

### Test administrator

This is usually the physician, exercise physiologist, physical therapist, respiratory therapist, or nurse who takes charge of the test and directs the test activities. The test administrator gives pretest instructions and monitors the subject throughout the test for signs and symptoms of exercise intolerance. The test administrator may also be responsible for blood pressure measurements and ECG monitoring.

### ECG technician

This person is in charge of preparing the subject for ECG electrodes, applying them, and recording the ECG during the test. A trained ECG technician will also monitor the ECG throughout the exercise test.

### Blood pressure monitor

This person is responsible for measuring the resting, warm-up, exercise, and recovery blood pressures.

**Table 3.15.** Reference values appropriate for resting conditions

| $f_C$ ($min^{-1}$) | $\dot{V}O_2$ ($ml \cdot min^{-1}$) | $\dot{V}CO_2$ ($ml \cdot min^{-1}$) | $R$ | $\dot{V}_E$ ($l \cdot min^{-1}$) | $P_{ET}O_2$ (mmHg) | $P_{ET}CO_2$ (mmHg) |
|---|---|---|---|---|---|---|
| 60–100 | 200–300 | 140–300 | 0.7–1.0 | 6–10 | 100–105 | 38–42 |

While this may be the function of a third person on the test team, when one is available, the test administrator or ECG technician can also monitor blood pressure.

### Metabolic cart operator

This person is in charge of calibrating and operating the metabolic cart, troubleshooting if necessary, and for providing end-of-test reports. This person will also ensure proper ergometer preparation, including appropriate adjustment for the subject in the case of leg or arm ergometry. Typically the metabolic cart operator is also responsible for application of the patient interface.

## Data acquisition

### Resting phase

Once the subject is comfortably seated on the cycle or standing on the treadmill, up to 4 min of baseline data should be acquired. The purpose of the baseline period is to observe patient responses in order to ensure proper calibration and performance of the metabolic measurement system. Key variables should be evaluated against expected values. Table 3.15 provides an example of key resting variables and their expected values. While there may be clinical explanations for departures from these baseline values, departures can usually be explained by pretest anxiety, leaks in the patient interface such as a poor-fitting mask or failure to apply the nose clip, or improper calibration of the metabolic measurement instruments. Anxiety typically increases $f_C > 80\,min^{-1}$, increases $R > 1.0$, increases $\dot{V}_E > 10\,l \cdot min^{-1}$, and decreases $P_{ET}CO_2 < 35$ mmHg. Leaking at the patient interface typically results in normal $f_C$ and $R$ values, whereas $\dot{V}_E$, $\dot{V}O_2$, and $\dot{V}CO_2$ are decreased in proportion to one another.

In addition to these variables, resting blood pressure and ECG should also be recorded.

### Warm-up phase

The warm-up phase consists of 3–4 min of unloaded cycling or treadmill walking at low speed and grade. This period allows the subject to accommodate to the ergometer, learning to maintain a fixed cycling cadence or establishing balance points on the treadmill. Care should be taken to ensure that the warm-up work rate is not so severe as to interfere with the completion of an 8–12-min exercise protocol. Warm-up work rates on the cycle ergometer are termed "unloaded" and represent the lowest work rate available, usually less than 10 W. Generally for CXT on a cycle ergometer, an unloaded pedaling warm-up phase of 3 min is utilized. This lends some consistency to clinical testing methods and facilitates comparison of data from different institutions. The approximate $\dot{V}O_2$ for unloaded pedaling in nonobese subjects is $500\,ml \cdot min^{-1}$. A speed of 0.1 m.p.h. on a horizontal treadmill predicts an oxygen uptake similar to that of unloaded cycling for a subject weighing 80 kg. Although this may seem quite slow, this speed provides appropriate warm-up for a clinically limited patient. Blood pressure and the ECG should be recorded near the end of this 3-min warm-up period.

### Exercise phase

The incremental work rate protocol begins immediately after the warm-up phase. Throughout the test, the subject should be carefully monitored for signs of intolerance as well as for abnormal ECG, $f_C$, and blood pressure responses that may necessitate early test termination (see indications for stopping a test in the section on safety considerations, below). Although sometimes overlooked in the course of administering an integrative exercise test, especially in apparently healthy individuals, blood pressure monitoring is essential as a safety measure to detect exercise-induced hypertension or hypotension and to calculate the rate pressure product (systolic BP multiplied by $f_C$). Blood pressure should be recorded every 2 or 3 min unless abnormal responses suggest more frequent measurement. For CXT, the ECG is continuously monitored throughout the test and recorded during the last 5–10 s of every other minute. Ratings of perceived exertion and breathlessness scores may also be obtained every 2 min during the exercise phase. Comments regarding events occurring during the test that may affect test interpretation should be recorded on the supplemental data sheet (see Appendix D).

### Recovery phase

Measurements of ECG, heart rate, and blood pressure should be made periodically for up to 10 min during recovery. Unless calculation of oxygen debt and deficit are desired, gas exchange variables need not be collected during this period.

Immediately upon test termination, the subject should be presented with psychometric scales such as the RPE scale and VAS for breathlessness with appropriate instructions for marking. At the same time, the subject should be asked, in a nonleading way, why he or she stopped exercise. The answer to this important question should be recorded, as it will be used later to assist with test interpretation.

## Generation of reports

As soon as feasible, tabular and graphical reports should be generated in preparation for test interpretation. See Chapter 5 for a description of the formatting and contents of these reports.

## Methodological considerations which enhance exercise test interpretation

An objective impression regarding subject performance as well as technical factors occurring during the test that might affect test interpretation should be recorded on the supplemental data sheet (Appendix D). These data further document test conditions, enhance test interpretation, and help ensure reliability of future tests. The supplemental data sheet along with the tabular and graphical results from the test will provide the practitioner with the necessary data for systematic interpretation of the test using the principles outlined in Chapter 5. Examples of objective impressions and technical factors that may affect test interpretation are given below.

### Objective impression

- Was the subject well motivated towards the test?
- Did the subject give an adequate effort (e.g., excellent, good, fair, or poor)?
- Has the subject exercised this hard recently?
- Did the subject require an unusually long recovery period?
- Was the test the best one for the subject in light of known medical problems?
- Will this test serve as a valid basis for subsequent comparison or exercise prescription?

### Technical issues

- Were all calibrations satisfactory?
- Were baseline measurements within expected limits?
- Were there problems with the patient interface (e.g., leaking mouthpiece)?
- Were there problems with ECG quality?
- Were there difficulties obtaining blood samples?
- What criteria were used to terminate the test?
- Was the $\dot{V}O_{2max}$ measured or estimated?
- What was the maximal tolerated work rate (symptom-limited test)?
- What was the maximal safe work rate (threshold

for angina, dysrhythmia, dyspnea, claudication, or other symptoms)?
- At what percent of $f_{Cmax}$, $\dot{V}O_{2max}$, or absolute $\dot{V}O_2$ did significant symptoms or dysrhythmia occur?
- What reference values are to be used for assessing the subject's response? Are these reference values appropriate for the work device and protocol used in the test?
- What medications is the subject taking? How long before the exercise test were the medications taken?

## Safety considerations

Standards and guidelines have been published for exercise-testing laboratories in health and fitness facilities (see Further Reading). Clinical facilities in the USA are likely to be bound by standards dictated by the Joint Commission for the Accreditation of Hospital Organizations (JCAHO). It is advisable that recommended standards be carefully interpreted and applied as appropriate to any XT setting. The following section summarizes some of the important safety considerations. The exercise-testing laboratory should be kept meticulously clean and free from clutter. In addition to instrumentation used in XT, emergency equipment and supplies should be available and well maintained (see below). The environment should be maintained with temperature, humidity, and air circulation controlled at 68–72 °F (20–21 °C), 60% or less relative humidity, and 8–12 air exchanges per hour, respectively. Illumination should be at least 50 foot-candles ($538\,\text{lm} \cdot \text{m}^{-2}$ at floor surface).

The XT laboratory should provide at least 100 square feet (9.3 square meters) of floor space. If carpeted, the material should be antistatic and treated with antifungal and antibacterial chemicals. Proper sterilization methods using one of the commercially available wet sterilization solutions should be employed for all equipment and supplies in direct contact with subjects. This includes mouthpieces, masks, nose clips, filters, breathing valves, flow transducers, and respiratory tubing.

**Table 3.16.** Absolute contraindications to exercise testing according to clinical history or ECG criteria

| Absolute contraindications based on clinical history | Absolute contraindications based on ECG criteria |
|---|---|
| Recent complicated myocardial infarction (unless patient is stable and painfree)[a] | Recent significant change in resting ECG suggesting infarction or other acute cardiac event |
| Unstable angina | Uncontrolled ventricular dysrhythmia |
| Unstable congestive heart failure | Uncontrolled atrial dysrhythmia that compromises cardiac function |
| Severe aortic stenosis | Third-degree atrioventricular heart block without pacemaker |
| Suspected or known dissecting aortic aneurysm | |
| Active or suspected myocarditis or pericarditis | |
| Active or suspected venous thromboembolic disease, including recent pulmonary embolism or intracardiac thrombus | |
| Acute infection | |
| Significant emotional distress (psychosis) | |

[a]Refer to relative contraindications.

Disposable supplies such as nose clips, filters, razors for ECG preparation, and even some flow transducers obviate the requirement for sterilization. Clearly, these should not be reused unless so designed and properly sterilized.

## Contraindications to exercise testing

### General considerations

The potential benefits of exercise testing must be carefully weighed against the risks of such testing in individuals presenting with certain conditions, signs, symptoms, or history. Those presenting with the absolute contraindications listed in Table 3.16

**Table 3.17.** Relative contraindications to exercise testing based on clinical history, ECG criteria, and blood pressure assessment

| Relative contraindications based on clinical history | Relative contraindications based on ECG criteria | Relative contraindications based on blood pressure |
|---|---|---|
| Moderate valvular heart disease | Frequent or complex ventricular ectopy | Resting arterial diastolic pressure >110 mmHg or resting arterial systolic pressure >200 mmHg |
| Known electrolyte abnormalities (hypokalemia, hypomagnesemia) | | |
| Fixed-rate pacemaker (rarely used) | | |
| Ventricular aneurysm | | |
| Uncontrolled metabolic disease (e.g., diabetes, thyrotoxicosis, or myxedema) | | |
| Chronic infectious disease (e.g., mononucleosis, hepatitis, AIDS) | | |
| Neuromuscular, musculoskeletal, or rheumatoid disorders that are exacerbated by exercise | | |
| Advanced or complicated pregnancy | | |

should not be tested until their condition is stabilized. Those with relative contraindications, listed in Table 3.17, may be tested if clinical judgment suggests a benefit that outweighs the risk of completing the exercise test. For ease of use, these contraindications can be organized into three categories: (1) contraindications based on clinical history; and (2) contraindications based on the ECG; and (3) contraindications based on blood pressure (see Tables 3.16 and 3.17).

### Absolute contraindications

Absolute contraindications generally include unstable cardiovascular disease, acute or active infection, and psychological instability. Exercise testing has been performed as early as 3 days after acute myocardial infarction. Maximal exercise testing can be safely performed soon after uncomplicated myocardial infarction, provided monitoring and safety criteria are strictly observed. However, submaximal testing may suffice to estimate aerobic capacity and to define thresholds for angina or dysrhythmia, thus enabling a safe and effective exercise prescription.

### Relative contraindications

Relative contraindications generally include less threatening or reversible conditions. These contraindications should be interpreted on a case-by-case basis with careful evaluation of the benefits and risks of exercise testing.

## Indications for stopping a test

The exercise practitioner should be aware of the several indications for terminating an exercise test. Although more commonly occurring at higher exercise intensity, these criteria may occur at any point during the exercise test, especially in patients with known cardiovascular or pulmonary disease. Table 3.18 provides indications for terminating an exercise test that is nondiagnostic and is being performed without physician supervision or ECG monitoring. Table 3.19 provides test termination criteria that are more specific and appropriate for use in clinical diagnostic XT with ECG monitoring and physician supervision. For this latter table, the decision to continue an exercise test in the presence of "relative" termination criteria should be based on the risk-to-benefit ratio and good clinical judgment.

**Table 3.18.** Exercise test termination criteria for nondiagnostic tests without ECG monitoring or physician supervision

| |
|---|
| Onset of angina or angina-like symptoms |
| Significant drop in arterial systolic blood pressure (>20 mmHg) |
| Failure of arterial systolic pressure to rise with increasing exercise intensity |
| Excessive increase in arterial systolic pressure to >250 mmHg or diastolic pressure to >115 mmHg |
| Signs of poor perfusion: lightheadedness, confusion, ataxia, pallor, cyanosis, nausea, or cold and clammy skin |
| Failure of an appropriate increase in heart rate with increased exercise intensity |
| New and significant change in cardiac rhythm |
| Physical or verbal manifestations of severe fatigue |
| Subject requests to stop |
| Failure of testing equipment |

## Emergency procedures

Every laboratory in which XT is conducted should have a documented and practiced emergency procedures plan appropriate to the setting. The desirable frequency for practicing such a plan is at least twice a year. The plan should provide for the following:

- Access to all areas of the facility.
- Controlling the environment, including bystanders.
- Reporting and documentation of the incident.
- Use and practice of specific procedures that effect the emergency plan.
- Methods for activating the emergency medical system (EMS).

As a basic minimum, exercise laboratory personnel should obtain training and certification in basic life support (BLS) such as that provided by the American Heart Association or American Red Cross. Personnel should know how to activate the emergency procedures plan, i.e., they should know how to place a telephone call to the appropriate EMS. This activation might require a 911 telephone call or pressing a "Code Blue" wall switch. Printed instructions at each laboratory phone location should remind the

**Table 3.19.** Exercise test termination criteria for diagnostic tests with ECG monitoring and physician supervision

| Absolute indications for exercise test termination | Relative indications for exercise test termination |
|---|---|
| Acute myocardial infarction or suspicion of myocardial infarction | Pronounced ECG changes from baseline (>2 mm of horizontal or downsloping ST segment depression, or >2 mm of ST segment elevation (except in aVR)). |
| Onset of moderate to severe angina | Changes in ST level are usually evaluated 80 ms beyond the J-point |
| Drop in arterial systolic pressure with increasing workload accompanied by signs or symptoms or drop below standing resting pressure | Any chest pain that is increasing |
| Serious dysrhythmias (e.g., second- or third-degree atrioventricular block, sustained ventricular tachycardia, or increasing premature ventricular contractions, atrial fibrillation with rapid ventricular response) | Physical or verbal manifestations of severe fatigue or shortness of breath |
| Signs of poor perfusion including pallor, or cold, clammy skin | Wheezing |
| Unusual or severe shortness of breath | Leg cramps or intermittent claudication (grade 3 on a four-point scale) |
| Central nervous system symptoms, including ataxia, vertigo, visual disturbance, paresthesia, gait problems, or confusion | Hypertensive response (systolic pressure >250 mmHg; diastolic pressure >115 mmHg) |
| Technical inability to monitor the ECG | Less serious dysrhythmias such as supraventricular tachycardia |
| Request of the subject | Exercise-induced bundle branch block that cannot be distinguished from ventricular tachycardia |

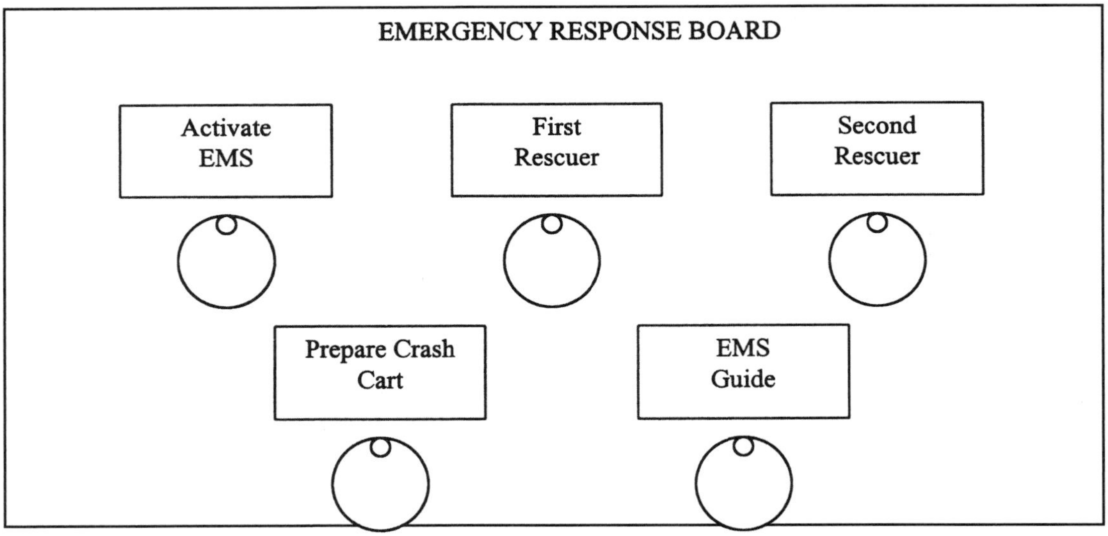


**Figure 3.6** An emergency response board. Emergency functions are labeled and permanently positioned. Tags with staff member names are positioned below an emergency function upon arrival in the laboratory or clinic, thus identifying staff member functions during an emergency.

caller of key information to be provided to the EMS. A typical example is as follows:

- EMS telephone number: ____________
- "This is ____________ (*your name*) at ____________ (*your facility*)."
- "We have an emergency."
- Describe the nature of the emergency, current action, and resuscitation equipment available.
- Describe location of the facility and how to get there.

> ***Note:*** *In some settings, this might require a laboratory staff member to meet the EMS personnel at an easily identified location and guide them into the facility.*

Laboratory personnel should know the location of all emergency equipment, know the responsibilities of all personnel for assisting in the emergency, and be able to prepare the equipment for trained emergency personnel or laboratory staff trained in advanced cardiac life support (ACLS).

One approach to effecting the emergency plan is to establish an emergency response board. This is a permanently mounted board with labels for emergency functions, below which are hung name tags for lab personnel on duty, as illustrated in Figure 3.6. It is important to remember that staff should only do what they are trained to do. Certification in BLS along with knowledge and practice of an appropriate emergency plan are basic requisites for every exercise-testing laboratory. In higher-risk settings, it is advisable to have one or more lab staff trained and certified in ACLS.

## Resuscitation equipment

Table 3.20 contains an abbreviated example of emergency resuscitation equipment that would be contained in a crash cart. Crash cart equipment and supplies should be regularly inspected for proper function and the expiration dates of emergency drugs. Further details of crash cart contents and arrangement are presented in Appendix D.

Aside from the oxygen tank that constitutes an

**Table 3.20.** Abbreviated example of crash cart equipment and supplies

| Equipment | Emergency drugs |
|---|---|
| Portable defibrillator (synchronized), patient cables, electrodes, and electrolyte gel | Sodium bicarbonate |
| Oxygen with two-stage regulator and tubing | Atropine |
| Airways (oral and endotracheal) | Isoproterenol |
| Laryngoscope and intubation equipment | Lidocaine |
| Ambu bag | Bretylium |
| Syringes and needles | Procainamide |
| Intravenous tubing and solutions | Epinephrine |
| Intravenous stand | Norepinephrine |
| Adhesive tape and gauze pads | Dopamine |
| Blood-drawing tubes (for arterial blood gases, chemistries) | Dobutamine |
| Suction devices and tubing | Nitroglycerine |
| Gloves | Sodium nitroprusside |
| | Furosemide |
| | Morphine sulfate |
| | Digoxin |

integral part of the resuscitation cart, an alternative supply of supplemental oxygen is helpful in the XT laboratory. This can be used to relieve subjects who experience chest pain or intense breathlessness. A short-acting bronchodilator inhaler should also be available to relieve EIB when it occurs, either coincidentally or as an anticipated response to an EIB study.

## FURTHER READING

ACC/AHA Task Force (1997). ACC/AHA guidelines for exercise testing: executive summary. A report of the American College of Cardiology/American Heart Association task force on practice guidelines (committee on exercise testing). *Circulation*, **96**, 345–54.

American College of Sports Medicine (1995). *ACSM's Guidelines for Exercise Testing and Prescription*, 5th edn. Baltimore: Williams & Wilkins.

Balady, G. J., Chaitman, B., Driscoll, D. et al. (1998). AHA/ACSM Scientific Statement: Recommendations for Cardiovascular Screening, Staffing, and Emergency Policies at Health/Fitness Facilities. *Circulation*, **97**, 2283–93.

Bruce, R. A. (1971). Exercise testing of patients with coronary artery disease. *Ann. Clin. Res.*, **3**, 323–32.

Bruce, R. A., & McDonough, J. R. (1969). Stress testing in screening for cardiovascular disease. *Bull. NY Acad. Med.*, **45**, 1288–305.

Cooper, K. H. (1982). *The Aerobics Program for Total Well-being.* New York: Bantam Books/M. Evans.

Cooper, K. H. (1985) *The Aerobics Program for Total Well Being. Exercise, Diet, Emotional Balance.* New York: Bantam, Doubleday, Dell.

Hansen, J. E., Sue, D. Y. & Wasserman, K. (1984). Predicted values for clinical exercise testing. *Am. Rev. Respir. Dis.*, **129**, S49–50.

Kline, G. M., Porcari, J. P., Hintermeister, R. et al. (1987). Estimation of $\dot{V}O_{2max}$ from one-mile track walk, gender, age and body weight. *Med. Sci. Sports Exerc.*, **19**, 253–9.

Lasko-McCarthey, P. & Davis, J. A. (1991). Protocol dependency of $\dot{V}O_{2max}$ during arm cycle ergometry in males with quadriplegia. *Med. Sci. Sports Exerc.*, **23**, 1097–101.

Léger, L. A. & Lambert, J. (1982). A maximal multistage 20-m shuttle run test to predict $\dot{V}O_{2max}$. *Eur. J. Appl. Physiol.*, **49**, 1–12.

McArdle, W. D., Katch, F. I., Pechar, G. S., Jacobson, L. & Ruck, S. (1972). Reliability and interrelationships between maximal oxygen uptake, physical work capacity, and step test scores in college women. *Med. Sci. Sports Exerc.*, **4**, 182–6.

McArdle, W. D., Pechar, G.S., Katch, F.I. & Magel, J.R. (1973). Percentile norms for a valid step test in college women. *Res. Q.*, **44**, 498–500.

McArdle, W. D., Katch, F. I. & Katch, V. L. (1986). *Exercise Physiology: Energy, Nutrition, and Human Performance*, 2nd edn. Philadelphia: Lea & Febiger.

Pollock, M., Roa, J., Benditt, J. & Celli, B. (1993). Estimation of ventilatory reserve by stair climbing. A study in patients with chronic airflow obstruction. *Chest*, **104**, 1378–83.

Siconolfi, S. F., Garber, C. E., Laster, T. M. & Carleton, R. A. (1985). A simple, valid step test for estimating maximal oxygen uptake in epidemiological studies. *Am. J. Epidemiol.*, **121**, 382–90.

Singh, S.J., Morgan, M.D.L., Scott, S., Walters, D. & Hardman, A.E. (1994). Development of a shuttle walking test of disability in patients with chronic airflow limitation. *Eur. Respir. J.*, **7**, 2016–20.

Sjostrand, T. (1947). Changes in the respiratory organs of workmen at an ore melting works. *Acta. Med. Scand.* (Suppl. 196), 687.

Storer, T. W., Davis, J. A. & Caiozzo, V. J. (1990). Accurate prediction of $\dot{V}O_{2max}$ in cycle ergometry. *Med. Sci. Sports Exerc.*, **22**, 704–12.

Tharrett, S. J. & Peterson, J. A. (eds) (1997) *ACSM's Health/Fitness Facility Standards and Guidelines*, 2nd edn. Champaign, IL: Human Kinetics.

Whipp, B. J. & Wasserman, K. (1969). Efficiency of muscular work. *J. Appl. Physiol.*, **26**, 644–8.

4

# Response variables

## Introduction

This chapter is a compendium of variables collected during different types of exercise test. Each variable is defined and its derivation and significance explained. For many of the variables, a normal data set is used to illustrate responses to the type of incremental protocol described in Figure 4.4 (A and B). Reference values are given for normal responses and various types of abnormal response are illustrated. The style of symbols used throughout this book is that recommended by the international scientific community. When new symbols are introduced they generally reflect established conventions. Some symbols represent a departure from previous usage but only when it seems necessary based on logic and consistency. A complete list of the recommended symbols can be found in Appendix A along with their definitions.

## Variables of the exercise response

### Endurance time ($t$)

#### Definition, derivation, and units of measurement

Endurance time quantifies exercise duration for defined constant and incremental work rate protocols as well as variable work rates such as walking and running tests. Endurance time represents the total time of exercise excluding the warm-up period and is often used with walking or running distance ($d_W$ or $d_R$) to calculate walking or running velocity (see below).

Time is one of the most important primary variables during exercise testing. The units of measurement are minutes or seconds.

#### Normal response

*Constant work rate exercise*
Endurance time for constant work rate exercise varies inversely with the percentage of maximum work rate used for that specific mode of exercise. No reference standards are available; however, $t$ is increased with endurance exercise training, weight loss, supplemental oxygen, pharmacological therapy, and other interventions, thus providing a simple measure of training progress and the efficacy of an intervention.

*Incremental exercise*
Endurance time for incremental exercise depends on the rate of increase in work rate. An optimal protocol results in $t$ of 8–12 min.

*Variable work rate exercise*
Endurance time for variable work rate exercise, such as walking or running tests, varies inversely with fitness level and degree of disability. Some walking and running tests require completion of a fixed distance with $t$ used as a criterion variable. In these applications, $t$ may be compared against quintile norms such as those contained in Tables C2 and C3 in Appendix C. Reference values for times in the Cooper 1.5-mile running test are included in Tables C7 and C9 in Appendix C. Since time is correlated

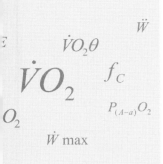

with $\dot{V}O_{2max}$, scores on these tests reflect the normalcy of aerobic capacity. A desirable fitness level should be considered as achieving the "good" category or above, as the lower limit of this quintile represents the 60th percentile. Fitness categories have been published for other performance tests as contained in Appendix C.

### Abnormal responses

*Constant work rate exercise*
Physical deconditioning, impaired oxygen delivery, ventilatory and gas exchange abnormalities will all reduce $t$ at the same absolute constant work rate.

*Incremental exercise*
Unduly short or excessively long tests (greater than 18 min) are undesirable and might result in a low $\dot{V}O_{2max}$.

*Variable rate exercise*
Performance on standardized walking (1 mile) or running (1.5 mile) tests may be compared to normal values contained in Appendix C, Tables C2 and C3. Scores below the "average" rating indicate performance at or below the 40th percentile and are thus considered abnormal.

## Walking and running distance ($d_W$ and $d_R$)

### Definition, derivation, and units of measurement

Distance completed in either walking or running tests is one of the criterion variables for the simple assessment of endurance performance. Examples include the 6- and 12-minute walk tests and the 12-minute run test (see Chapter 3).

The units of measurement are meters; however, the data may also be expressed as a velocity ($m \cdot min^{-1}$) when $d_W$ or $d_R$ is divided by time in minutes. This velocity can then be used with standard equations in order to estimate the intensity of the activity or the caloric expenditure rate (see Chapter 2).

### Normal response

The normal relaxed human walking speed is 67–80 $m \cdot min^{-1}$ (2.5–3.0 m.p.h.), hence it is reasonable to expect a $d_W$ to be greater than 800 m for 12 min or greater than 400 m for 6 min of relaxed walking.

Running times or speeds are greatly variable between individuals and mainly influenced by physical training. Orthopedic limitations notwithstanding, most healthy individuals are able to run for at least short distances, particularly in youth.

### Abnormal responses

Factors affecting cardiovascular and ventilatory endurance such as physical deconditioning or abnormalities in oxygen delivery and gas exchange will decrease walking or running distance and decrease their corresponding velocities. Scores below the "average" category on standardized tests represent percentile rankings at or below the 40th percentile and are thus considered abnormal.

## Six-minute walking distance ($d_{W6}$)

### Definition, derivation, and units of measurement

- The 6-minute walking test is a popular example of a timed distance test that is used extensively in clinical research and rehabilitation. The criterion variable is the distance walked by an individual, at his or her own chosen pace, in a predetermined time (6 min). This distance is recorded without regard to the number and duration of stops to rest.
- When used for clinical investigation, the 6-minute walking test should be standardized. Approved methods include tape-recorded instructions (see Appendix D, Standard instructions), repeated testing by the same exercise practitioner, identical levels of encouragement, and having the observer walk behind the subject. A premarked track is advantageous. The environment should be controlled, i.e., it is preferable to use an enclosed, level track that is free of obstacles. Often the walking distance is recorded as a number and

a fraction of circuits of the premarked track.

- The preferred units of measurement for $d_{W6}$ are meters (m).

### Normal response

Published data for $d_{W6}$ indicate an approximate value of 600 m at age 40 years, declining by about 50 m per decade, thus reaching 400 m at age 80 years (Figure 4.1). These values equate to normal walking speeds of 3–5 m.p.h. depending on stride length. It is most important with certain types of XT to recognize that a learning effect can occur. This implies that the same subject, repeating identical XT protocols over a relatively short time frame, will demonstrate increased performance which is unrelated to any true physiological changes. An example of this effect is shown for 10 patients with chronic obstructive pulmonary disease who performed 6-minute walking tests on three consecutive days (Figure 4.2). The mean difference was 8% between days 1 and 2 and 11% between days 1 and 3. Other investigators have shown that the learning effect tends to plateau after about three attempts.

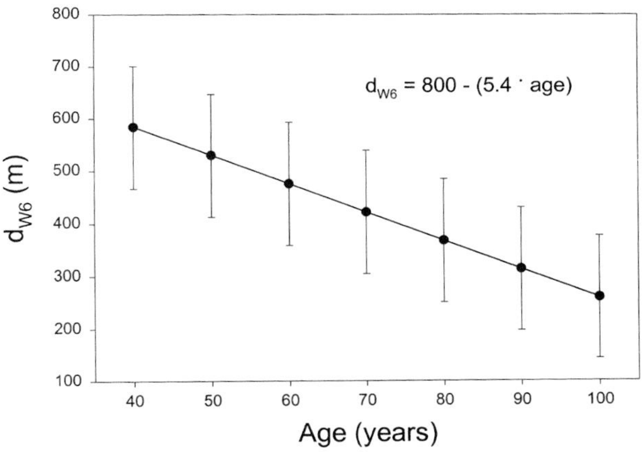


**Figure 4.1** Reference values for 6-min walking distance related to age. These data are derived from the results reported by Enright, P. L. & Sherrill, D. L. (1998). Reference equations for the six-minute walk in healthy adults. *Am. J. Respir. Crit. Care Med.*, **158**, 1384–7.

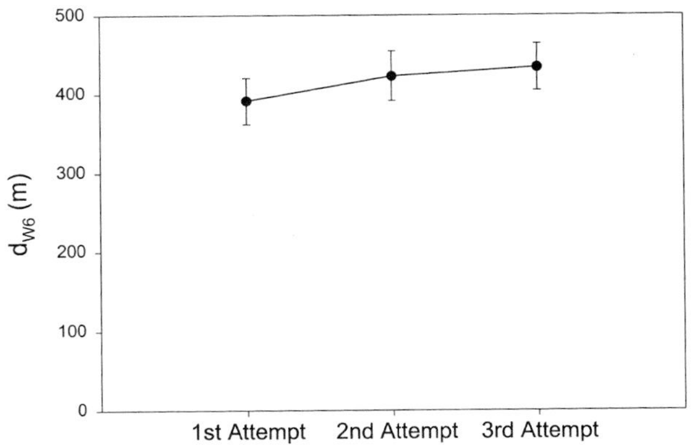


**Figure 4.2** Learning effect for the 6-min walking test demonstrated in 10 patients with chronic obstructive pulmonary disease performing identical walks on three consecutive days.

### Abnormal responses

Some individuals with severe chronic pulmonary disease might walk less than 400 m in 6 min (as shown in Figure 4.2). In this type of patient $d_{W6}$ correlates well with $\dot{V}o_{2max}$, thus validating the walking test as a meaningful measure of functional capacity.

## Shuttle test speed

### Definition, derivation, and units of measurement

- Shuttle test speed is the maximum speed over the ground achieved by a subject performing one of the standard shuttle field tests between two markers.
- The shuttle test is performed according to audible cues from a prerecorded tape. In performance exercise testing a 20-m shuttle run is used whereas in clinical exercise testing a 10-m shuttle walk might be preferred. Each shuttle stage defines a specific speed, as described in the methods section of Chapter 3. For a given individual, the highest shuttle stage achieved during the test defines

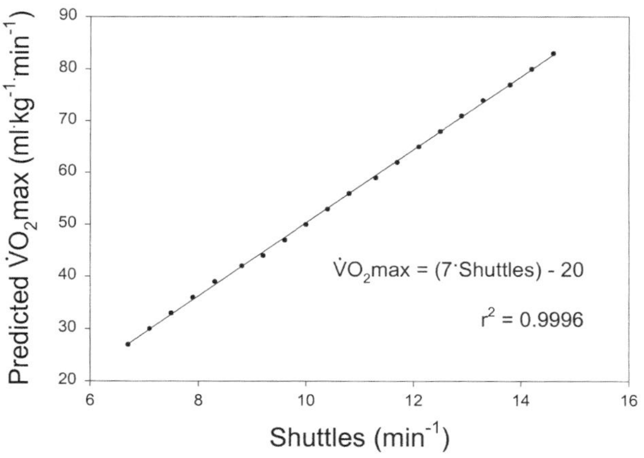


**Figure 4.3** Prediction of $\dot{V}O_{2max}$ from a multistage 20-m shuttle run test for aerobic fitness. Data obtained with permission from Léger, L. A., Mercier, D., Gadoury, C. & Lambert, J. (1988). The multistage 20 meter shuttle run test for aerobic fitness. *J. Sports Sci.*, **6**, 93–101.

the maximum speed or number of shuttles per minute. Both of these measures can be used to estimate $\dot{V}O_{2max}$.

- The units of shuttle test speed are kilometers per hour ($km \cdot h^{-1}$) or alternatively speed may be expressed as shuttles per minute.

### Normal response (Table 3.6 and 3.11; Figure 4.3)

A reference value for $\dot{V}O_{2max}$ in a given individual can be used retrogressively to predict a normal shuttle test speed using data such as those shown in Tables 3.6 and 3.11 or regression equations 3.4 and 3.13, shown in Chapter 3.

### Abnormal responses

A maximum shuttle test speed that falls below the expected value predicts a reduced aerobic capacity or reduced $\dot{V}O_{2max}$. The interpretation of a reduced $\dot{V}O_{2max}$ is described in the following section. In patients with chronic obstructive pulmonary disease, performance on a shuttle walking test correlates with performance on a 6-minute walking test ($r = 0.68$).

## Maximum oxygen uptake ($\dot{V}O_{2max}$)

### Definition, derivation, and units of measurement

- Maximum oxygen uptake is the highest value for oxygen uptake, which can be attained and measured during an incremental exercise protocol for a specific exercise mode. Attainment of $\dot{V}O_{2max}$ generally necessitates the use of large muscle groups over 5–15 min – so-called aerobic exercise. Hence, $\dot{V}O_{2max}$ is also called aerobic capacity.

*Terminology*

*Confusion has arisen over terminology for the highest value of oxygen uptake. Maximal oxygen uptake is the highest value attainable by a given individual. Maximal oxygen uptake is therefore dependent upon the exercise mode, age, gender, and body weight. Maximum oxygen uptake is used to describe the highest value measured (Figure 4.4A). Hence, the highest value measured for a given individual performing a specific exercise task might not be the highest value that individual could attain. Observation of a plateau value for oxygen uptake during an incremental exercise protocol is evidence of true maximal oxygen uptake (Figure 4.4B). Maximal oxygen uptake can be attained during constant work rate exercise of sufficient intensity to cause a relentless upward drift of oxygen uptake (Figure 4.4C and D). In these circumstances the constant work rate will be tolerated only as long as it takes for* $\dot{V}O_2$ *to reach* $\dot{V}O_{2max}$. *Hence, a higher constant work rate results in earlier attainment of* $\dot{V}O_{2max}$, *as shown in Figure 4.4D.*

*Generally, when performing XT, it is preferable to use the term maximum oxygen uptake (*$\dot{V}O_{2max}$*). The term* $\dot{V}O_{2peak}$ *is sometimes used synonymously with* $\dot{V}O_{2max}$. *It is a superfluous term and only serves to add to the confusion surrounding this nomenclature.*

*Another important issue of terminology needs to be clarified. That is the distinction between oxygen uptake and oxygen consumption. Oxygen uptake is the correct term for non-steady-state measurements obtained from expired gas analysis. Oxygen consumption refers to that quantity of oxygen used*

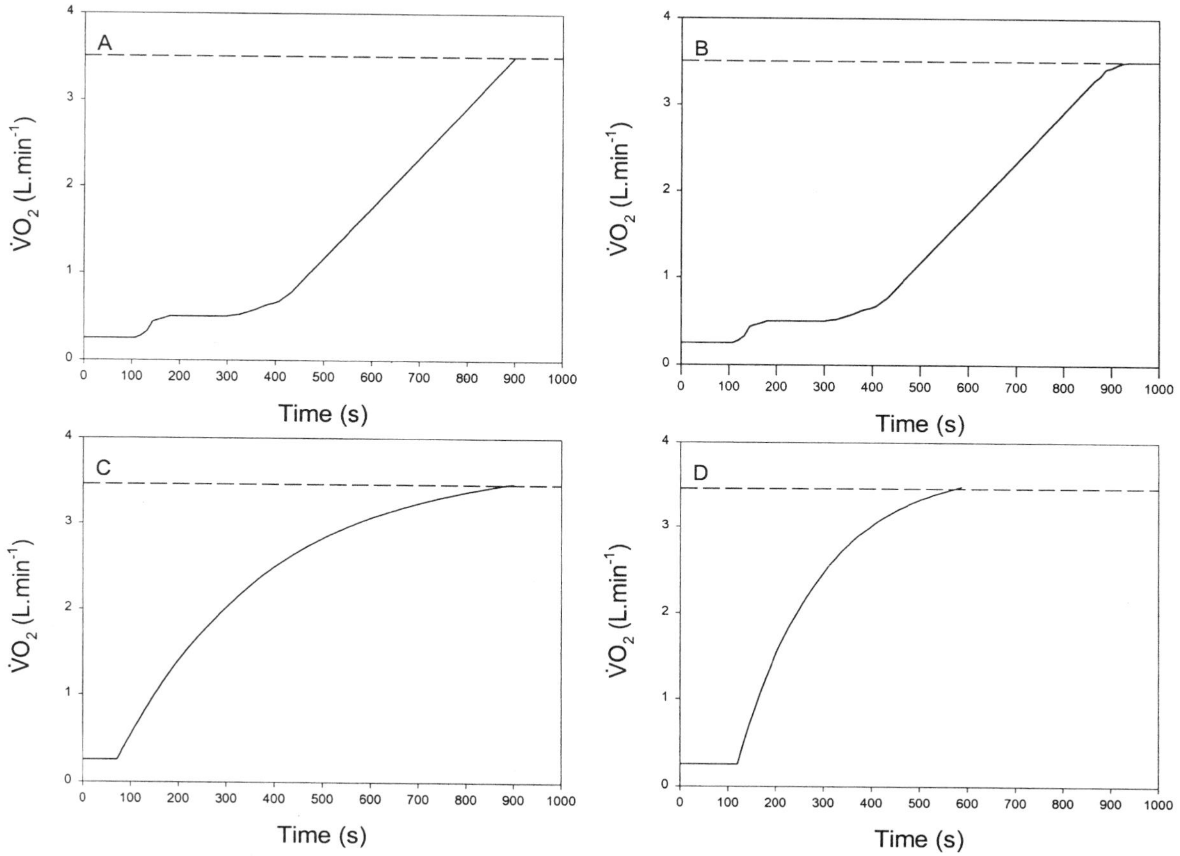


**Figure 4.4** Increases in oxygen uptake in response to various exercise test protocols. (A and B) Responses to rest, then unloaded pedaling followed by an incremental work rate. (C and D) Responses to high and very high constant work rates respectively. Only (B) shows definite evidence of maximal oxygen uptake because a plateau is seen just before exercise termination.

*in metabolic processes at a cellular level. Similar distinctions apply to carbon dioxide output and carbon dioxide production. For example, tissues might produce a certain amount of carbon dioxide but not all of this carbon dioxide is necessarily evolved through the lung or measured as carbon dioxide output. Carbon dioxide output should approximate tissue carbon dioxide production when the body is in steady state.*

- $\dot{V}o_{2max}$ is a primary variable normally measured near the end of an incremental exercise protocol. The method for selecting $\dot{V}o_{2max}$ from a matrix of data needs to be addressed. Towards the end of an incremental exercise test $\dot{V}o_2$ might reach a plateau, in which case determination of $\dot{V}o_{2max}$ is simplified. Alternatively, $\dot{V}o_2$ might reach a maximum and then begin to decline even before the end of the exercise phase is marked. This is commonly due to failure to maintain pedaling cadence or keep up with the increasing power output demanded by the ergometer. To allow for this possibility, $\dot{V}o_{2max}$ can be selected as the highest value of $\dot{V}o_2$ recorded during the last 30 s of an

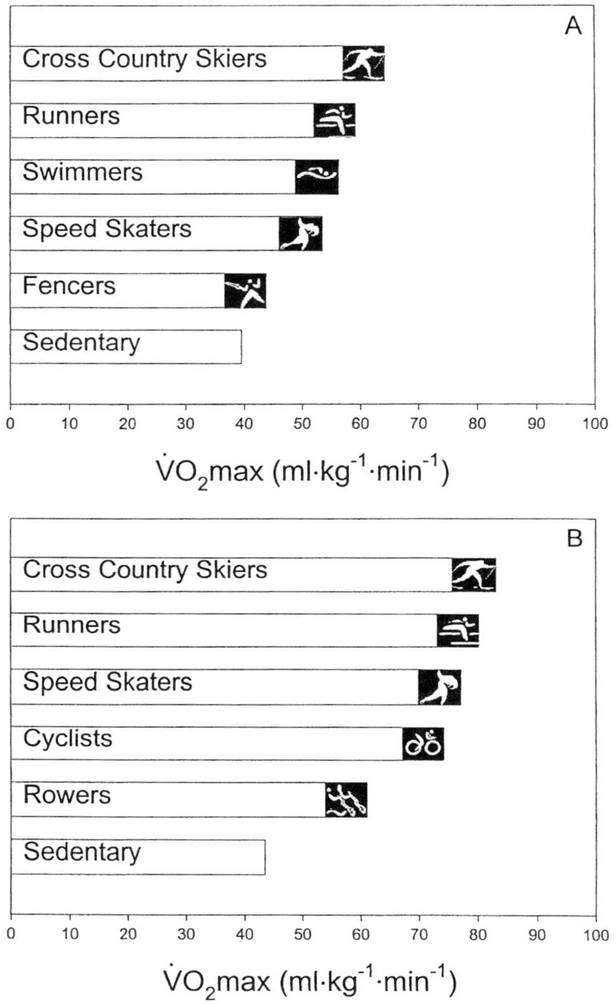


**Figure 4.5** Typical values for $\dot{V}O_{2max}$ recorded in (A) female and (B) male athletes. Endurance sports utilizing greater muscle mass tend to elicit higher values for $\dot{V}O_{2max}$.

incremental protocol. $\dot{V}O_2$ rarely increases beyond the end of a symptom-limited exercise test.

Unquestionably, breath-by-breath data give the most detailed profile of oxygen uptake at end exercise. However, there is marked variability in breath-by-breath data and an averaging method is needed. Any averaging method introduces a timing error, which has a greater impact when the primary variable is rapidly changing. Retrograde time averaging (e.g., mean $\dot{V}O_2$ for the preceding 20 s) is commonly used. This method tends to underestimate $\dot{V}O_{2max}$. An alternative method is the rolling average of a defined number of breaths (e.g., mean $\dot{V}O_2$ for a given breath plus the preceding four breaths, usually known as the five-breath rolling average). This method is appealing since the time for five breaths shortens progressively with increasing exercise intensity and the timing error is thus minimized.

- The absolute units of measurement of $\dot{V}O_{2max}$ are liters per minute ($l \cdot min^{-1}$) or milliliters per minute ($ml \cdot min^{-1}$). Also, oxygen uptake is frequently related to an individual's body weight and expressed as milliliters per kilogram per minute ($ml \cdot kg^{-1} \cdot min^{-1}$). The MET is an imprecise unit which refers to an arbitrary resting metabolic rate of $3.5\ ml \cdot kg^{-1} \cdot min^{-1}$ (1 MET). In some applications oxygen uptake is related to the resting level by being expressed as a number of METs.

### Normal response (Figures 4.4, 4.5, and 4.6A)

A healthy but sedentary adult male might have a $\dot{V}O_{2max}$ of $35\ ml \cdot kg^{-1} \cdot min^{-1}$. In a normal individual performing incremental exercise, $\dot{V}O_2$ can increase by as much as 16-fold: from $0.25\ l \cdot min^{-1}$ at rest to a $\dot{V}O_{2max}$ of $4.00\ l \cdot min$. $\dot{V}O_{2max}$ is clearly related to the mode of exercise performed. Figure 4.5 shows values of $\dot{V}O_{2max}$ obtained from élite athletes performing different sports. The variation in values for $\dot{V}O_{2max}$ reflects the different muscle mass used for different tasks. Women generally have $\dot{V}O_{2max}$ values about 10% less than men for the same reason (Figure 4.5). $\dot{V}O_{2max}$ declines with increasing age and varies with body size.

The prediction of normal $\dot{V}O_{2max}$ should therefore take into account exercise mode, gender, age, and body size. Reference values are available for $\dot{V}O_{2max}$ (see Tables C1–3 and Figures C2–4 in Appendix C). In Table C1 the values reported by Shvartz & Reibold (1990) were obtained from an extensive literature review of studies in which $\dot{V}O_{2max}$ was measured directly in healthy untrained subjects. Their

**Table 4.1.** Common convention used to relate measured values to reference values

| Measured value/ reference value (%) | Interpretation |
|---|---|
| >80 | Normal |
| 71–80 | Mildly reduced |
| 51–70 | Moderately reduced |
| ≤50 | Severely reduced |

data include 98 samples of males and 43 samples of females, aged 6–75 years, reported in a total of 62 studies conducted in the USA, Canada, and seven European countries. The values reported by Jones & Campbell (1982) are also derived from data obtained in Europe, Scandinavia, and North America. The values predicted by Hansen et al. (1984) were obtained from a group of male shipyard workers in California of mean age 54 years. Obviously, one must exercise caution in applying reference values to the general population. The most important consideration is whether the subject being studied matches the population from which the reference values were derived. For a more complete discussion of reference values, see Chapter 5.

The normal profile of increase in $\dot{V}O_2$ for a maximal incremental XT is shown in Figure 4.6A.

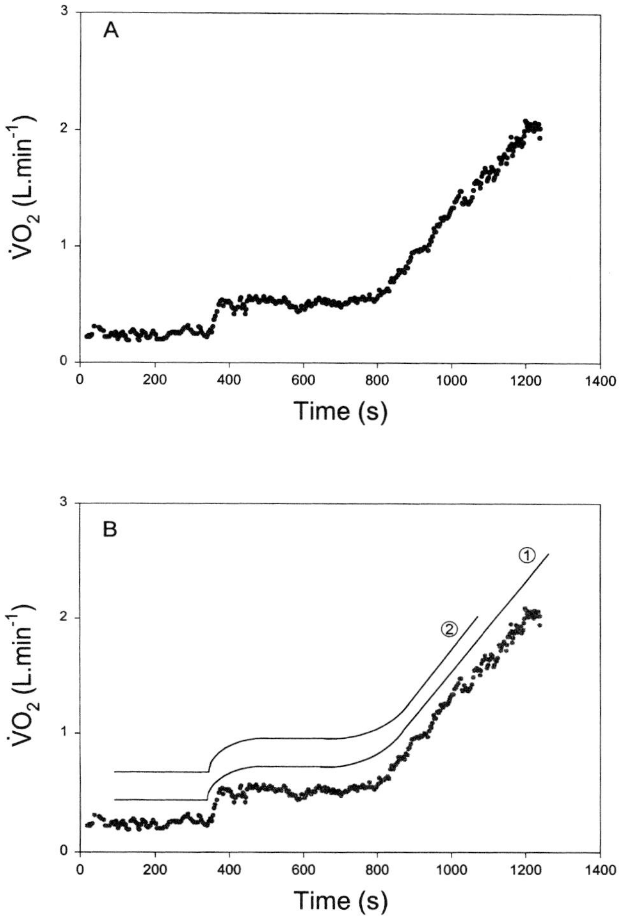


**Figure 4.6** Relationship between $\dot{V}O_2$ and time during an incremental work rate XT. (A) Normal response. (B) Abnormal responses for ① moderate obesity and ② severe obesity.

### Abnormal responses (Figure 4.6B)

The variability of $\dot{V}O_{2max}$ is estimated to be 10%. Therefore an individual $\dot{V}O_{2max}$ less than 80% of the predicted value is likely to be abnormal in 95% of cases. Table 4.1 shows a convention which can be used to categorize $\dot{V}O_{2max}$ based on selected reference values, using 80% as the lower limit of normality.

A healthy adult male might have a $\dot{V}O_{2max}$ of 35 ml · kg$^{-1}$ · min$^{-1}$. A person with simple physical deconditioning could have a $\dot{V}O_{2max}$ of 25 ml · kg$^{-1}$ · min$^{-1}$ (75% of normal) without functional impairment. The cardiology literature suggests that persons with a $\dot{V}O_{2max}$ less than 20 ml · kg$^{-1}$ · min$^{-1}$ (60% of normal) have disability which can be classified as mild disability ($\dot{V}O_{2max}$ of 15–20 ml · kg$^{-1}$ · min$^{-1}$), moderate disability ($\dot{V}O_{2max}$ of 10–15 ml · kg$^{-1}$ · min$^{-1}$), and severe disability ($\dot{V}O_{2max}$ less than 10 ml · kg$^{-1}$ · min$^{-1}$).

Table 4.2 and Table 4.3 show two common approaches to the classification of cardiovascular disease with corresponding values of $\dot{V}O_{2max}$ expressed in ml · kg$^{-1}$ · min$^{-1}$.

Obesity increases oxygen uptake at rest and during unloaded pedaling. Reference values for resting oxygen uptake are not usually applied during exercise testing. However, the oxygen uptake for

**Table 4.2.** New York Heart Association (NYHA) classification of cardiovascular impairment based on functional capacity[a] alongside estimates of maximum oxygen uptake and oxygen pulse

| NYHA class | Functional capacity[a] | $\dot{V}O_{2max}$ (ml · kg$^{-1}$ · min$^{-1}$)[b] | $\dot{V}O_2/f_{Cmax}$ (% of reference) |
|---|---|---|---|
| I | No impairment | 26–35 | 90 |
| II | Minimal impairment | 21–25 | 75 |
| III | Moderate impairment | 16–20 | 55 |
| IV | Severe impairment | <15 | 45 |

[a]The Criteria Committee of the New York Heart Association, 1994.
[b]Modified from Riley, M., Porszasz, J., Stanford, C. F. & Nicholls, D. P. (1994). Gas exchange responses to constant work rate exercise in chronic cardiac failure. *Br. Heart J.*, **72**, 150–5.

**Table 4.3.** Weber classification of cardiovascular impairment based on maximum oxygen uptake[a] alongside estimates of stroke volume at rest and at maximum exercise

| Functional class | $\dot{V}O_{2max}$ (ml · kg$^{-1}$ · min$^{-1}$)[a] | Resting SV[b] (ml) | Maximum SV[b] (ml) |
|---|---|---|---|
| A | >20 | 80 | 120 |
| B | 16–20 | 60 | 90 |
| C | 10–15 | 50 | 70 |
| D | <10 | 40 | 50 |

[a]Weber, K. T., Kinasewitz, G. T., Janicki, J. S. & Fishman, A. P. (1982). Oxygen utilization and ventilation during exercise in patients with chronic cardiac failure. *Circulation*, **65**, 1213–23.
[b]Weber, K. T. & Janicki, J. S. (1985). Cardiopulmonary exercise testing for evaluation of chronic cardiac failure. *Am. J. Cardiol.*, **55**, 22A–31A.

unloaded pedaling on a cycle ergometer can be interpreted with regard to body weight, being increased by 5.8 ml · min$^{-1}$ for every kilogram of excess body weight (Figure 4.6B). Obesity complicates the interpretation of $\dot{V}O_{2max}$. An obese relatively fit subject might have a high absolute value for $\dot{V}O_{2max}$ but spuriously low value when expressed as ml · kg$^{-1}$ · min$^{-1}$ (see Figures C3 and C4 in Appendix C).

Reduced $\dot{V}O_{2max}$ can occur due to many different types of limitation, as described in Chapter 5. A normal $\dot{V}O_{2max}$ excludes exercise impairment and generally excludes a serious, or at least an advanced, disease process.

## Work efficiency ($\eta$, $\eta^{-1}$)

### Definition, derivation, and units of measurement

- Work efficiency ($\eta$) is a measure of the metabolic cost of performing external work. Hence, work efficiency is calculated by dividing the caloric value of the external work performed by the metabolic cost of the work in terms of the caloric value of the oxygen uptake.

$$\eta = \frac{\delta \dot{W} \cdot 0.01433}{\delta \dot{V}O_2 \cdot 4.95} \quad (4.1)$$

- For incremental exercise the "efficiency" is often expressed as the slope of the relationship between $\dot{V}O_2$ and work rate. This slope represents the reciprocal of $\eta$ or $\eta^{-1}$.

$$\eta^{-1} = \frac{\delta \dot{V}O_2}{\delta \dot{W}} \quad (4.2)$$

- Being a ratio of caloric values, $\eta$ is often expressed as a percentage. The units of measurement of $\eta^{-1}$ are ml · min$^{-1}$ · W$^{-1}$.

### Normal response (Figure 4.7A)

The $\dot{V}O_2$–$\dot{W}$ slope has remarkable linearity and consistency for normal subjects, being 10.3 ml · min$^{-1}$ · W$^{-1}$ (Figure 4.7A). The standard deviation of this measurement is 1.0 ml · min$^{-1}$ · W$^{-1}$, meaning that 95% of normal values lie between 8.3 and 12.3 ml · min$^{-1}$ · W$^{-1}$.

The remarkable linearity and consistency of the

$\dot{V}O_2$–$\dot{W}$ slope is explained by the rigid physiological coupling of these parameters below the metabolic threshold (see Figure 1.1 in Chapter 1). In normal subjects it is likely happenstance that the $\dot{V}O_2$–$\dot{W}$ relationship remains linear above the metabolic threshold. There is no obvious physiological explanation why the relationship should remain linear above this point. Increasing reliance on anaerobic metabolism would tend to reduce the slope whilst increased body temperature, circulating catecholamines, and the oxygen cost of lactate disposal have been postulated to contribute to increasing the slope.

The lower section of the $\dot{V}O_2$–$\dot{W}$ slope is thought to reflect the physiological mechanisms described in Chapter 1, whereas the upper section of the $\dot{V}O_2$–$\dot{W}$ relationship appears to be influenced by oxygen delivery to exercising muscles.

### Abnormal responses (Figure 4.7B)

Inadequate oxygen delivery to exercising muscles lowers the slope of the $\dot{V}O_2$–$\dot{W}$ relationship, particularly above the metabolic threshold. Paradoxically, a lower slope might be taken to indicate better work efficiency. However, like the engine that strains at low revolutions, an unduly low slope is considered abnormal.

Some athletes exhibit increased $\dot{V}O_2$–$\dot{W}$ slopes. Commonly this is due to a faster pedaling cadence on the cycle and recruitment of greater muscle bulk for the exercise task. This phenomenon is commonly seen when an exercising subject rises out of the saddle and contributes arm power to accomplish the increasing work rate. It is tempting to interpret this as reduced work efficiency, like an engine overrevving, but of course the reduced work efficiency is a consequence of the increased oxygen uptake unrelated to the external work performed on the ergometer.

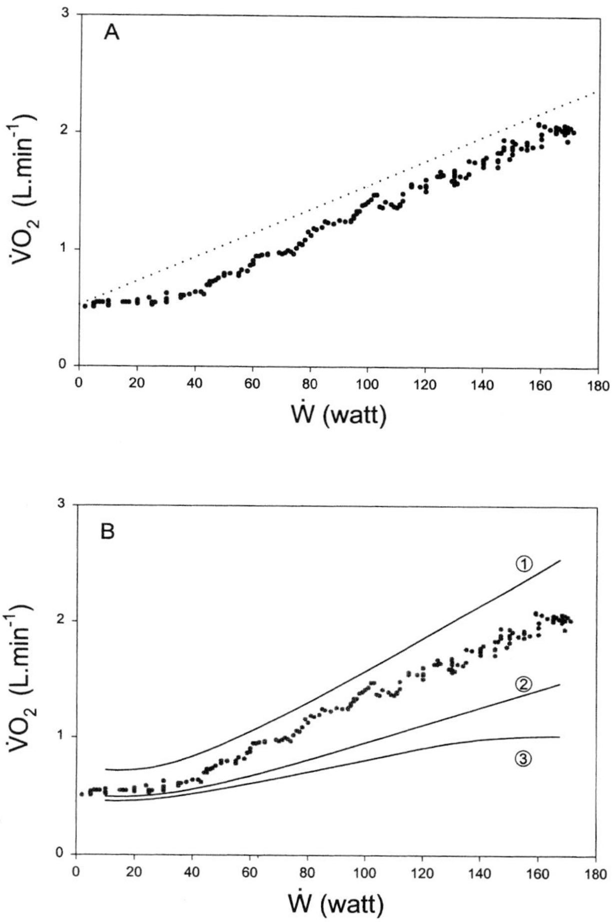


**Figure 4.7** Relationship between $\dot{V}O_2$ and $\dot{W}$ during an incremental work rate XT. (A) Normal response: dotted reference line with a slope of 10.3 ml · min$^{-1}$ · W$^{-1}$. (B) Abnormal responses for ① high pedaling cadence followed by an alteration in work efficiency at higher exercise intensity; ② a slope of 8.3 ml · min$^{-1}$ · W$^{-1}$; and ③ impaired oxygen delivery due to cardiomyopathy.

## Metabolic, gas exchange, or lactic acid threshold ($\dot{V}O_2\theta$)

### Definition, derivation, and units of measurement

- There exist two distinct domains of exercise intensity. At lower work rates, metabolism is predominantly aerobic and can be continued for a prolonged time in physiological steady state. Above a certain work rate for a given individual, aerobic metabolism is supplemented by anaerobic ATP regeneration with the accumulation of lactic acid in the contracting muscles and circulating blood. At work rates higher than this "threshold," prolonged exercise is not possible and fatigue will eventually ensue. The existence of two domains of exercise intensity is indisputable but physiologists have long debated the nature of the transition and its proper terminology. Whilst accepting that the threshold is imprecise, i.e., that a gradual transition exists from one domain to the other, it is helpful nevertheless, in the understanding and interpretation of human exercise responses, to ascribe a single value of oxygen uptake to the threshold ($\dot{V}O_2\theta$).

*Terminology*
*The terminology for* $\dot{V}O_2\theta$ *is fraught with controversy. The term "anaerobic threshold" is most widely known and has a certain logical appeal. However, the appearance of lactic acid at low work rates is testimony to the fact that aerobic and anaerobic metabolism coexist at all stages of exercise intensity. One basic principle helps resolve some of the controversy surrounding threshold terminology: that is, to describe the threshold using the terms with which it has been identified. Thus, when the threshold is detected by noninvasive gas exchange measurements it is appropriate to call it the "gas exchange threshold." Only when the threshold has been defined by sequential blood lactate measurements should it be called the "lactate threshold."*

- $\dot{V}O_2\theta$ is a secondary variable but its derivation is complex. The most popular and reliable way to identify the gas exchange threshold is by plotting $\dot{V}CO_2$ against $\dot{V}O_2$ for incremental exercise. After about 2 min, whilst body $CO_2$ stores are increasing, the $\dot{V}CO_2$–$\dot{V}O_2$ relationship adopts a slope of approximately 1.0 (Figure 4.8A). Like the $\dot{V}O_2$–$\dot{W}$ relationship, this slope has remarkable consistency for normal, nonfasted individuals. This lower slope (S1) of 1.0 represents utilization of carbohydrate as the dominant metabolic substrate (see section on muscle respiratory quotient, later in this chapter). When lactic acid begins to accumulate, the $\dot{V}CO_2$–$\dot{V}O_2$ relationship exhibits a steeper slope (S2) due to the evolution of "additional $CO_2$" derived from bicarbonate buffering of lactic acid. Usually, when an incremental test is of optimal duration (8–12 min), the inflection point can be clearly identified by fitting straight lines to the $\dot{V}CO_2$–$\dot{V}O_2$ plot. Drawing a line of identity from the origin (45° on a square plot) can also be helpful in identifying S1 (Figure 4.8A).
  Another traditional method for identifying $\dot{V}O_2\theta$ employs plots of ventilatory equivalents and end-tidal gas tensions against time, work rate or $\dot{V}O_2$ (Figure 4.9). As discussed in Chapter 1, $\dot{V}O_2\theta$ signals the onset of alveolar hyperventilation with respect to oxygen uptake. Therefore, $\dot{V}_E/\dot{V}O_2$ and $P_{ET}O_2$ are both expected to increase systematically beyond this point. At the same time, since ventilation remains coupled to $CO_2$ output, $\dot{V}_E/\dot{V}CO_2$, and $P_{ET}CO_2$ remain constant. The identification of an inflection in the $\dot{V}_E/\dot{V}O_2$ plot whilst $\dot{V}_E/\dot{V}CO_2$ remains constant, or an inflection in the $P_{ET}O_2$ plot whilst $P_{ET}CO_2$ remains constant, is know as the "dual criteria" for the identification of $\dot{V}O_2\theta$. Alveolar hyperventilation with respect to *both* oxygen and carbon dioxide exchange does not occur until there is ventilatory compensation for metabolic acidosis. At this point (see section on ventilatory threshold, below), $\dot{V}_E/\dot{V}CO_2$ increases and $P_{ET}CO_2$ decreases simultaneously.
  In our laboratory, experienced observers choose the threshold with agreement and consistency. Inexperienced observers with a rudimentary training of exercise physiology do not. We have found that an autodetection method programmed into a commercially available metabolic cart was generally reliable but needed to be over-read by an experienced observer to avoid occasional erroneous results and conclusions.
- The units of $\dot{V}O_2\theta$ are clearly the same as those for oxygen uptake, i.e., $l \cdot min^{-1}$ or $ml \cdot kg^{-1} \cdot min^{-1}$.

### Normal response (Figure 4.8A)

Reference values for $\dot{V}O_2\theta$ can be calculated using published algorithms (see Appendix C, Metabolic threshold). $\dot{V}O_2\theta$ should be interpreted in relation to

**Table 4.4.** Interpretation of the metabolic threshold in relation to the reference value for maximum oxygen uptake

| $\dot{V}o_2\theta$/ reference $\dot{V}o_{2max}$ (%) | Interpretation |
|---|---|
| 80–60 | Athletic |
| 60–50 | Sedentary |
| 50–40 | Deconditioned |
| <40 | Diseased |

predicted $\dot{V}o_{2max}$ (Table 4.4). Comparison with measured $\dot{V}o_{2max}$ can produce serious errors of interpretation in the case of a suboptimal effort and noncardiovascular limitation.

Normal sedentary individuals exhibit $\dot{V}o_2\theta$ around 50% of $\dot{V}o_{2max}$. With successful physical training, the threshold increases both as an absolute value and also as a percentage of $\dot{V}o_{2max}$ (Figure 4.10). Hence, with endurance training $\dot{V}o_2\theta$ can increase from 50% to 80% or more of the measured $\dot{V}o_{2max}$.

### Abnormal responses (Figure 4.8B)

Experience in laboratories with precise data-collecting capabilities has shown that when $\dot{V}o_2\theta$ is less than 40% of the reference value for $\dot{V}o_{2max}$, serious pathology can be expected. Values of $\dot{V}o_2\theta$ between 40 and 50% of the reference value for $\dot{V}o_{2max}$ could be explained by physical deconditioning. However, early cardiovascular or muscular disease can result in values of $\dot{V}o_2\theta$ within the same range. The inevitable overlap in physiological responses between deconditioning and early pathology frequently causes a dilemma in exercise test interpretation. The response to judicious exercise prescription is one way to distinguish these two possibilities (see Chapter 5).

Patients with McArdle's syndrome (myophosphorylase deficiency), who fail to develop a lactic acidosis during exercise, should not exhibit a true $\dot{V}o_2\theta$ (Figure 4.8B). Chapter 5 explains more about the exercise response patterns in patients with different types of myopathy.

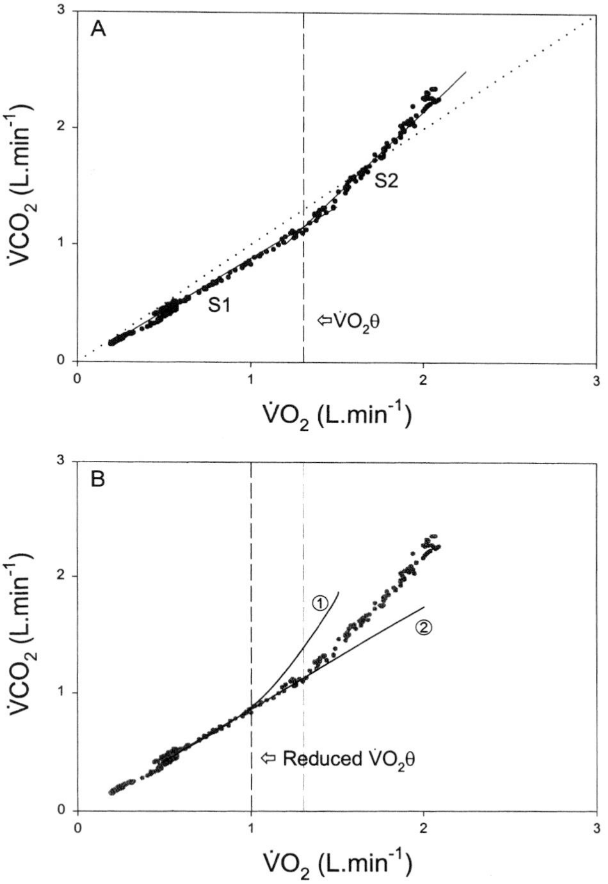


**Figure 4.8** Relationship between $\dot{V}co_2$ and $\dot{V}o_2$ during an incremental work rate XT. (A) Normal response: dotted reference line with a slope of 1.0. The intersection of the lower slope (S1) and upper slope (S2) determines $\dot{V}o_2\theta$. (B) Abnormal responses for ① physical deconditioning and ② McArdle's disease.

## Time constant of oxygen uptake ($\tau\dot{V}o_2$)

### Definition, derivation, and units of measurement

- With the introduction of a constant exercise stimulus, oxygen uptake increases in a predictable pattern that can be described conveniently by first-order kinetics with an exponential function (Figure 4.11). There is debate about the

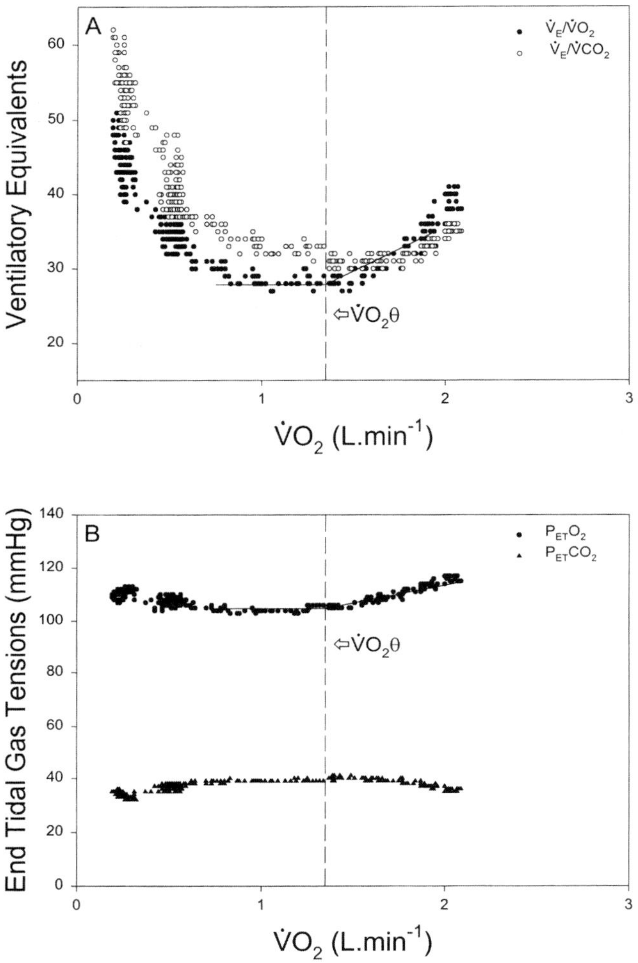


**Figure 4.9** Determination of $\dot{V}o_2\theta$ using the dual criteria. (A) Relationships between the ventilatory equivalents ($\dot{V}_E/\dot{V}o_2$ and $\dot{V}_E/\dot{V}co_2$) and $\dot{V}o_2$. (B) Relationship between the end-tidal gas tensions ($P_{ET}o_2$ and $P_{ET}co_2$) and $\dot{V}o_2$. $\dot{V}o_2\theta$ is identified as the point at which $\dot{V}_E/\dot{V}o_2$ and $P_{ET}o_2$ both begin to rise whilst $\dot{V}_E/\dot{V}co_2$ and $P_{ET}co_2$ remain constant.

exact nature of this function and whether or not there are time delays or multiple exponential components. However, for practical purposes, i.e., performance or clinical XT, the kinetic increase of oxygen uptake with the onset of exercise can be conveniently described by a monoexponential function with a time constant, $\tau\dot{V}o_2$. This time constant is defined in the standard equation for a "wash-in" exponential function.

$$\dot{V}o_{2(t)} = \delta\dot{V}o_2(1 - e^{-t/\tau}) \tag{4.3}$$

where $\dot{V}o_{2(t)}$ is the oxygen uptake at a given time ($t$), $\delta\dot{V}o_2$ is the total increase in oxygen uptake and $e$ is the base of natural logarithms.

Based on the monoexponential model, after one time constant ($\tau\dot{V}o_2$), the increase in $\dot{V}o_2$ will be 63% of the total increase to the new steady-state value and after four time constants, the increase in $\dot{V}o_2$ will be 98% of the total increase. Direct interpolation of the data set to derive the time when $\dot{V}o_2$ has reached 63% of the eventual increase gives a value called the mean response time which is an estimate of $\tau\dot{V}o_2$.

$\tau\dot{V}o_2$ is important because, along with $\dot{V}o_{2max}$, $\eta$ and $\dot{V}o_2\theta$, it is one of the fundamental parameters of aerobic function. Above $\dot{V}o_2\theta$, the determination of $\tau\dot{V}o_2$ is more complex because of the continuing upward drift of $\dot{V}o_2$ even for constant work rate exercise.

- $\tau\dot{V}o_2$ is best derived from a constant work rate XT with a baseline warm-up phase followed by imposition of a square wave of moderate-intensity work rate for at least 6 min. During this type of test, $\dot{V}o_2$ is expected to increase to a new steady state after about 3 min (Figure 4.12). Exponential curve-fitting software can be used to derive $\tau\dot{V}o_2$. Alternatively, if the oxygen deficit ($\dot{V}o_{2def}$) is derived using more complex mathematical methods, then $\tau\dot{V}o_2$ can be calculated from the following formula:

$$\tau\dot{V}o_2 = \frac{\dot{V}o_{2def}}{\delta\dot{V}o_2} \tag{4.4}$$

- Being a time constant, the units of $\tau\dot{V}o_2$ are seconds.

### Normal response (Figure 4.12A)

The normal value for $\tau\dot{V}o_2$, derived according to Equation 4.3, in young sedentary subjects is 38 s with a standard deviation of 5 s. $\tau\dot{V}o_2$ is reduced by physical training, e.g., 30 days of endurance training can reduce $\tau\dot{V}O_2$ by about 10 s. $\tau\dot{V}O_2$ can be as short as 20 s in athletes. $\tau\dot{V}O_2$ is shorter when measured immediately following prior exercise. Presumably, this is due to priming of the mechanisms that enable oxygen delivery and utilization by contracting muscle. By contrast, $\tau\dot{V}O_2$ becomes prolonged with physical deconditioning. This is presumed to be due to suboptimal functioning of the mechanisms that enable oxygen delivery and utilization by contracting muscle.

### Abnormal responses (Figure 4.12B)

Patients with cardiovascular disease have prolonged $\tau\dot{V}O_2$. Patients with chronic pulmonary disease also have prolonged $\tau\dot{V}O_2$. Partly, this is due to deconditioning since physical training in patients with chronic obstructive pulmonary disease has been shown to shorten $\tau\dot{V}O_2$. An additional factor influencing $\tau\dot{V}O_2$ in cardiovascular and pulmonary disease is likely to be hypoxemia. Experiments in normal subjects breathing hypoxic gas mixtures (e.g., 14% $F_IO_2$) slowed $\tau\dot{V}O_2$ by as much as 6 s. Finally, $\tau\dot{V}O_2$ might be slowed by abnormal pulmonary vascular conductance in certain chronic pulmonary diseases.

## Respiratory exchange ratio (*R*)

### Definition, derivation, and units of measurement

- The respiratory exchange ratio is the ratio of carbon dioxide output over oxygen uptake, both measured at the mouth. Essentially, *R* is a non-steady-state measurement that can vary from breath to breath as well as from time to time depending on physiological circumstances.
- *R* is simply derived from instantaneous measurements of $\dot{V}CO_2$ and $\dot{V}O_2$.

$$R = \frac{\dot{V}CO_2}{\dot{V}O_2} \tag{4.5}$$

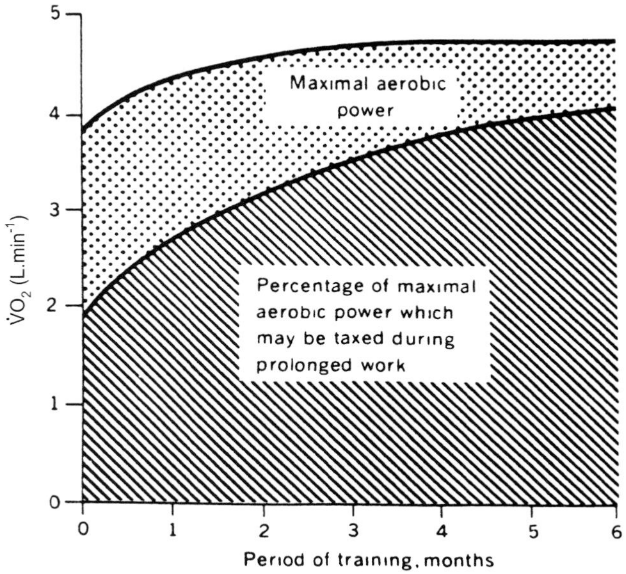


**Figure 4.10** Increases of $\dot{V}O_{2max}$ and $\dot{V}O_2\theta$ in normal subjects with 6 months of physical training. Reproduced with permission from Åstrand, P.-O. & Rodahl, K. (1986). *Textbook of Work Physiology*, 3rd edn. London: McGraw-Hill.

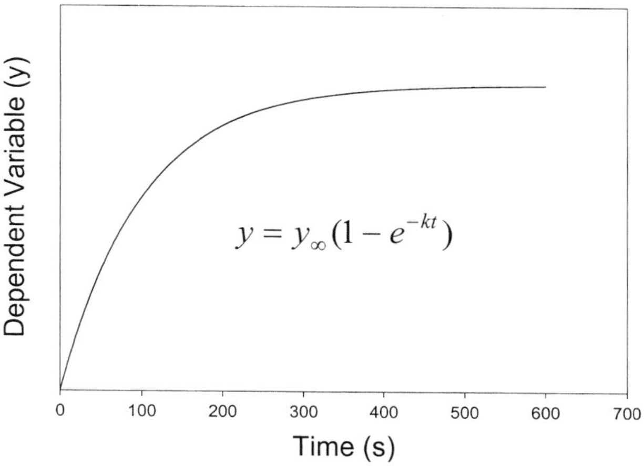


**Figure 4.11** "Wash-in" exponential function where the rate of change of the dependent variable (*y*) in relation to time is proportional to the instantaneous value of *y*. The time constant ($\tau$) is the reciprocal of the constant k in the equation. After one $\tau$, *y* will have risen to 63% of its final value. After four $\tau$, *y* will have risen to 98% of its final value.

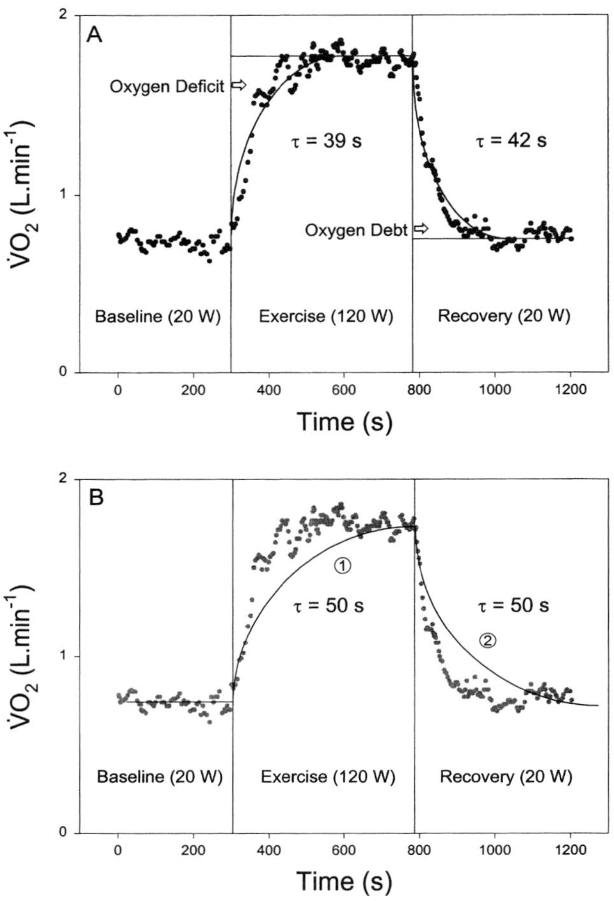


**Figure 4.12** Relationship between $\dot{V}O_2$ and time during a constant work rate XT. (A) Normal response with a similar time constant (τ) for exercise onset and recovery. The oxygen deficit and oxygen debt are shown. (B) Abnormal responses for ① the on-transit, and ② the off-transit, which can be seen in cardiovascular and pulmonary disease.

*Terminology*

*An important distinction must be made between the respiratory exchange ratio which is a non-steady-state measure derived from instantaneous values of $\dot{V}CO_2$ and $\dot{V}O_2$, and respiratory quotient (RQ), which is normally derived from steady-state measures of $\dot{V}CO_2$ and $\dot{V}O_2$. R applies to the whole body, whereas RQ can apply to the whole body or be related to individual organs such as liver or muscle. Determination of an organ RQ necessitates isolation of the organ and measurement of its oxygen consumption and carbon dioxide production over time. Importantly, these measures reflect tissue metabolism and are influenced by metabolic substrate. If the metabolic substrate is purely carbohydrate, then the RQ value is 1.0. When the metabolic substrate is predominantly fat, the RQ approaches 0.7. Thus, RQ values differ for different organs and whole-body RQ represents the summation of many different organ system RQ values. Measurement of whole-body RQ demands steady-state conditions and so during XT this measurement is only applicable to constant work rate exercise of sufficient duration (at least 4 min) below the metabolic threshold. However, allowing for certain considerations, an estimate of the RQ of contracting muscle can be obtained during incremental exercise from the increases of oxygen uptake and carbon dioxide output above baseline values (see next section).*

- Since $\dot{V}CO_2$ and $\dot{V}O_2$ both have units of liters per minute, *R* has no units.

### Normal response (Figure 4.13A)

Resting *R* is typically 0.7–0.95, indicating that overall body metabolism utilizes a mixture of carbohydrate and fat. Resting *R* is influenced by the nutritional state of the subject. Hence, normally nourished subjects who have taken no food for about 4 h prior to testing should have an average *R* value of 0.85. Prolonged fasting lowers resting *R* whereas recent carbohydrate ingestion tends to elevate its value towards 1.0.

When first measured breathing through a mouthpiece, *R* tends to increase due to hyperventilation, which increases $\dot{V}CO_2$ whilst having relatively little effect on $\dot{V}O_2$. During XT, when precision is important, it is necessary to allow long enough for the subject to acclimatize to the mouthpiece before obtaining baseline values. An *R* value greater than 1.0 at rest is a certain indication of hyperventilation.

With the onset of exercise, *R* decreases. This transient phase occurs because of the important differences in the dynamic changes of $\dot{V}O_2$ and $\dot{V}CO_2$. Measured at the mouth, $\dot{V}O_2$ increases more rapidly than $\dot{V}CO_2$. This phenomenon is thought to be due to the greater solubility of $CO_2$, causing some of the $CO_2$ from increased muscle metabolism to load into body stores rather than to appear immediately in the exhaled breath. A reverse phenomenon is observed when exercise ends. In this situation the body continues to eliminate excess carbon dioxide until body stores have normalized. Consequently there is a transient increase in *R* after exercise cessation.

During incremental exercise, particularly after adjustment of body carbon dioxide stores, *R* increases steadily. Above the metabolic threshold, when additional carbon dioxide is derived from bicarbonate buffering of lactic acid, *R* increases more rapidly, resulting in the inflection on the $\dot{V}CO_2$–$\dot{V}O_2$ plot that is used to determine $\dot{V}O_2\theta$. Again it is important to note that *R* should be less than 1.0 at the metabolic threshold, as shown in Figure 4.8.

End-exercise *R* has been advocated as a measure of maximal effort. Although there is some logic to this approach, it is not to be recommended. End-exercise *R* can vary considerably between individuals (e.g., 1.1–1.5) and hyperventilation for various reasons can elevate *R* independently of effort. *R* should not be used as a criterion for stopping a maximal incremental exercise test.

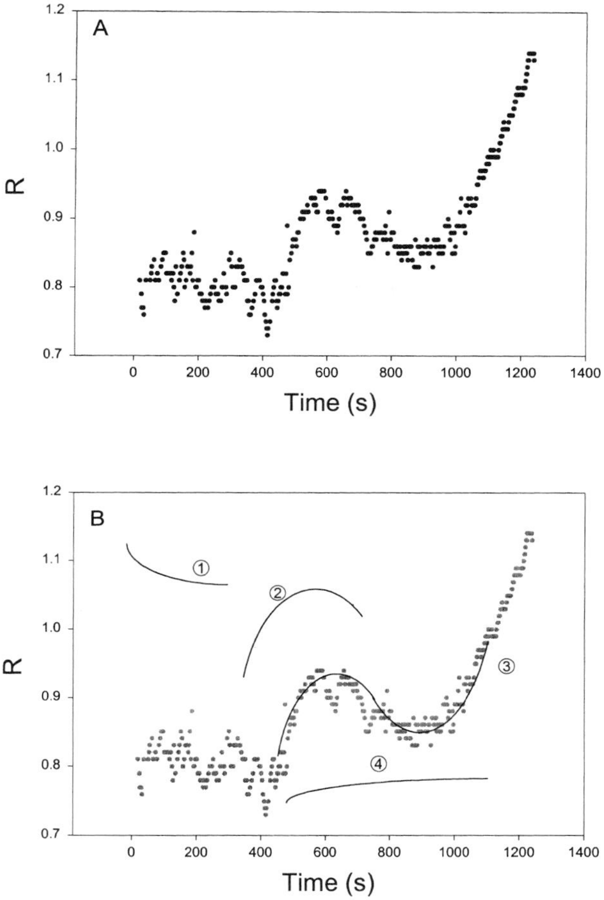


**Figure 4.13** Relationship between *R* and time during an incremental work rate XT. (A) Normal response. Note that *R* decreases with exercise onset at 300 s. (B) Abnormal responses for ① hyperventilation at rest; ② hyperventilation with exercise onset; ③ suboptimal effort; and ④ McArdle's disease.

## Abnormal responses (Figure 4.13B)

The most frequent factor adversely increasing *R* is hyperventilation. This can be acute during rest, exercise, and recovery, or chronic related to underlying metabolic acidosis or psychological factors. Pain or anxiety might cause acute hyperventilation during exercise. Hyperventilation, by definition, is characterized by an inappropriate increase in minute ventilation as well as high ventilatory equivalents (see the section on ventilatory equivalents later in Chapter 4). Individuals with chronic hyperventilation develop compensatory reductions in plasma bicarbonate levels that tend to normalize pH. Conceivably, this could reduce lactic acid-buffering capacity during exercise.

Patients with McArdle's disease (myophosphorylase deficiency) do not generate lactic acid during exercise. Their metabolic responses are abnormal in several respects, including low *R* values at rest and maximum exercise.

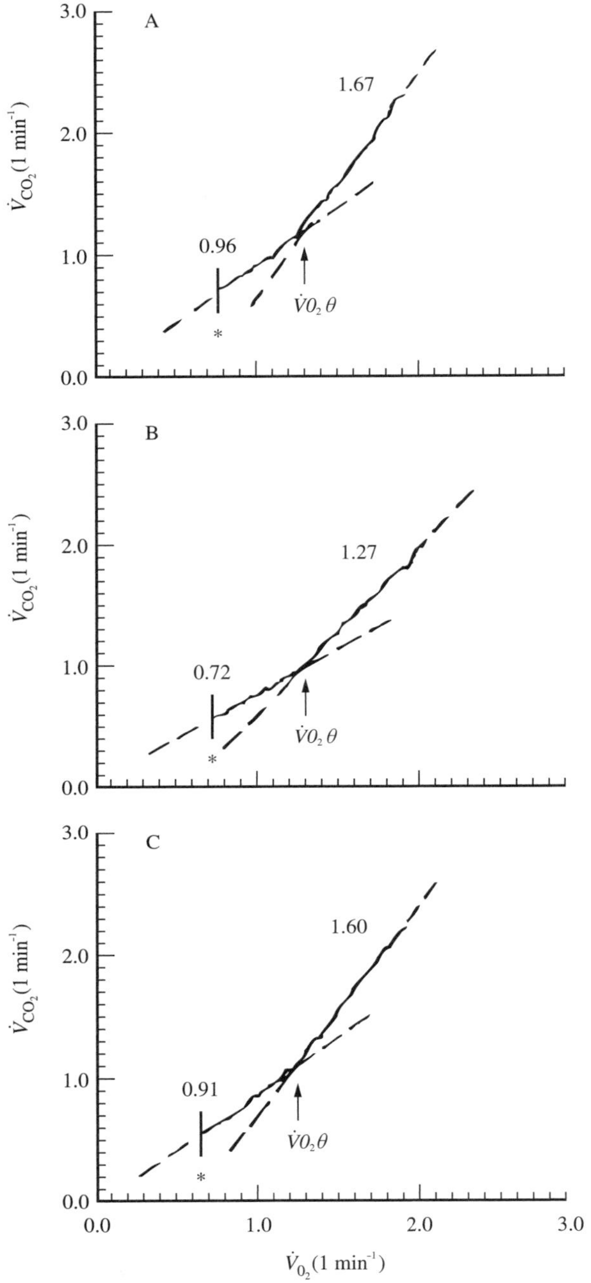


## Muscle respiratory quotient ($RQ_{mus}$)

### Definition, derivation, and units of measurement

- During incremental exercise, the respiratory quotient of exercising muscle ($RQ_{mus}$) is represented by the increase in muscle $CO_2$ production divided by the concomitant increase in muscle $O_2$ consumption.

  Once body carbon dioxide stores have stabilized, further increases in $\dot{V}CO_2$ and $\dot{V}O_2$, measured by expired gas analysis, predominantly reflect the increasing metabolism of exercising muscle. This will be true until additional nonmetabolic $CO_2$ begins to be evolved from bicarbonate buffering of lactic acid.
- $RQ_{mus}$ is derived from the lower slope (S1) of the $\dot{V}CO_2$–$\dot{V}O_2$ relationship for incremental exercise.

$$RQ_{mus} = \frac{\delta \dot{V}CO_2}{\delta \dot{V}O_2} \tag{4.6}$$

- Since $\dot{V}CO_2$ and $\dot{V}O_2$ both have units of liters per minute, $RQ_{mus}$ has no units.

### Normal response

In normal individuals the lower slope (S1) of the $\dot{V}CO_2$–$\dot{V}O_2$ relationship has a value close to 1.0 (Figure 4.14). This indicates that the metabolic substrate for the exercising muscle must be almost entirely carbohydrate.

**Figure 4.14** Relationships between $\dot{V}CO_2$ and $\dot{V}O_2$ during incremental work rate XTs for a group of normal subjects. Day 1 shows the initial control response. Day 2 shows the same subjects after glycogen depletion. Day 3 shows reversion to the normal resonse following glycogen repletion. The asterisk indicates the beginning of the slope analysis. Reproduced with permission from Cooper, C. B., Beaver, W. L., Cooper, D. M. & Wasserman, K. (1992). Factors affecting components of the alveolar $CO_2$ output–$O_2$ uptake relationship during incremental exercise in man. *Exp. Physiol.*, **77**, 51–64.

### Abnormal responses

S1 can be manipulated in normal individuals by prolonged fasting combined with prior depletion of muscle glycogen by endurance exercise. In these circumstances $RQ_{mus}$ can be closer to 0.7, the respiratory quotient of fat. Figure 4.14 shows the effects of intentional glycogen depletion on $RQ_{mus}$. S1 is reduced in McArdle's disease, where lack of muscle phosphorylase prevents normal utilization of muscle glycogen.

## Maximum heart rate ($f_{Cmax}$)

### Definition, derivation, and units of measurement

- Maximum heart rate is the highest value of the heart rate or pulse rate which can be attained and measured during incremental exercise.
- $f_{Cmax}$ is a primary variable best measured from the R-R intervals of a continuous electrocardiogram during incremental exercise. Newer technologies allow $f_{Cmax}$ to be measured using telemetric monitoring. Alternatively, $f_{Cmax}$ can be calculated from 10-s pulse rate in a field test or by auscultation.
- The units of $f_{Cmax}$ are beats per minute or $min^{-1}$.

### Normal response

Every individual has a theoretical maximum heart rate, which declines with increasing age. Figure 4.15 shows the prediction of $f_{Cmax}$ according to data collected by Åstrand et al. (1973). There are two formulae commonly used for calculation of predicted $f_{Cmax}$. Both are shown in Figure 4.15 and the reader can draw his or her own conclusions about their reliability in relationship to this data set:

$$\text{pred}f_{Cmax} = 220 - \text{age} \quad (4.7)$$

$$\text{pred}f_{Cmax} = 210 - (\text{age} \cdot 0.65) \quad (4.8)$$

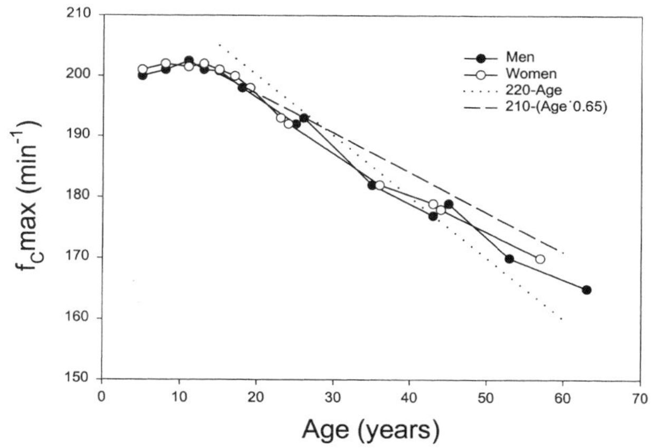


**Figure 4.15** Age-related decline in $f_{Cmax}$. Actual data are derived from Åstrand, I., Åstrand, P.-O., Hallbäck, I. & Kilbom, Å. (1973). Reduction in maximal oxygen uptake with age. *J. Appl. Physiol.*, **35**, 649–54. Commonly used prediction equations are superimposed.

As with any physiological entity, there is variability among the normal population (see Chapter 5). The standard deviation for $f_{Cmax}$ is estimated to be $10\,min^{-1}$. Hence, for 95% of individuals of a specific age, $f_{Cmax}$ will be included in a calculated range of $40\,min^{-1}$. Whilst predicted $f_{Cmax}$ values are useful in exercise testing and interpretation, clearly the methods of prediction have their limitations. It is far preferable to measure $f_{Cmax}$ in the context of an incremental exercise test with an adequate physical effort. The same problems occur when attempting to use predicted $f_{Cmax}$ in conjunction with submaximal $\dot{V}O_2$ and heart rate data, to calculate $\dot{V}O_{2max}$. The range of normal $f_{Cmax}$ is too great to make this method reliable.

Some individuals exhibit a plateau at maximum heart rate, similar to the plateau which can be seen at $\dot{V}O_{2max}$. When this occurs, the observer can be reasonably certain that a true $f_{Cmax}$ is being exhibited.

### Abnormal responses

Noncardiovascular limitations of various types prevent attainment of true $f_{Cmax}$. Recognition of these different response patterns will be discussed further in Chapter 5.

Certain drugs, which interfere with cardiac conduction, slow heart rate and reduce $f_{Cmax}$. These

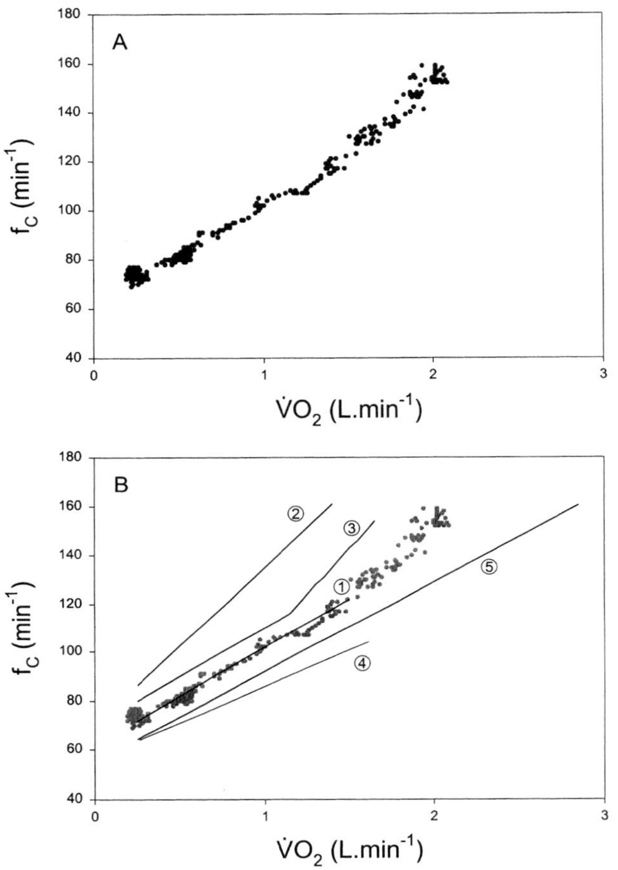


**Figure 4.16** Relationship between $f_C$ and $\dot{V}o_2$ during an incremental work rate XT. (A) Normal response. (B) Abnormal responses for ① suboptimal effort; ② cardiomyopathy; ③ myocardial ischemia developing at $f_C$ of 115 min$^{-1}$; and ④ chronotropic incompetence. ⑤ Normal trained response.

drugs include $\beta$-sympathomimetic antagonists like propranolol and metoprolol, calcium channel antagonists like verapamil and diltiazem, and digoxin. Rarely, individuals with coronary artery disease fail to exhibit a normal heart rate response to incremental exercise. This phenomenon, called chronotropic incompetence, can occur without overt signs of myocardial ischemia. Failure of heart rate to increase appropriately is presumed to be due to ischemic dysfunction of the sinoatrial node. The result is a low $f_{C\max}$.

## Slope of the cardiovascular response ($\delta f_C / \delta \dot{V}o_2$)

### Definition, derivation, and units of measurement

- $\delta f_C / \delta \dot{V}o_2$ is the slope of the relationship between heart rate and $\dot{V}o_2$ during incremental exercise. The relationship has remarkable linearity, as shown in Figure 4.16. The robustness of this relationship is due to its derivation from the Fick equation:

$$\dot{V}o_2 = \dot{Q}_C \cdot C_{(a-\bar{v})}o_2 \quad (4.9)$$

where $\dot{Q}_C$ is cardiac output and $C_{(a-\bar{v})}o_2$ is the difference in oxygen content between arterial and mixed venous blood.

The following considerations lead to an equation for the slope of the cardiovascular response. Since:

$$\dot{Q}_C = f_C \cdot SV \quad (4.10)$$

where SV is cardiac stroke volume, then:

$$\dot{V}o_2 = f_C \cdot SV \cdot C_{(a-\bar{v})}o_2 \quad (4.11)$$

or:

$$f_C = \dot{V}o_2 \cdot \frac{1}{SV \cdot C_{(a-\bar{v})}o_2} \quad (4.12)$$

i.e.

$$\frac{f_C}{\dot{V}o_2} = \frac{1}{SV \cdot C_{(a-\bar{v})}o_2} \quad (4.13)$$

Hence the slope $\delta f_C / \delta \dot{V}o_2$ is related to stroke volume and the difference in oxygen content between arterial and mixed venous blood.

- $\delta f_C / \delta \dot{V}o_2$ is derived by linear regression analysis of a plot of $f_C$ versus $\dot{V}o_2$ during incremental exercise. An alternative, reasonably accurate and simpler method for calculating this slope uses resting and maximal values for both variables:

$$\delta f_C / \delta \dot{V}o_2 = \frac{f_{C\max} - f_{C\text{rest}}}{\dot{V}o_{2\max} - \dot{V}o_{2\text{rest}}} \quad (4.14)$$

As a measure of cardiovascular efficiency, $\delta f_C / \delta \dot{V}o_2$ is closely related to the oxygen pulse (see below). An important difference is that oxygen pulse is derived from instantaneous values of $\dot{V}O_2$ and $f_C$, and therefore changes as a rising exponential during incremental exercise. In fact, $\delta f_C/\delta \dot{V}O_2$ is the reciprocal of the asymptotic oxygen pulse.

- The units of $\delta f_C/\delta \dot{V}O_2$ are $l^{-1}$.

### Normal response (Figure 4.16A)

The normal value for $\delta f_C/\delta \dot{V}O_2$ in a given individual can be calculated using the Equation 4.14 above with assumed or measured resting values and predicted maximum values for $f_C$ and $\dot{V}O_2$. A plot of $f_C$ versus $\dot{V}O_2$ gives an excellent visual representation of $\delta f_C/\delta \dot{V}O_2$, especially if the physiological boundaries of the normal response ($f_{Cmax}$ and $\dot{V}O_{2max}$) are drawn on the graph. The relationship between $f_C$ and $\dot{V}O_2$ thus has a target point corresponding to predicted $f_{Cmax}$ and predicted $\dot{V}O_{2max}$. The data published by Spiro et al. in 1974 suggest reference values of $\delta f_C/\delta \dot{V}O_2$ of 42–43 $l^{-1}$ for men and 63–71 $l^{-1}$ for women.

### Abnormal responses (Figure 4.16B)

Equation 4.13 above illustrates that the slope $\delta f_C/\delta \dot{V}O_2$ is related to cardiac stroke volume and arterial–venous oxygen difference. Alterations of $\delta f_C/\delta \dot{V}O_2$ can therefore be helpfully interpreted in terms of these underlying physiological parameters.

Physical training, which increases SV, and also $C_{(a-\bar{v})}O_2$, will predictably reduce $\delta f_C/\delta \dot{V}O_2$, allowing an individual to attain a higher $\dot{V}O_{2max}$ at $f_{Cmax}$ (Figure 4.16). The traditional concept of the training response having both central (SV) and peripheral ($C_{(a-\bar{v})}O_2$) components fits well with this analytical approach.

Conversely, conditions that reduce SV or impair peripheral oxygen extraction (reducing $C_{(a-\bar{v})}O_2$) increase $\delta f_C/\delta \dot{V}O_2$, resulting in a lower $\dot{V}O_{2max}$ at $f_{Cmax}$ (Figure 4.16).

Typical cardiac conditions causing a steeper $\delta f_C/\delta \dot{V}O_2$ would include congestive heart failure, coronary artery disease resulting in myocardial dysfunction, and valvular heart disease. Typical peripheral conditions would include deconditioning and certain types of myopathy.

## Oxygen pulse ($\dot{V}O_2/f_C$)

### Definition, derivation, and units of measurement

- $\dot{V}O_2/f_C$ is a measure of cardiovascular efficiency indicating what metabolic value in terms of oxygen uptake derives from every heart beat. Hence, $\dot{V}O_2/f_C$ is a secondary variable calculated by dividing instantaneous oxygen uptake by the heart rate.

$$\text{Oxygen pulse} = \frac{\dot{V}O_2}{f_C} \qquad (4.15)$$

- $\dot{V}O_2/f_C$ is intricately related to cardiac stroke volume (SV) and can be used to estimate stroke volume at various stages of incremental exercise. Recalling the Fick equation:

$$\dot{V}O_2 = Q_C \cdot (C_{(a-\bar{v})}O_2) \qquad (4.16)$$

where $Q_C$ is cardiac output and $(C_{(a-\bar{v})}O_2)$ is arteriovenous difference in oxygen content, since:

$$Q_C = f_C \cdot \text{SV} \qquad (4.17)$$

then:

$$\frac{\dot{V}O_2}{f_C} = \text{SV} \cdot C_{(a-\bar{v})}O_2 \qquad (4.18)$$

or:

$$\text{SV} = \frac{\dot{V}O_2/f_C}{C_{(a-\bar{v})}O_2} \qquad (4.19)$$

where $\dot{V}O_2/f_C$ is the oxygen pulse.

Using this equation and making several assumptions, we can estimate SV during incremental exercise. At rest, arterial oxygen content is close to 20 ml per 100 ml of blood ($0.20\ ml \cdot ml^{-1}$), whereas mixed venous oxygen content is close to 15 ml per 100 ml of blood ($0.15\ ml \cdot ml^{-1}$). Hence, $C_{(a-\bar{v})}O_2$ is $0.05\ ml \cdot ml^{-1}$. At rest:

$$\text{SV} = \dot{V}O_2/f_C \cdot 20 \qquad (4.20)$$

Throughout exercise, in normal individuals, arterial oxygen content remains close to 20 ml per 100 ml of blood ($0.20\ ml \cdot ml^{-1}$). In a sedentary person, mixed venous oxygen content typically falls

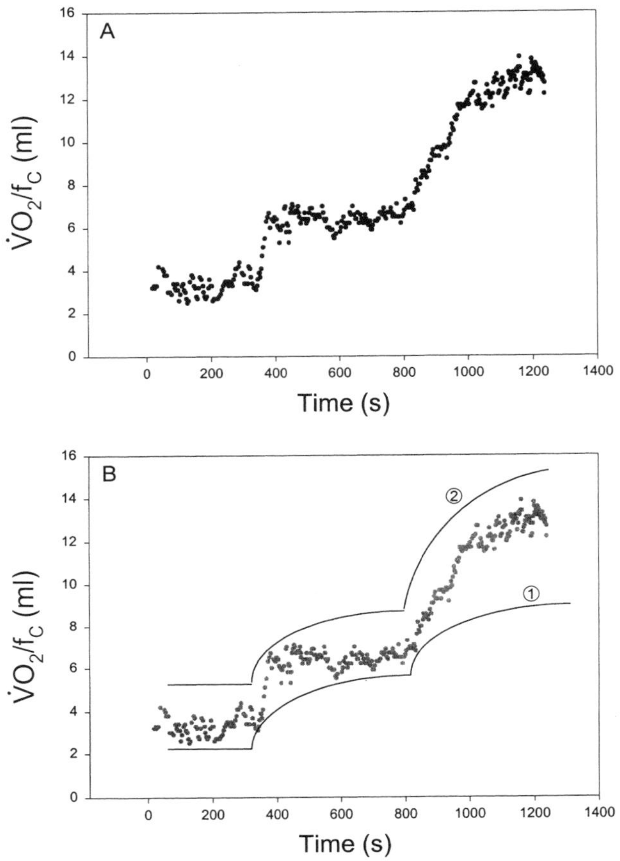


**Figure 4.17** Relationship between $\dot{V}o_2/f_C$ and time during an incremental work rate XT. (A) Normal response. (B) Typical responses for ① cardiovascular disease and ② physical training.

to 8 ml per 100 ml of blood (0.08 ml · ml$^{-1}$). Hence $C_{(a-\bar{v})}o_2$ is 0.12 ml · ml$^{-1}$. At maximal exercise:

$$SV = \dot{V}o_2/fc \cdot 8.3 \quad (4.21)$$

In an athlete, mixed venous oxygen content can fall to 5 ml per 100 ml of blood (0.05 ml · ml$^{-1}$). Hence $C_{(a-\bar{v})}o_2$ is 0.15 ml · ml$^{-1}$. At maximal exercise:

$$SV = \dot{V}o_2/f_C \cdot 6.8 \quad (4.22)$$

Using the same reasoning, it follows that if an individual could extract all the oxygen from circulating blood, the theoretical maximum $C_{(a-\bar{v})}o_2$ would be 0.20 ml · ml$^{-1}$. At maximal exercise:

$$SV = \dot{V}o_2/f_C \cdot 5 \quad (4.23)$$

where $\dot{V}o_2/f_C$ is the asymptotic oxygen pulse.

- The units of $\dot{V}o_2/f_C$ are milliliters per beat or ml.

### Normal response (Figure 4.17A)

The normal resting $\dot{V}o_2/f_C$ is 3.5–4.5 ml, corresponding to a cardiac stroke volume of 70–90 ml. Maximum $\dot{V}o_2/f_C$ depends upon fitness level. A sedentary 20-year-old individual has a maximum $\dot{V}o_2/f_C$ of 12–15 ml, corresponding to a cardiac stroke volume of 100–120 ml (Figure 4.17). An athlete can have a maximum $\dot{V}o_2/f_C$ of 16–20 ml, corresponding to a cardiac stroke volume of 120–140 ml.

### Abnormal responses (Figure 4.17B)

Maximum $\dot{V}o_2/f_C$ is reduced in physical deconditioning, noncardiovascular limitation, and all forms of cardiovascular limitation or disease. Studies of maximal exercise responses in patients with cardiac failure reveal a relationship between maximum $\dot{V}o_2/f_C$ and the NYHA classification of cardiac failure (Table 4.2).

Typical $\dot{V}o_2/f_C$ response patterns for cardiovascular disease and physical training are shown in Figure 4.17.

## Electrocardiogram (ECG)

### Definition, derivation, and units of measurement

- The ECG is a summation of electrical vectors occurring during the cardiac cycle and being measured at the body surface by certain configurations of skin electrodes.
- During a performance exercise test (PXT) the heart rate is typically derived from a three-lead ECG. This method shows cardiac rhythm but gives limited diagnostic information. A clinical exercise test (CXT) should include full 12-lead ECG with analysis of rhythm, mean frontal plane

axis, and P, QRS, and T-wave configuration. During field exercise tests heart rate is usually palpated from the pulse or recorded using a pulse rate monitor. In these circumstances ECG information is not available. ECG interpretation is a complex subject. For the purposes of this book we will merely state important normal and abnormal features.

- The conventional 12-lead ECG is measured on standard recording paper with a speed of $25\,mm \cdot s^{-1}$. Hence, each millimeter on the horizontal axis represents 0.04 s and the heart rate can be quickly estimated by dividing 300 by the number of centimeters between R waves. Standard calibration sets the amplitude at 10 mm per millivolt (mV). Hence, each millimeter on the vertical axis represents 0.1 mV.

### Normal response

The normal ECG should exhibit sinus rhythm with a rate between 60 and 100 $min^{-1}$ at rest (Figure 4.18A). Sinus rhythm can be confirmed by marking the R–R′ intervals of several QRS complexes on the edge of a piece of paper and then sliding this paper along the ECG to confirm that the QRS complexes are equally spaced.

There is a small variation in R–R′ interval during respiration causing heart rate to fluctuate – usually less than 10 $min^{-1}$ – called sinus arrhythmia (Figure 4.18B). The heart rate quickens during inspiration and slows during expiration due to variation in vagal tone. Occasionally exaggerated sinus arrhythmia is observed in normal individuals.

At rest a heart rate less than 60 $min^{-1}$ is sinus bradycardia. A rate greater than 100 $min^{-1}$ is sinus tachycardia. Sinus bradycardia occurs as a result of intensive physical training and rates less than 50 $min^{-1}$ are not unusual. Sinus tachycardia at rest is commonly associated with anxiety.

Occasional (less than 6 $min^{-1}$), premature atrial or ventricular contractions (PACs and PVCs) can be normal, particularly if they disappear with exercise.

The mean frontal plane axis is derived from the QRS complex. The normal axis lies between –30° and +90°. Thus, a normal axis can be easily recognized when the QRS is predominantly positive in both leads I and II. Right axis deviation occurs in 5% of normal individuals.

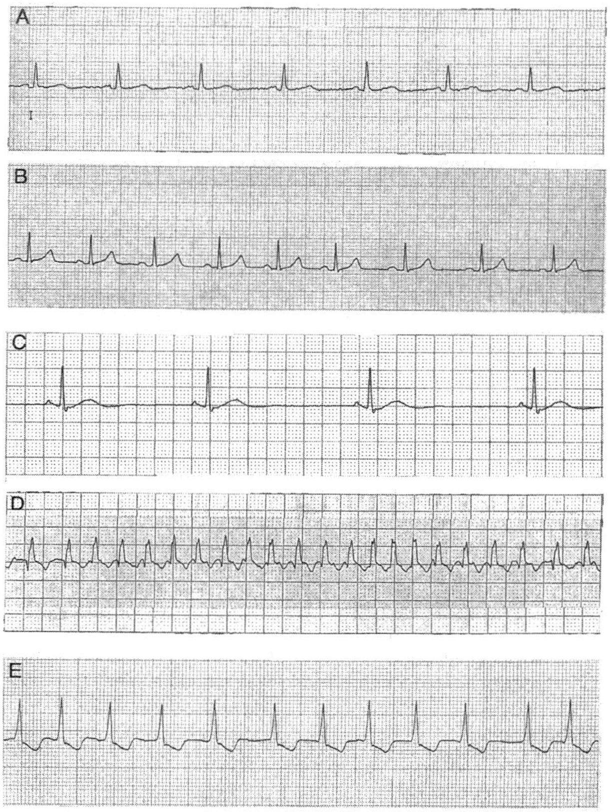


**Figure 4.18** Electrocardiographic recordings showing normal variations and common supraventricular dysrhythmias. (A) Normal sinus rhythm. (B) Sinus arrhythmia. (C) Sinus bradycardia. (D) Supraventricular tachycardia. (E) Atrial fibrillation.

The normal P-R interval is 0.12–0.20 ms (3–5 mm on a conventional ECG tracing). The normal QRS voltage (maximum R plus maximum S in the precordial leads) is less than 35 mV (35 mm on a conventional ECG tracing). QRS voltage sometimes appears increased in a lean individual with a thin chest wall.

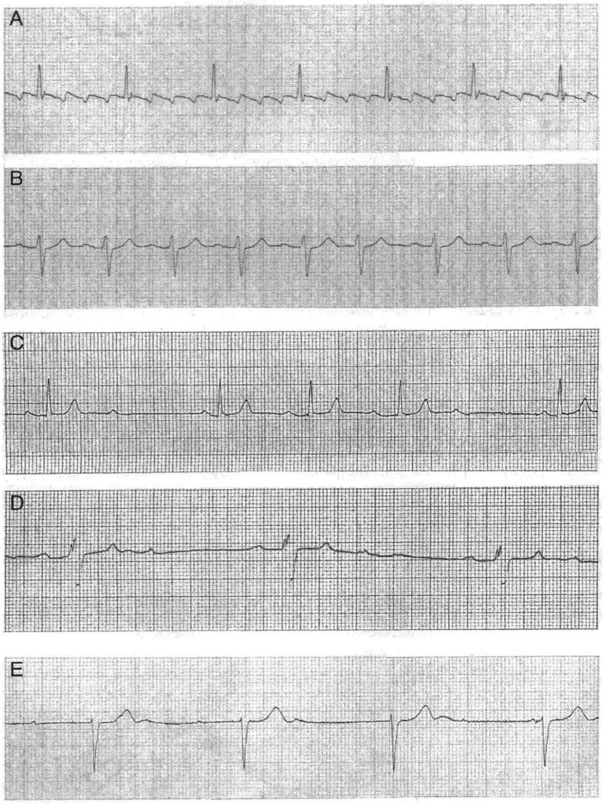


**Figure 4.19** Electrocardiographic recordings showing common dysrhythmias. (A) Atrial flutter. (B) First-degree heart block with a premature atrial contraction. (C) Second-degree heart block (Möbitz type I). (D) Second-degree heart block (Möbitz type II). (E) Third-degree (complete) heart block.

## Abnormal responses

The intention of this book is to help the exercise practitioner to recognize normal variations of the ECG and to identify significant abnormalities, since the development of ECG abnormalities is among the important contraindications to exercise testing and indications for stopping an exercise test (see Chapter 3). The ECG appearances of the common dysrhythmias are presented in Figures 4.18–4.20 and an approach to the identification of ECG changes that suggest myocardial ischemia is shown in Figure 4.21. For more information, the reader is advised to consult a detailed text on ECG interpretation and to confer with a cardiologist.

*Cardiac dysrhythmias (Figures 4.18–4.20)*

Any cardiac rhythm other than those discussed in the foregoing section is abnormal, including frequent PACs ($>6\,min^{-1}$), frequent PVCs ($>30\%$ of all ventricular complexes), atrial fibrillation, atrial flutter, supraventricular tachycardia, and paroxysmal ventricular tachycardia or ventricular fibrillation. An incremental exercise test can be conducted in the presence of atrial fibrillation and in patients with cardiac pacemakers. A clinical setting is clearly recommended and the cardiovascular responses must be interpreted with caution.

*Other common abnormalities*

Left axis deviation (LAD) more than –30° and new right axis deviation (RAD) more than +90° are abnormal. A P-R interval less than 0.12 ms can be indicative of preexcitation. One longer than 0.20 ms indicates first-degree heart block. A QRS complex wider than 0.22 ms indicates bundle branch block. A combined QRS voltage greater than 35 mV indicates ventricular hypertrophy. The criteria for left ventricular hypertrophy (LVH), as seen in significant cases of hypertension, are LAD, QRS $>$ 0.22 ms and $>$35 mV. In addition, ST depression can be seen in lateral leads indicating relative myocardial ischemia – the so-called strain pattern.

*Myocardial ischemia (Figure 4.21)*

The classical features of myocardial ischemia on the ECG are horizontal, downsloping, or rounded ST depression of 0.1 mV observed $>$80 ms past the J-point. Upsloping ST depression $>$0.1 mV occurring $>$80 ms past the J-point is suspicious but less conclusive. ST changes often present a consistent pattern in the anterior, lateral, or inferior leads. However, in practice, the distribution of ST changes does not necessarily predict the location of ischemia or the coronary artery involved. In subjects with left bundle branch block, ST segment depression cannot be used to diagnose myocardial ischemia. Also certain medications such as digoxin affect the ST segment and confound the diagnosis of myocardial ischemia. Rarely, ST segment elevation can be seen as a result of myocardial ischemia during exercise. The reliability of the exercise ECG for the identification of myocardial ischemia has been evaluated by comparison with coronary angiography, using 50% stenosis of at least one coronary artery as the "gold standard." The *sensitivity*, i.e., the percentage of individuals with coronary artery disease who will have a positive test, is approximately 70%. The *specificity*, i.e., the percentage of individuals without coronary artery disease who will have a negative test, is 80%.

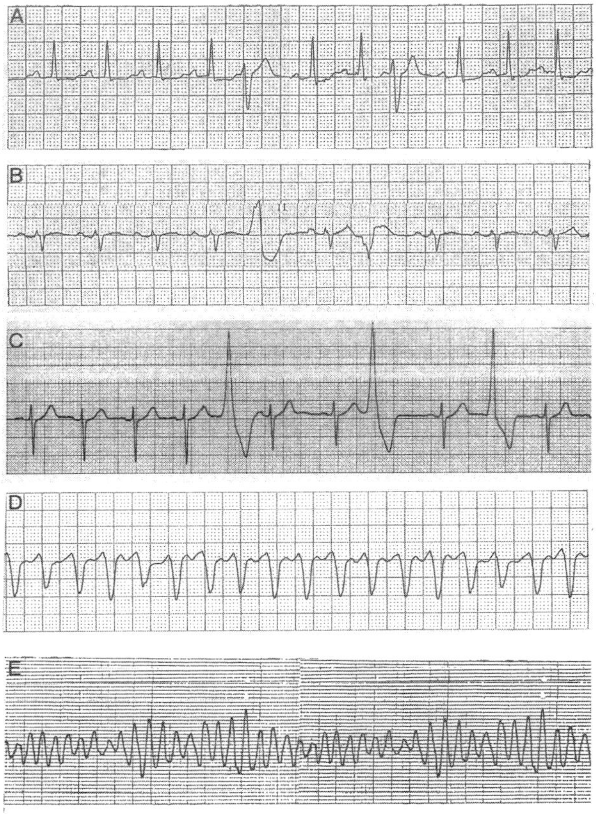


**Figure 4.20** Electrocardiographic recordings showing common ventricular dysrhythmias. (A) Unifocal premature ventricular contractions. (B) Multifocal premature ventricular contractions. (C) Trigemini becoming bigemini. (D) Ventricular tachycardia. (E) Ventricular fibrillation.

## Arteriovenous difference in oxygen content ($C_{(a-\bar{v})}O_2$)

### Definition, derivation, and units of measurement

- The arteriovenous difference in oxygen content ($C_{(a-\bar{v})}O_2$) is the absolute difference in content of oxygen in arterial and mixed venous blood from the systemic circulation. Hence, $C_{(a-\bar{v})}O_2$ represents the amount of oxygen extracted from blood circulating in the systemic circulation by all body tissues. During exercise $C_{(a-\bar{v})}O_2$ is substantially influenced by the increased oxygen extraction of exercising muscles. Under steady-state conditions, the oxygen content of the systemic arterial blood is equal to the oxygen content of the pulmonary venous blood and the oxygen content of systemic mixed venous blood is equal to the oxygen content of the pulmonary arterial blood. Hence, $C_{(a-\bar{v})}O_2$ also represents the amount of oxygen taken up by the blood in the lungs.
- $C_{(a-\bar{v})}O_2$ is a secondary variable which must be derived by simultaneous sampling of both systemic arterial and systemic mixed venous blood. The former requires discrete puncture or catheterization of a radial, brachial, or femoral artery. The latter requires placement of a flow-directed central venous catheter in the right atrium or the main pulmonary artery outflow tract. Obviously these procedures are not straightforward and can only be accomplished with experienced personnel in a laboratory setting.
- The traditional units of $C_{(a-\bar{v})}O_2$ are milliliters of oxygen per deciliter of blood ($ml \cdot dl^{-1}$). However, when used in equations to calculate cardiac output or cardiac stroke volume $C_{(a-\bar{v})}O_2$ must be expressed with like units, i.e., milliliters per milliliter or liters per liter.

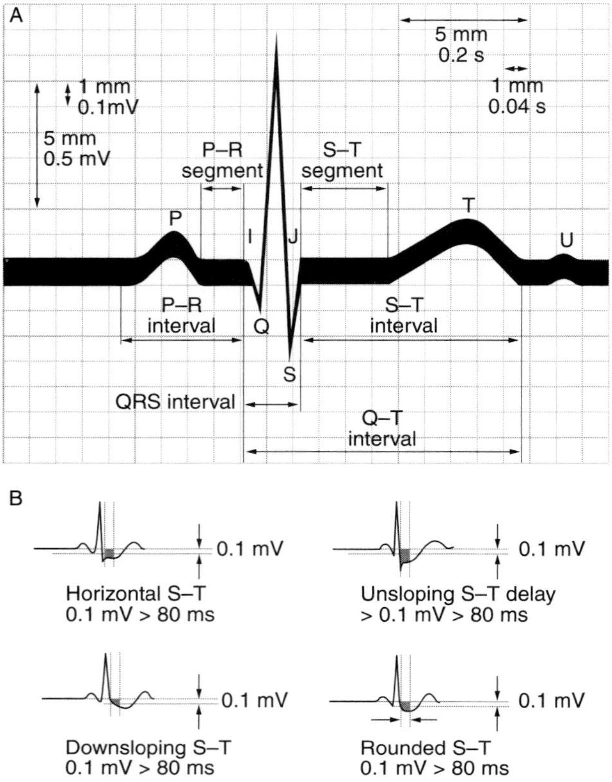


**Figure 4.21** Normal ECG configuration and criteria for the diagnosis of myocardial ischemia. (A) Normal P, QRS, T and U wave configurations with normal values for amplitudes and intervals. (B) Four different patterns seen in myocardial ischemia, including horizontal, downsloping, and rounded ST depression of 0.1 mV occurring 80 ms after the J-point as well as upsloping ST depression >0.1 mV occurring 80 ms after the J-point.

### Normal response

Systemic arterial oxygen content is reasonably constant in normal individuals, being $20\,ml \cdot dl^{-1}$ or $0.20\,ml \cdot ml^{-1}$. At rest, mixed venous oxygen content is typically about $15\,ml \cdot dl^{-1}$ or $0.15\,ml \cdot ml^{-1}$. Hence, $C_{(a-\bar{v})}O_2$ is $5\,ml \cdot dl^{-1}$ or $0.05\,ml \cdot ml^{-1}$. Thus, at rest, about 25% of available oxygen is extracted from the circulating systemic blood. During exercise the extraction of oxygen may approach 75%, depending on the level of fitness of the individual.

Fortuitously, $C_{(a-\bar{v})}O_2$ has a predictable relationship with relative exercise intensity, i.e., the percentage of predicted $\dot{V}O_{2max}$. This relationship was elegantly demonstrated for normal subjects and is illustrated in Figure 4.22. The following equation, derived from these data, can be used to estimate $C_{(a-\bar{v})}O_2$ from relative exercise intensity:

$$C_{(a-\bar{v})}O_2 = 5.72 + (0.1 \cdot \%ref\,\dot{V}O_{2max}) \qquad 4.24$$

where $C_{(a-\bar{v})}O_2$ is the difference in oxygen content between arterial and mixed venous blood expressed in $ml \cdot dl^{-1}$ and $\%ref\,\dot{V}O_{2max}$ is the relative exercise intensity, i.e., the instantaneous $\dot{V}O_2$ expressed as a percentage of reference or predicted $\dot{V}O_{2max}$.

Experimental data in general, and application of Equation 4.24 in particular, show that for maximal exercise in normal individuals, $C_{(a-\bar{v})}O_2$ approaches $15\,ml \cdot dl^{-1}$ or $0.15\,ml \cdot ml^{-1}$. In a sedentary person, mixed venous oxygen content typically falls to $8\,ml \cdot dl^{-1}$ or $0.08\,ml \cdot ml^{-1}$. Hence $C_{(a-\bar{v})}O_2$ is $0.12\,ml \cdot ml^{-1}$. Values for mixed venous oxygen content of $0.03\,ml \cdot ml^{-1}$ have been observed in highly trained athletes, giving a value for $C_{(a-\bar{v})}O_2$ of $0.17\,ml \cdot ml^{-1}$.

### Abnormal responses

Compromised oxygen delivery due to inadequate blood flow or cardiac output results in relatively higher $C_{(a-\bar{v})}O_2$ compared with relative exercise intensity. This pattern of abnormality might be expected with cardiac failure due to a variety of causes. By contrast, impaired ability of exercising muscle to extract oxygen would result in lower $C_{(a-\bar{v})}O_2$ and also lower $\dot{V}O_2$. The relationships between $C_{(a-\bar{v})}O_2$, $\dot{V}O_2$, and cardiac output are further considered in the following section on cardiac output.

## Cardiac output ($\dot{Q}_C$)

### Definition, derivation, and units of measurement

- The cardiac output ($\dot{Q}_C$) is the total circulating

blood flow. Averaged over time, the blood flow through the systemic and pulmonary circulations must be equal.

- Several techniques are available for determining cardiac output. Cardiac output is most reliably measured by cardiac catheterization, although estimates can be obtained using echocardiography. One approach is to measure $\dot{V}O_2$, arterial oxygen content, and mixed venous oxygen content and then to apply the direct Fick principle.

$$\dot{Q}_C = \frac{\dot{V}O_2}{C_{(a-\bar{v})}O_2} \quad (4.25)$$

Knowledge of the predictable relationship between $C_{(a-\bar{v})}O_2$ and relative exercise intensity, i.e., the percentage of reference $\dot{V}O_{2max}$, shown in Equation 4.25, allows us to express $\dot{Q}_C$ in terms of the instantaneous $\dot{V}O_2$.

$$\dot{Q}_C = \left( \frac{\dot{V}O_2}{0.0572 + (0.001 \cdot \%ref\,\dot{V}O_{2max})} \right) \quad (4.26)$$

where $\dot{Q}_C$ and $\dot{V}O_2$ are both expressed in $l \cdot min^{-1}$ and $\%ref\,\dot{V}O_{2max}$ is the relative exercise intensity, i.e., the instantaneous $\dot{V}O_2$ expressed as a percentage of reference or predicted $\dot{V}O_{2max}$.

The ability to predict $\dot{Q}_C$ based on noninvasive measures such as $\dot{V}O_2$ has definite appeal. This approach is reasonable in normal subjects; however, it is likely to be subject to inaccuracies in disease states.

An alternative invasive approach is to determine $\dot{Q}_C$ by cardiac catheterization using an indicator dilution technique and then applying the indirect Fick principle.

- The units of $\dot{Q}_C$ are liters per minute ($l \cdot min^{-1}$).

## Normal response (Figure 4.23A)

Resting cardiac output is about $5\,l \cdot min^{-1}$. Younger healthy subjects performing maximal exercise can achieve values of $\dot{Q}_C$ about $25\,l \cdot min^{-1}$, representing an approximate fivefold increase. Figure 4.23A shows the hypothetical relationship between $\dot{Q}_C$ and $C_{(a-\bar{v})}O_2$ based on Equation 4.24. This relationship can be seen to be nonlinear. In normal subjects, the metabolic threshold is known to occur approximately when $C_{(a-\bar{v})}O_2$ exceeds $10\,ml \cdot dl^{-1}$, i.e., when $\dot{Q}_C$ is about $15–20\,l \cdot min^{-1}$.

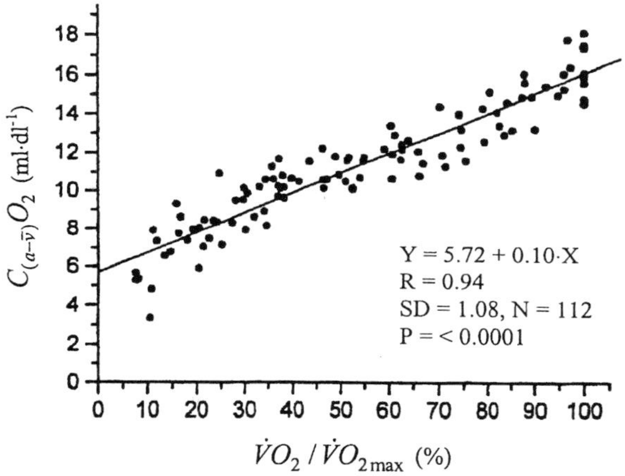


**Figure 4.22** Relationship between arteriovenous difference in oxygen content and percentage of measured maximum oxygen uptake. Data were determined from systemic arterial and pulmonary arterial (equivalent to systemic mixed venous) blood that was simultaneously sampled each minute during 10 incremental exercise tests in 5 subjects. Reproduced with permission from Stringer, W. W., Hansen, J. E. & Wasserman, K. (1997). Cardiac output estimated non-invasively from oxygen uptake during exercise. *J. Appl. Physiol.*, **82**, 908–12.

## Abnormal responses (Figure 4.23B)

Various cardiac diseases result in compromised $\dot{Q}_C$, particularly during exercise. Whenever $\dot{Q}_C$ is inappropriately low during incremental exercise, tissue oxygen consumption tends to be maintained by increased oxygen extraction from the blood. As a result, $C_{(a-\bar{v})}O_2$ increases more rapidly at relatively lower levels of exercise. The effect on the relationship between $\dot{Q}_C$ and $C_{(a-\bar{v})}O_2$ is shown in Figure 4.23B. Data from Weber and Janicki (Table 4.3) can be plotted on Figure 4.23 to illustrate this phenomenon and how it progresses through the different stages of severity of congestive heart failure. Theoretically, in cases of myopathy, the hemodynamic response to incremental exercise should be different, as

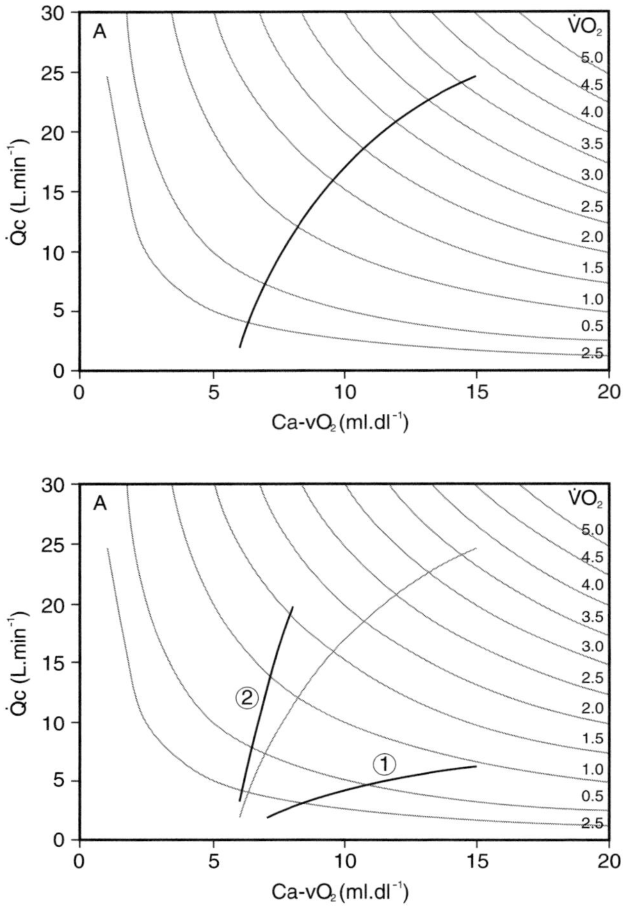


**Figure 4.23** Hypothetical relationship between $\dot{Q}_C$ and $C_{(a-\bar{v})}O_2$ for incremental exercise. Isopleths represent levels of $\dot{V}O_2$. The normal response shown in (A) was derived using Equation 4.24. (B) Abnormal responses for ① cardiac failure and ② skeletal myopathy.

illustrated in Figure 4.23B. One might expect normal or even exaggerated increases in cardiac output to occur while oxygen extraction fails to increase appropriately. The predicted effect on the relationship between $\dot{Q}_C$ and $C_{(a-\bar{v})}O_2$ is shown in Figure 4.23B. However, sufficient data do not yet exist to substantiate this concept.

## Cardiac stroke volume (SV)

### Definition, derivation, and units of measurement

- Cardiac stroke volume is the volume of blood ejected by either the left or right ventricle with each systolic contraction. Averaged over time, the left- and right-sided SV must be equal.
- Precise measurement of SV necessitates determination of cardiac output. SV is then calculated knowing the heart rate:

$$SV = \frac{\dot{Q}_C}{f_C} \qquad (4.27)$$

  Several techniques are available for determining cardiac output and hence deriving SV. Cardiac output is most reliably measured by cardiac catheterization, although estimates can be obtained using echocardiography. One approach is to measure $\dot{V}O_2$, arterial oxygen content, and mixed venous oxygen content and then apply the direct Fick principle. Alternatively, cardiac output can be determined by cardiac catheterization using an indicator dilution technique and applying the indirect Fick principle.
- The units of SV are milliliters.

### Normal response

Normal resting cardiac stroke volume is about 70 ml. During incremental exercise SV increases due to increased venous return to the heart, increased end-diastolic volume, and sympathetic nervous system stimulation of myocardial contractility. SV increases during the early phase of incremental exercise, approaching a plateau at about 50% of maximum cardiac output or 40% of $\dot{V}O_{2max}$ (Figure 4.24). In a sedentary adult, SV reaches 100–120 ml whereas in the athlete the increase can reach 120–140 ml.

### Abnormal response

Cardiac diseases, including coronary artery disease, cardiomyopathy, valvular heart disease and congenital heart disease, typically result in a low cardiac stroke volume. In some cases end-diastolic volume

**Table 4.5.** Sphygmomanometry: tonal qualities of the Korotkoff sounds and their interpretation

| Korotkoff sound | Tonal qualities | Interpretation |
|---|---|---|
| I | Onset of sounds, metallic tapping that increases in intensity | Peak systolic blood pressure |
| II | Swishing sound or murmur, occasionally absent and referred to as auscultatory gap | |
| III | Increased intensity with crisper, sharper sounds | |
| IV | Sudden and distinct muffling of sound | Diastolic blood pressure |
| V | Disappearance of sounds | Return of laminar flow |

is increased but SV is low due to impaired myocardial contractility. In the case of mitral regurgitation, the left ventricle becomes dilated and left ventricular stroke volume might actually be increased, at least in early disease. However, it must be remembered that a fraction of the stroke volume is retrograde flow through the regurgitant mitral valve. Hence, the effective forward SV is actually reduced.

Table 4.3 shows estimated values for SV at rest and maximum exercise based on the Weber classification of cardiovascular impairment alongside the familiar classification of functional capacity advocated by the New York Heart Association (NYHA).

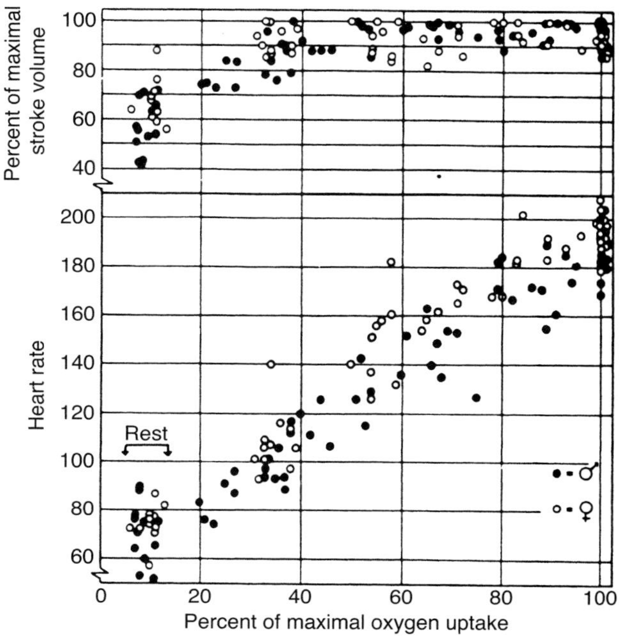


**Figure 4.24** Relationship between SV and $\dot{V}o_2$ as percentages of maximum during an incremental work rate XT. SV reaches a plateau value at approximately 40% of $\dot{V}o_{2max}$. Reproduced with permission from Åstrand, P.-O., Cuddy, T. E., Saltin, B. & Stenberg, J. (1964). Cardiac output during submaximal and maximal work. *J. Appl. Physiol.*, **20**, 268–74.

## Systemic arterial pressure

### Definition, derivation, and units of measurement

- Most exercise professionals are familiar with systemic arterial pressure. Systemic systolic blood pressure coincides with left ventricular contraction whereas systemic diastolic blood pressure coincides with left ventricular relaxation immediately before systole.
- During exercise testing systemic arterial pressure is usually measured by manual or automated sphygmomanometer and occasionally by indwelling arterial catheter connected to a pressure transducer. Measurement techniques are discussed in Chapter 3. The Korotkoff sounds that are heard during sphygmomanometry are reviewed in Table 4.5.

Mean arterial pressure ($P\bar{a}$), which represents the average force of the blood against arterial walls, can be derived by electronic averaging of the pressure signal. Alternatively, $P\bar{a}$ can be estimated using a simple formula that assumes the mean pressure is at a level one-third of the way from diastolic pressure to systolic pressure:

$$P\bar{a} = \frac{Pa_{sys} + (2 \cdot Pa_{dia})}{3} \tag{4.28}$$

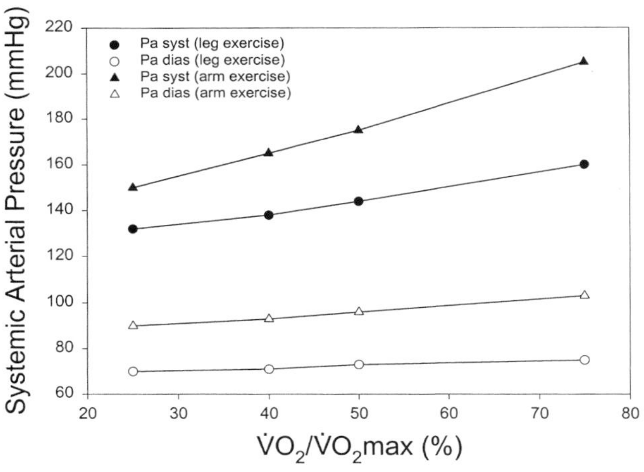


**Figure 4.25** Relationship between systemic arterial pressure and $\dot{V}O_2$ as a percentage of maximum during an incremental work rate XT. Normal responses are shown for systolic and diastolic pressures during leg and arm exercise. Adapted with permission from Åstrand, P.-O., Ekblom, B., Messin, R., Saltin, B. & Stenberg, J. (1965). *J. Appl. Physiol.*, **20**, 253–6.

where $Pa_{sys}$ is systemic arterial systolic pressure and $Pa_{dia}$ is systemic arterial diastolic pressure.

- The traditional units of systemic arterial pressure are millimeters of mercury (mmHg).

## Normal response

During exercise, heart rate and blood pressure increase in response to increased sympathetic tone and circulating catecholamines. Systemic arterial systolic pressure often increases by about 10 mmHg in anticipation of performing an XT. During incremental exercise $Pa_{sys}$ increases by 7–10 mmHg for every MET increase in $\dot{V}O_2$. With maximal exercise, normal subjects exhibit an increase in systemic arterial systolic pressure of 50–70 mmHg and a decrease in systemic arterial diastolic pressure of 4–8 mmHg. Normal responses are shown in Figure 4.25. Note that systemic arterial pressure increases more for arm work compared with leg work. The reduced diastolic pressure during leg work is attributable to reduced peripheral vascular resistance. The increase in systolic pressure during exercise is slightly potentiated by reduced body temperature. Normally, after the termination of exercise, systemic arterial pressure falls rapidly. This phenomenon might lead to relative hypotension in some individuals.

## Abnormal responses

Criteria for abnormal systemic arterial pressures are not easy to define. Undoubtedly, they increase with advancing age – a phenomenon probably explained by reduced systemic vascular compliance with the stiffening of arterial walls. As a result of the increased peripheral vascular resistance, older persons require higher perfusion pressures to maintain adequate tissue blood flow. Notwithstanding these considerations, systemic arterial pressures at rest that are greater than 140/90 mmHg are generally regarded as abnormal.

Several studies indicate that an exaggerated increase in arterial systolic pressure during exercise is predictive of the development of systemic hypertension in later life. Hence, individuals who develop an arterial systolic pressure above 200 mmHg during incremental exercise have a two- to threefold increased risk of developing resting hypertension. Similarly, individuals with untreated hypertension tend to develop arterial systolic pressures over 200 mmHg during exercise. A similar discriminatory value should exist for arterial diastolic pressure and, although one has not been reported, 100 mmHg seems appropriate. Certainly, increases in arterial diastolic pressure during exercise of greater than 15 mmHg have been associated with arteriosclerosis. During maximal incremental exercise, systemic arterial pressures greater than 250/115 mmHg are regarded as indications for stopping the exercise test, as described in Chapter 3.

Arterial systolic pressure normally falls towards maximal exercise by as much as 20 mmHg. This is probably explained by reduced cardiac stroke volume due to inadequate diastolic filling. A convincing fall of systemic arterial systolic pressure of more than 20 mmHg towards end-exercise is suspicious for cardiac dysfunction, either inadequate time for diastolic filling or the development of myocardial ischemia and consequent impairment of contractility. Furthermore, when a fall of this magnitude is observed, the exercise practitioner should consider terminating the test.

Systemic arterial pressures should fall rapidly during the recovery phase immediately after exercise has ceased. When this expected change does not occur, an association with hypertension can be suspected. Routine measurement of blood pressure after 2 min of recovery is helpful in making this determination.

## Pulmonary arterial pressure (*Ppa*)

### Definition, derivation, and units of measurement

- Pulmonary arterial pressure is the cyclical pressure in the pulmonary outflow tract and main pulmonary arteries. The pressure waveform becomes dampened and the mean pressure decreases as blood flows across the pulmonary circulation.
- Pulmonary arterial pressure is best measured using a balloon flotation pulmonary artery catheter which has been inserted via a central vein such as the jugular, subclavian, or femoral vein. When the intention is to measure *Ppa* during exercise, then a long line can be inserted from a vein in the antecubital fossa. Doppler echocardiography offers an alternative method of estimating pulmonary arterial pressure when significant tricuspid regurgitation is present.

$$Ppa_{sys} = Pra + 4 \cdot (\dot{V}_{TR})^2 \qquad (4.29)$$

  where *Pra* is the mean right atrial pressure and $\dot{V}_{TR}$ is peak tricuspid regurgitation velocity measured by echocardiography. *Pra* is assumed to be 5 mmHg if the superior vena cava (SVC) completely collapses during inspiration, 10 mmHg if the SVC partially collapses, and 15 mmHg if the SVC does not collapse.

  Mean pulmonary arterial pressure is derived similarly to mean systemic arterial pressure, as shown in Equation 4.28. Thus:

$$P\overline{pa} = \frac{Ppa_{sys} + (2 \cdot Ppa_{dia})}{3} \qquad (4.30)$$

  where $Ppa_{sys}$ is pulmonary arterial systolic pressure and $Ppa_{dia}$ is pulmonary arterial diastolic pressure.
- The traditional units of pulmonary arterial pressure are millimeters of mercury (mmHg).

### Normal response

Generally, pressures within the pulmonary circulation are about one-sixth of corresponding pressures in the systemic circulation. Therefore, normal resting *Ppa* is approximately 20/10 mmHg, with a mean value of 13 mmHg. Exercise produces modest increases in *Ppa* as shown in Figure 4.26. The increase is more evident in the supine versus upright posture. Provided that the pulmonary circulation is normal, *Ppa* might actually revert to resting levels during prolonged moderate-intensity exercise. The fact that *Ppa* increases so little despite substantial increases in cardiac output during exercise is testimony to the fact that the pulmonary vascular resistance falls dramatically due to extensive recruitment of the pulmonary capillary bed.

### Abnormal responses

Pulmonary vascular disease, either primary or secondary to chronic pulmonary or cardiovascular disease, results in increased *Ppa*. In primary pulmonary hypertension, *Ppa* can be as high as 80/40 mmHg. In pulmonary hypertension secondary to chronic pulmonary disease, $Ppa_{sys}$ is rarely greater than 45 mmHg and $P\overline{pa}$ is rarely greater than 35 mmHg. During exercise *Ppa* will be further increased in patients with resting pulmonary hypertension. When pulmonary vascular disease is severe, the high pulmonary vascular resistance can prevent an adequate increase in cardiac output during exercise. This could result in systemic arterial hypotension in the presence of peripheral vasodilatation. For this reason patients with pulmonary vascular disease must be exercised with caution and careful hemodynamic monitoring.

The development of hypoxemia during exercise will cause reflex pulmonary vasoconstriction and

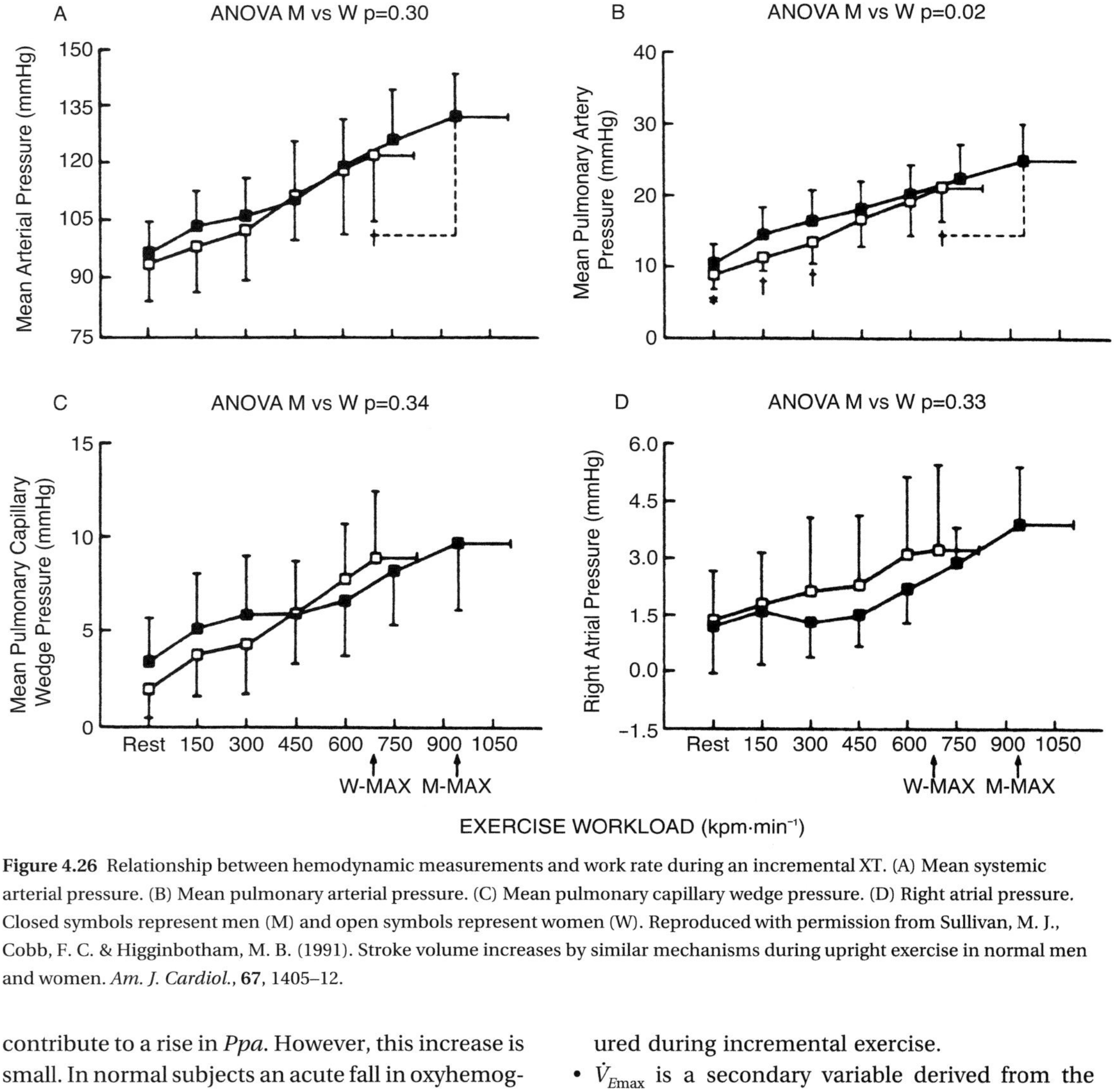


**Figure 4.26** Relationship between hemodynamic measurements and work rate during an incremental XT. (A) Mean systemic arterial pressure. (B) Mean pulmonary arterial pressure. (C) Mean pulmonary capillary wedge pressure. (D) Right atrial pressure. Closed symbols represent men (M) and open symbols represent women (W). Reproduced with permission from Sullivan, M. J., Cobb, F. C. & Higginbotham, M. B. (1991). Stroke volume increases by similar mechanisms during upright exercise in normal men and women. *Am. J. Cardiol.*, **67**, 1405–12.

contribute to a rise in *Ppa*. However, this increase is small. In normal subjects an acute fall in oxyhemoglobin saturation to 77% has been reported to increase *Ppa* by only 5 mmHg.

## Maximum minute ventilation ($\dot{V}_{E\max}$)

### Definition, derivation, and units of measurement

- Maximum minute ventilation is the highest value of ventilation which can be attained and measured during incremental exercise.
- $\dot{V}_{E\max}$ is a secondary variable derived from the product of tidal volume and respiratory rate. During an incremental exercise test, using a metabolic cart, minute ventilation can be calculated this way with each breath. Alternatively, exhaled gas can be collected over a specific time interval (e.g., 1 min) and ventilation measured using a conventional spirometer. Both methods produce variability, the former due to breath-by-breath variations in $V_T$ and $f_R$, the latter due to errors in

interval sampling according to the number of breaths or partial breaths collected. $\dot{V}_{Emax}$ should be determined over a short time interval at end exercise, preferably using an averaging technique, as discussed in Chapter 2. The rolling average of nine breaths that would typically represent 10–15 s at maximum exercise is ideal.

- The units of $\dot{V}_{Emax}$ are $l \cdot min^{-1}$.

### Normal response

With symptom-limited incremental exercise, minute ventilation typically increases from a resting value of 5–8 $l \cdot min^{-1}$ up to 100–150 $l \cdot min^{-1}$, i.e., a 20–30-fold increase. The response is nonlinear (Figure 4.27).

Every individual has a theoretical ventilatory capacity ($\dot{V}_{Ecap}$). $\dot{V}_{Ecap}$ can be measured in the laboratory using a maneuver called maximum voluntary ventilation (MVV). The subject is asked forcibly to increase tidal volume and respiratory rate during 12 or 15 s of a maximal ventilatory effort. The MVV maneuver is clearly effort-dependent and should not be considered to correspond physiologically to maximum exercise ventilation. In particular, hyperventilation induces hypocapnia, which can provoke reflex bronchoconstriction. By contrast, exercise increases circulating catecholamines, which cause bronchodilation. Thus, the mechanics of the respiratory system are different in these two situations. Notwithstanding these shortcomings, MVV measurement is currently the preferred method for estimating $\dot{V}_{Ecap}$.

An alternative method is to estimate $\dot{V}_{Emax}$ from the forced expired volume in one second ($FEV_1$). This is obtained by spirometry during a single forced expiration and has the obvious advantage that it is quick and easy to perform. When a spirometer is not available, $FEV_1$ can be predicted using nomograms (see Appendix C, figures C6–C9). Two equations are commonly used to estimate $\dot{V}_{Ecap}$ from $FEV_1$:

$$\dot{V}_{Ecap} = FEV_1 \cdot 40 \quad (4.31)$$

$$\dot{V}_{Ecap} = FEV_1 \cdot 35 \quad (4.32)$$

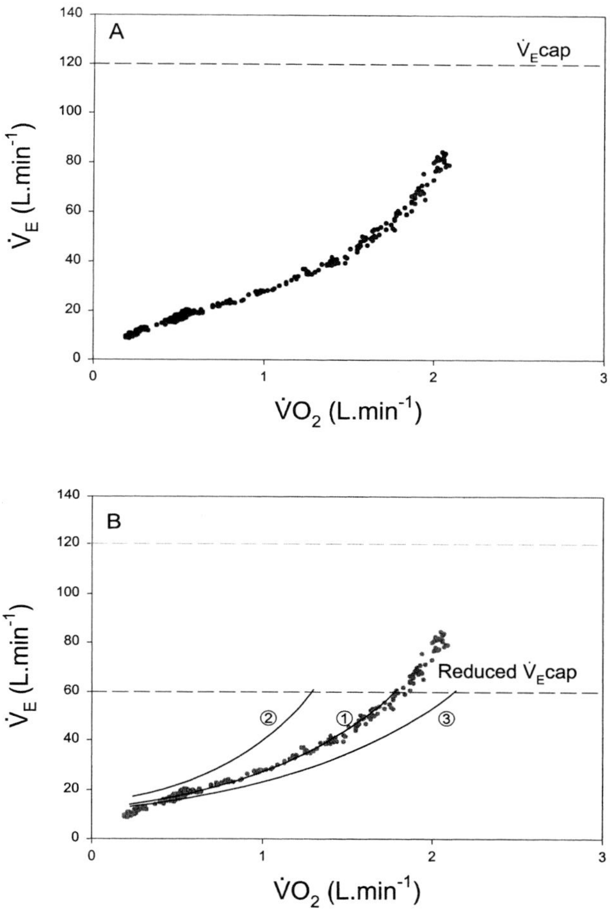


**Figure 4.27** Relationship between $\dot{V}_E$ and $\dot{V}o_2$ during an incremental work rate XT. (A) Normal response where $\dot{V}_{Emax}$ is about 70% of $\dot{V}_{Ecap}$. (B) Abnormal responses for ① reduced $\dot{V}_{Ecap}$ due to obstructive or restrictive mechanical abnormalities; ② increased $\delta\dot{V}_E/\delta\dot{V}o_2$ due to increased $R$, decreased $Paco_2$ or increased $V_D/V_T$; and ③ decreased $\delta\dot{V}_E/\delta\dot{V}o_2$ due to decreased $R$, increased $Paco_2$, or decreased $V_D/V_T$.

Figure 4.28 shows the relationship between $FEV_1$ and $\dot{V}_{Emax}$ for several groups of subjects. Lines representing Equations 4.31 and 4.32 are indicated on this graph. Neither of these equations is accurate over a wide range of $FEV_1$ values. Interestingly, the

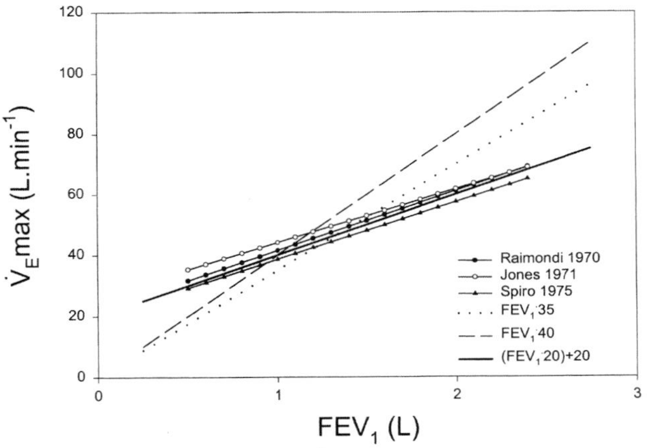


**Figure 4.28** Prediction of $\dot{V}_{Emax}$ during exercise from $FEV_1$. Regression lines are shown from three published studies, along with commonly used prediction equations.

available data are best fitted with the following equation, which is also indicated on Figure 4.28:

$$\dot{V}_{Emax} = (FEV_1 \cdot 20) + 20 \quad (4.33)$$

A normal individual uses 50–75% of his or her ventilatory capacity at maximum exercise. Thus, a normal individual is not expected to exhibit ventilatory limitation. Athletes who have successfully extended their cardiovascular fitness use a higher proportion of their ventilatory capacity at maximum exercise. Although not strictly limited by the mechanical considerations of $\dot{V}_{Emax}$, athletes might experience expiratory flow limitation at maximum exercise (see below).

### Abnormal responses

Mechanical abnormalities of the respiratory system such as obstructive or restrictive lung disease, respiratory muscle weakness, or reduced chest wall compliance all reduce ventilatory capacity. If sufficiently severe, such abnormalities could result in true ventilatory limitation at maximum exercise with a reduced $\dot{V}_{Emax}$. True ventilatory limitation is defined as occurring when the ventilatory requirement for maximum exercise ($\dot{V}_{Emax}$) reaches the ventilatory capacity ($\dot{V}_{Ecap}$) (Figure 4.27).

## Slope of the ventilatory response ($\delta\dot{V}_E/\delta\dot{V}o_2$)

### Definition, derivation, and units of measurement

- $\delta\dot{V}_E/\delta\dot{V}o_2$ is the slope of the relationship between minute ventilation and $\dot{V}o_2$ during incremental exercise. The relationship is nonlinear and increases throughout incremental exercise (Figure 4.27). Sometimes, three phases of the response can be discerned which conform to the concepts of the underlying physiological determinants of the response. During the first phase, ventilation is coupled to the increasing $\dot{V}o_2$. During the second phase, ventilation is coupled to the increasing $\dot{V}co_2$, including carbon dioxide derived from bicarbonate buffering of lactic acid. During the third phase, acidemia acting via the carotid body stimulates ventilation.
- The $\delta\dot{V}_E/\delta\dot{V}o_2$ relationship is determined from the Bohr equation:

$$\dot{V}co_2 = \dot{V}_A \cdot F_Aco_2 \quad (4.34)$$

where $\dot{V}co_2$ is carbon dioxide output, $\dot{V}_A$ is alveolar ventilation, and $F_Aco_2$ is the fractional concentration of alveolar carbon dioxide. Substituting $(\dot{V}_E - \dot{V}_D)$ for $\dot{V}_A$ and $(\dot{V}o_2 \cdot R)$ for $\dot{V}co_2$, then:

$$\dot{V}_E - \dot{V}_D = \dot{V}o_2 \cdot \frac{R}{F_Aco_2} \quad (4.35)$$

where $\dot{V}_E$ is minute ventilation, $\dot{V}_D$ is dead space ventilation, and $R$ is the respiratory exchange ratio.

$$F_Aco_2 = \frac{Paco_2}{P_B - 47} \quad (4.36)$$

where $Paco_2$ is partial pressure of arterial carbon dioxide which is presumed to equal the alveolar partial pressure of carbon dioxide, $P_B$ is the barometric pressure and 47 represents the partial pressure of saturated water vapor at body temperature.

$$\dot{V}_D = \dot{V}_E \cdot \left(1 - \frac{V_D}{V_T}\right) \quad (4.37)$$

where $\dot{V}_D$ is the dead space volume and $V_T$ is the tidal volume.

$$\dot{V}_E = \dot{V}O_2 \cdot \frac{R}{PaCO_2 \cdot (1 - V_D/V_T)} \quad (4.38)$$

Hence, the slope $\delta\dot{V}_E/\delta\dot{V}O_2$ is related to three important factors: (1) the respiratory exchange ratio, which in turn is related to metabolic substrate; (2) the level at which arterial carbon dioxide tension is regulated; and (3) the dead space/tidal volume ratio, a measure of ventilatory efficiency.

- The $\delta\dot{V}_E/\delta\dot{V}O_2$ slope has no units.

### Normal response

The value for $\delta\dot{V}_E/\delta\dot{V}O_2$ changes throughout incremental exercise. There is little information regarding reference values for $\delta\dot{V}_E/\delta\dot{V}O_2$. However, Spiro et al. (1974) report values of 23–26 for men and 27 for women. Some commercial exercise systems display a normal zone for the $\delta\dot{V}_E/\delta\dot{V}O_2$ response, taking into account an arbitrary range of variation.

### Abnormal responses

Equation 4.38 above illustrates that $\delta\dot{V}_E/\delta\dot{V}O_2$ is related to the $R$, $PaCO_2$, and $V_D/V_T$. Alterations of $\delta\dot{V}_E/\delta\dot{V}O_2$ can therefore be helpfully interpreted in terms of these underlying physiological parameters. With reference to Figure 4.27, consider the following circumstances which illustrate important influences on the ventilatory response pattern during incremental exercise:

1. Ingestion of carbohydrate prior to exercise increases $R$ and would thus tend to increase $\delta\dot{V}_E/\delta\dot{V}O_2$. By contrast, ingestion of a higher-fat, lower-carbohydrate diet would tend to decrease $\delta\dot{V}_E/\delta\dot{V}O_2$. These considerations form the basis of the rationale for recommending a higher-fat, lower-carbohydrate diet for patients with chronic lung disease with the hope of reducing ventilatory requirement for exercise. Although rigorous scientific justification for this approach is lacking, it is known that excessive carbohydrate ingestion impairs exercise performance in such patients, presumably by increasing ventilatory requirement.

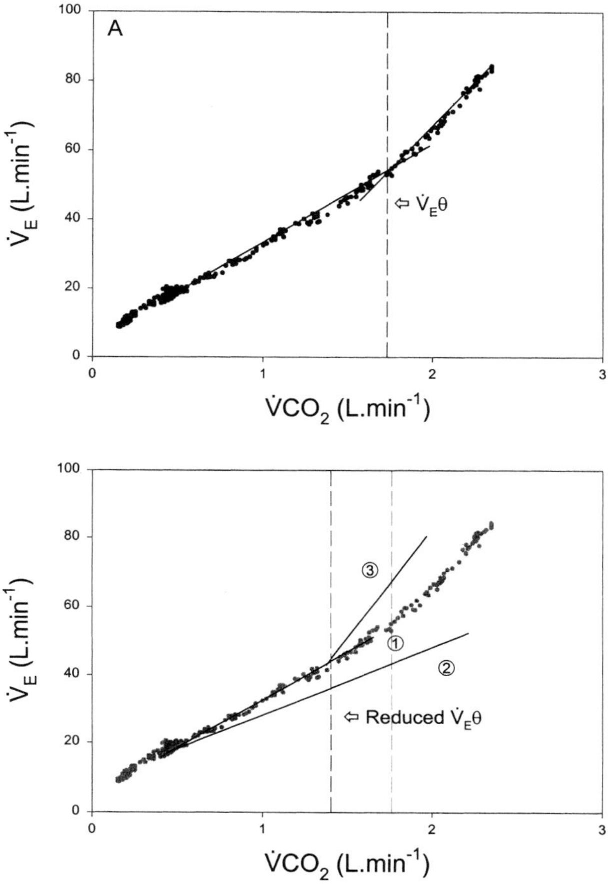


**Figure 4.29** Relationship between $\dot{V}_E$ and $\dot{V}CO_2$ during an incremental work rate XT. (A) Normal response, with $\dot{V}_E\theta$ identified. (B) Abnormal responses for ① suboptimal effort, ② abnormal ventilatory response to carbon dioxide, and ③ depleted bicarbonate-buffering capacity.

2. Disturbances of ventilatory control which result in higher or lower than normal $PaCO_2$ can be expected to alter the ventilatory response to exercise. For example, anxiety causing alveolar hyperventilation results in a low $PaCO_2$. Maintenance of a low $PaCO_2$ increases $\delta\dot{V}_E/\delta\dot{V}O_2$ during incremental exercise. This situation is seen in many patients with chronic lung disease who display anxiety, fear, and marked breathlessness.

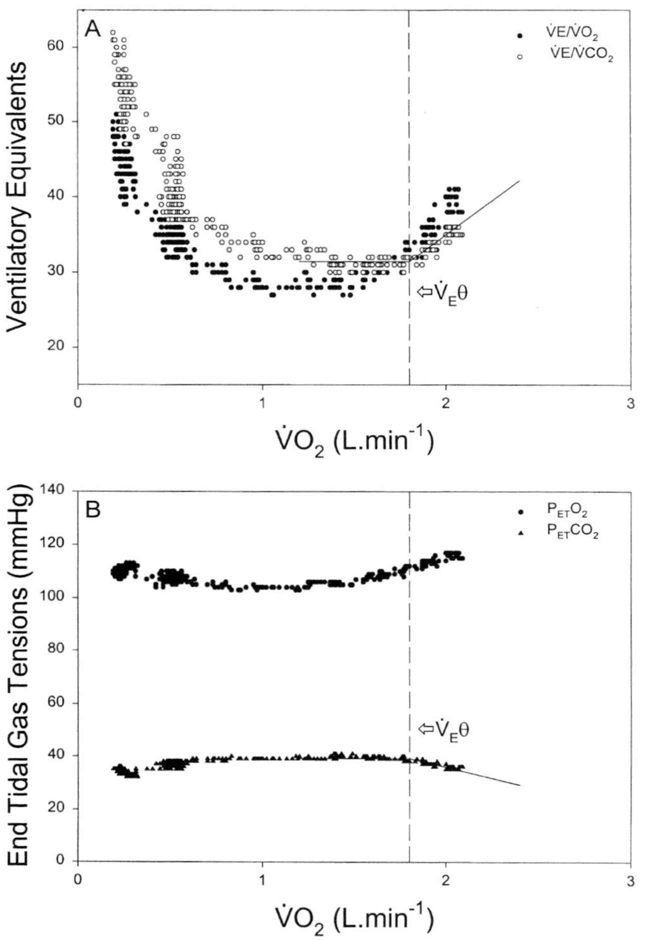


**Figure 4.30** Alternative method for the determination of $\dot{V}_E\theta$ using the dual criteria graphs. (A) Relationships between the ventilatory equivalents ($\dot{V}_E/\dot{V}O_2$ and $\dot{V}_E/\dot{V}CO_2$) and $\dot{V}O_2$. (B) Relationship between the end-tidal gas tensions ($P_{ET}O_2$ and $P_{ET}CO_2$) and $\dot{V}O_2$. $\dot{V}_E\theta$ is identified as the point at which $\dot{V}_E/\dot{V}CO_2$ rises and $P_{ET}CO_2$ falls. $\dot{V}_E/\dot{V}O_2$ and $P_{ET}O_2$ are noted to have begun rising earlier at $\dot{V}_E\theta$ (see Figure 4.9).

These patients have been called "pink puffers" because their exaggerated ventilatory drive is manifest in breathlessness and maintenance of normal oxygenation. Notably, some patients with chronic lung disease tolerate an increased $Paco_2$ (alveolar hypoventilation). Along with the increased $Paco_2$ there is often a reduced $Pao_2$ (hypoxemia). These patients have been called "blue bloaters." Although they appear to have a diminished respiratory drive during exercise, paradoxically they require a lower level of ventilation to excrete a given amount of carbon dioxide. Reference to Figure 4.27 shows that tolerance of a higher $Paco_2$ reduces $\delta\dot{V}_E/\delta\dot{V}O_2$. "Blue bloaters" are noticeably less breathless than "pink puffers."

3. Lastly, breathing efficiency, as demonstrated by the ratio of dead space to tidal volume, has predictable effects on ventilatory requirement. High $V_D/V_T$, as seen in chronic lung diseases, particularly emphysema and pulmonary vascular disease, results in a steeper $\delta\dot{V}_E/\delta\dot{V}O_2$.

In summary, any physiological mechanism which tends to increase $\delta\dot{V}_E/\delta\dot{V}O_2$ will result in a higher ventilatory requirement for all levels of exercise. Furthermore, if ventilatory capacity is significantly reduced, a steeper $\delta\dot{V}_E/\delta\dot{V}O_2$ will result in earlier exercise termination due to ventilatory limitation. Conversely, any physiological mechanism which tends to reduce $\delta\dot{V}_E/\delta\dot{V}O_2$ will result in a lower ventilatory requirement for all levels of exercise. For individuals with ventilatory limitation, such a change would be expected to increase exercise capacity (Figure 4.27).

## Ventilatory threshold, respiratory compensation point ($\dot{V}_E\theta$)

### Definition, derivation, and units of measurement

- During incremental exercise minute ventilation increases ever more rapidly towards its maximum (Figure 4.27). However, throughout lower- and moderate-intensity exercise, $\dot{V}_E$ is coupled appropriately to the $\dot{V}CO_2$, as shown in Figure 4.29. At higher-intensity exercise, a point exists when $\dot{V}_E$ becomes dissociated from $\dot{V}CO_2$. This point is usually easily identified during XT and can be termed the ventilatory threshold ($\dot{V}_E\theta$).

*Terminology*
*The definition of ventilatory threshold needs clarification since it has often been used synonymously with lactate threshold and anaerobic threshold. A ventilatory threshold can only truly be described when minute ventilation is being measured. The question then arises as to what constitutes a distinct and meaningful threshold in the ventilatory response. At and immediately above the metabolic threshold (see* $\dot{V}O_2\theta$*),* $\dot{V}_E$ *remains coupled to* $\dot{V}CO_2$ *and is therefore appropriately geared to metabolism, including buffering. It is only when acidemia stimulates ventilation independently via the carotid bodies that* $\dot{V}_E$ *increases independently. This is a distinct physiological entity that is well illustrated by plotting the relationship between* $\dot{V}_E$ and $\dot{V}CO_2$ *(see section on normal response, below). Furthermore, human subjects appreciate this point as the moment when ventilation increases noticeably. Therefore it is logical to designate this point as the ventilatory threshold (*$\dot{V}_E\theta$*) to distinguish it from the metabolic threshold (*$\dot{V}O_2\theta$*). Others have referred to this entity as the respiratory compensation point, wishing to acknowledge that it represents ventilatory compensation for lactic acidemia.*

- Given that $\dot{V}_E\theta$ represents the dissociation of $\dot{V}_E$ from $\dot{V}CO_2$, this threshold can be best identified by plotting these two variables (Figure 4.29). This relationship remains linear as long as $\dot{V}_E$ is coupled to $\dot{V}CO_2$ but increases more steeply at $\dot{V}_E\theta$. This method yields a value for $\dot{V}CO_2$ at which $\dot{V}_E\theta$ occurs. However, in order to relate $\dot{V}_E\theta$ to exercise intensity, and to compare it with $\dot{V}O_2\theta$, it is often desirable to relate $\dot{V}_E\theta$ to the level of $\dot{V}O_2$ at which it occurs. The value of $\dot{V}O_2$ which corresponds with the value of $\dot{V}CO_2$ at $\dot{V}_E\theta$ can be found quite simply by reference to tabulated values of $\dot{V}O_2$ and $\dot{V}CO_2$ or to the plot of $\dot{V}CO_2$ versus $\dot{V}O_2$. An alternative method exists for deriving $\dot{V}_E\theta$ using the ventilatory equivalents and end-tidal gas tensions in a way that is similar to the method used for the derivation of $\dot{V}O_2\theta$ (Figure 4.9). The dual criteria for detection of $\dot{V}O_2\theta$ stipulate that $\dot{V}_E/\dot{V}O_2$ and $P_{ET}O_2$ begin to increase whilst $\dot{V}_E/\dot{V}CO_2$ and $P_{ET}CO_2$ remain constant. The same plots can be used to identify the point, later in the study, when $\dot{V}_E/\dot{V}CO_2$ begins to increase and $P_{ET}CO_2$ begins to decrease simultaneously (Figure 4.30). This point represents $\dot{V}_E\theta$.
- The units of $\dot{V}_E\theta$ are the same as those for oxygen uptake, i.e., $l \cdot min^{-1}$ or $ml \cdot kg^{-1} \cdot min^{-1}$.

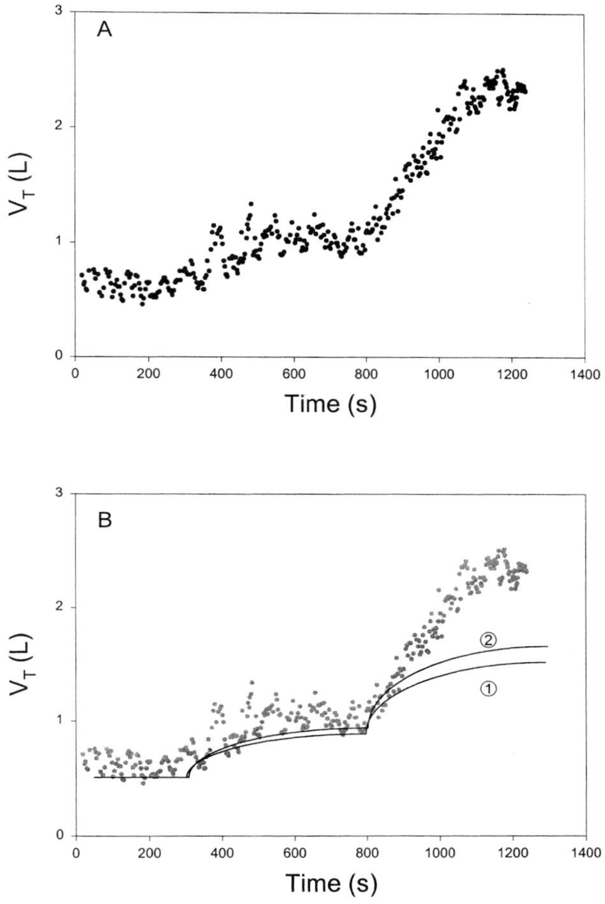


**Figure 4.31** Relationship between $V_T$ and time during an incremental work rate XT. (A) Normal response. (B) Abnormal responses for ① obstructive pulmonary disease and ② restrictive pulmonary disease.

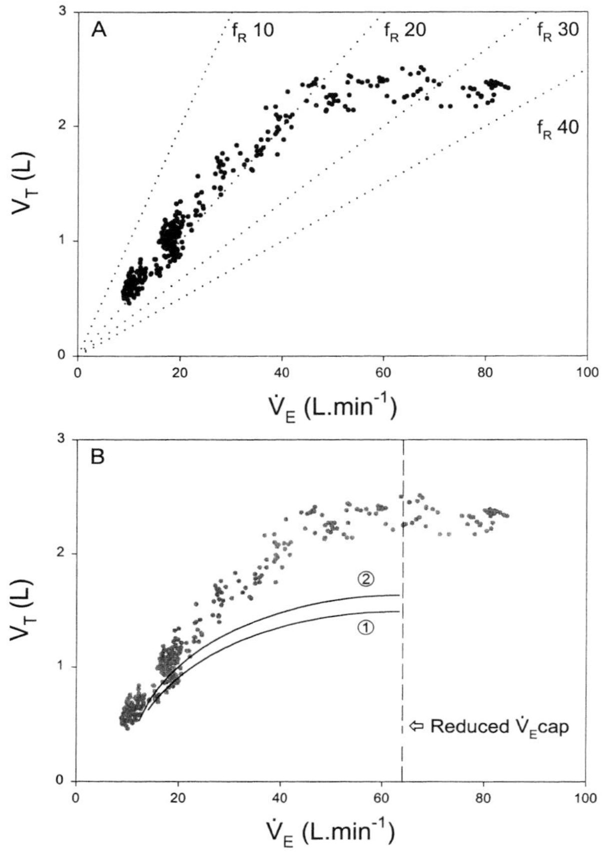


**Figure 4.32** Relationship between $V_T$ and $\dot{V}_E$ during an incremental work rate XT. (A) Normal response with isopleths representing different respiratory rates. (B) Abnormal responses for ① obstructive pulmonary disease and ② restrictive pulmonary disease. Also the consequences of reduced ventilatory capacity are illustrated.

### Normal response (Figure 4.29A)

$\dot{V}_E\theta$ occurs at 80–90% of $\dot{V}O_{2max}$. The identification of $\dot{V}_E\theta$ during XT is a reliable indicator that the subject is close to maximal effort. $\dot{V}_E\theta$ has not been systematically studied and therefore little more can be said about its normal value.

### Abnormal responses (Figure 4.29B)

When $\dot{V}_E\theta$ cannot be identified from the plot of $\dot{V}_E$ versus $\dot{V}CO_2$, this typically indicates a submaximal effort or premature test termination. Conditions which deplete bicarbonate-buffering capacity such as chronic metabolic acidosis might result in a lower $\dot{V}_E\theta$ but also a lower $\dot{V}O_{2max}$. An unusual group of patients who had carotid body resection in the 1960s to alleviate breathlessness no longer exhibited $\dot{V}_E\theta$. Also, rare individuals with abnormalities of ventilatory control fail to respond to lactic acidemia and therefore do not exhibit $\dot{V}_E\theta$.

## Tidal volume ($V_T$)

### Definition, derivation, and units of measurement

- $V_T$ is the volume of a single breath.
- By convention, $V_T$ is expressed as the expired volume and is derived by volumetric displacement or by integration of the expiratory flow signal with respect to time. Several factors cause the expired volume to be slightly different from the inspired volume, notably temperature, humidity, and the altered composition of expired gas that result from exchange of oxygen and carbon dioxide in the lungs. Typically the expired volume is slightly greater than the inspired volume. During integrative XT it is common to measure $V_E$. However, both $V_I$ and $V_E$ must be known in order to calculate oxygen uptake (see Appendix B, Equation B30). $V_I$ and $V_E$ are interrelated by the Haldane equation which assumes that the volume of nitrogen expired is equal to the volume inspired:

$$V_I \cdot F_I N_2 = V_E \cdot F_E N_2 \quad (4.39)$$

The inspired nitrogen concentration ($F_I N_2$) is assumed to be 0.7903. The expired nitrogen concentration ($F_E N_2$) can either be measured, e.g., using a mass spectrometer, or calculated, assuming that the expired concentrations of $O_2$, $CO_2$ and $N_2$ add up to 100%, i.e.:

$$F_E N_2 = (1 - F_E O_2 - F_E CO_2) \quad (4.40)$$

- The units of $V_T$ are liters or milliliters.

### Normal response (Figure 4.31A)

Normal resting $V_T$ varies according to body size and

also varies from breath to breath. A simple estimate of normal resting $V_T$ of 10 ml per kg of body weight can be used to set a mechanical ventilator on the intensive care unit. In other words, for a 70-kg man, resting $V_T$ would be 700 ml. Note that $V_T$ measured during integrative XT is influenced by the dead space of the breathing apparatus.

During exercise $V_T$ increases in a nonlinear fashion reaching a plateau value equal to approximately 50–60% of vital capacity at about 70% of $\dot{V}O_{2max}$ (Figure 4.31). The pattern of increase in $V_T$ is often studied in relation to $\dot{V}_E$, as described by the Hey plot ($\dot{V}_E$ versus $V_T$) or its reciprocal ($V_T$ versus $\dot{V}_E$), as shown in Figure 4.32. The isopleths shown in Figure 4.32A represent respiratory rate ($f_R$).

### Abnormal responses (Figure 4.31B)

Human breathing patterns vary considerably, particularly when first breathing through a mouthpiece at rest. However, during exercise one expects to see a more regular breathing pattern established. A persistent, erratic breathing pattern, with undue variability of $V_T$, occurs with anxiety and is often a feature of hyperventilation.

Patients with chronic pulmonary disease, both restrictive and obstructive, have reduced $V_T$ during exercise along with a compensatory increase in breathing frequency (see below). There may be subtle differences between these two types of patients but in practice they are difficult to distinguish (Figure 4.31 and Figure 4.32). Generally, restrictive patients achieve their maximum $V_T$ early during incremental exercise and then rely on increasing breathing frequency to increase $\dot{V}_E$.

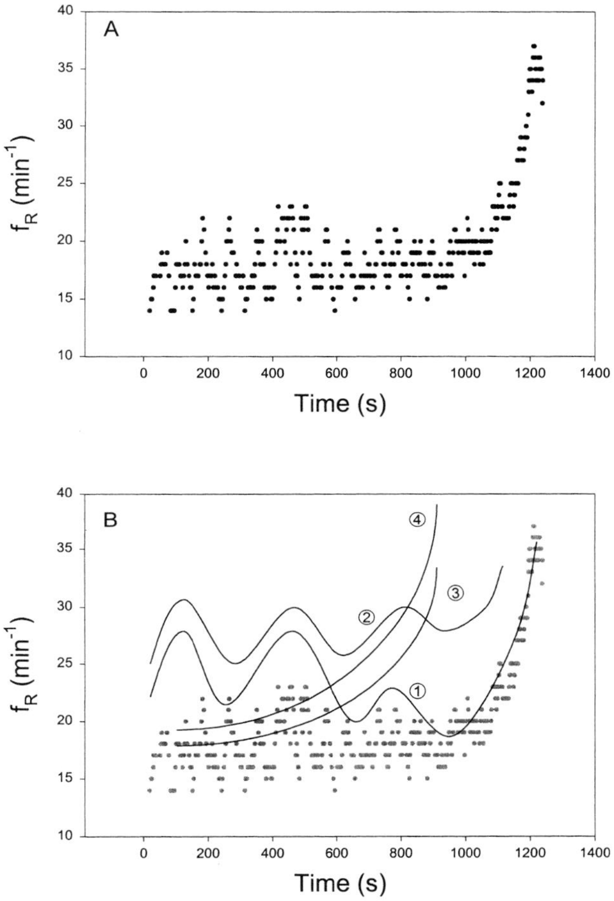


**Figure 4.33** Relationship between $f_R$ and time during an incremental work rate XT. (A) Normal response. (B) Abnormal responses for ① hyperventilation which normalizes at higher exercise intensity; ② hyperventilation which persists throughout the study; ③ obstructive pulmonary disease; and ④ restrictive pulmonary disease.

## Respiratory rate ($f_R$)

### Definition, derivation, and units of measurement

- The respiratory rate is the number of breaths taken per minute.
- $f_R$ is a primary variable. In a field XT, the number of breaths taken per minute can be counted by visual inspection of chest wall movements. During integrative XT with exhaled gas analysis, the derivation of $f_R$ depends upon accurate breath detection. Metabolic measurement systems usually rely on cessation of expiratory flow or measurement of a sustained inspiratory flow to determine the onset of a new breath phase. However, owing to the variability of flow patterns, criteria must be developed to reject erroneous signals that would not truly represent an actual breath. This is certainly one of the challenges of

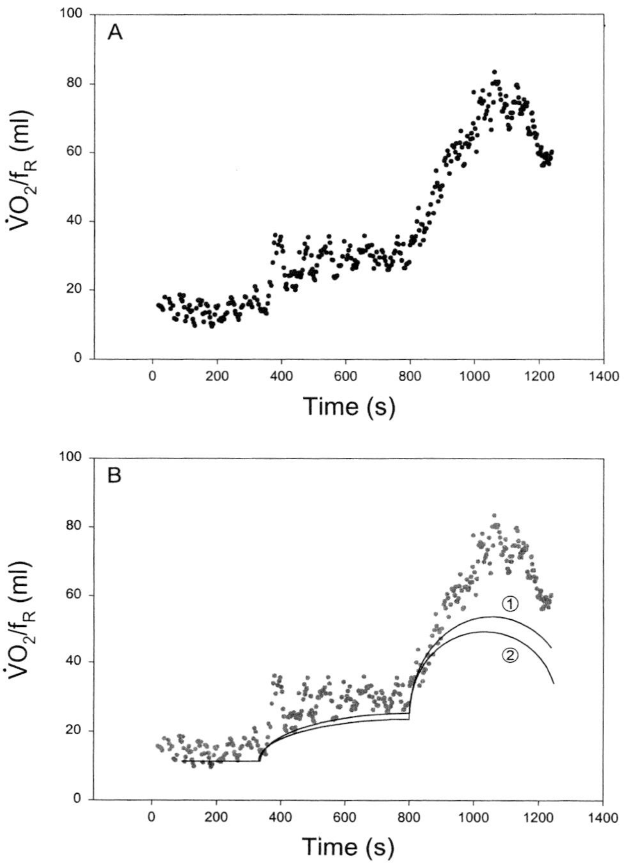


**Figure 4.34** Relationship between $\dot{V}O_2/f_R$ and time during an incremental work rate XT. (A) Normal response. (B) Abnormal responses for ① obstructive pulmonary disease and ② restrictive pulmonary disease.

integrative XT. Once a new breath has been detected, $f_R$ can be calculated using the time interval from the preceding breath or, preferably, the new breath interval can be factored in with several preceding breaths to obtain a more consistent measure of $f_R$.

- The units of $f_R$ are breaths per minute or $min^{-1}$.

### Normal response (Figure 4.33A)

The normal resting $f_R$ is 8–12 $min^{-1}$. Typically, when subjects first breathe through a mouthpiece, $f_R$ increases, e.g., up to 20 $min^{-1}$. $f_R$ can be used to assess stability at rest before proceeding with the next phase of XT. However, it is not unusual for $f_R$ to remain high at rest in certain individuals.

Characteristically, $f_R$ increases steadily to a maximum value of 30–40 $min^{-1}$. $f_{Rmax}$ rarely exceeds 50 $min^{-1}$. However, some élite athletes may exhibit $f_R$ values as high as 80 $min^{-1}$ at maximum exercise.

### Abnormal responses (Figure 4.33B)

A clear distinction between normal and abnormal responses for $f_R$ during exercise does not exist. However, it is unusual for $f_R$ to remain above 20 $min^{-1}$ at rest or to exceed 50 $min^{-1}$ at maximum exercise, with the possible exception of élite athletes.

Patients with restrictive pulmonary disease are generally unable to increase $V_T$ adequately during exercise; therefore they depend upon increasing $f_R$ to meet their ventilatory requirement. These patients might exhibit values of $f_R$ at maximum exercise greater than 50 $min^{-1}$.

Hyperventilation, for example as a result of anxiety, might also cause $f_R$ to be greater than 50 $min^{-1}$. Unlike patients with restrictive disease, cases of primary hyperventilation are often associated with erratic breathing patterns, i.e., marked variations in $\dot{V}_E$ and $V_T$ from breath to breath, and characteristic changes in ventilatory equivalents and end-tidal gas tensions (see below).

## Oxygen breath ($\dot{V}O_2/f_R$)

### Definition, derivation, and units of measurement

- The oxygen breath is a measure of breathing efficiency indicating what metabolic value derives from each breath. In the same way that the oxygen pulse is an indirect measure of cardiac stroke volume, the $\dot{V}O_2/f_R$ is related to alveolar tidal volume. The $\dot{V}O_2/f_R$ can be tracked during incremental exercise to illustrate how breathing efficiency might change at differing work intensities.
- $\dot{V}O_2/f_R$ is a secondary variable calculated by dividing the instantaneous oxygen uptake by the respiratory rate:

$$\text{Oxygen breath} = \frac{\dot{V}o_2}{f_R} \quad (4.41)$$

- The units of oxygen breath are milliliters per breath or ml.

### Normal response (Figure 4.34A)

The resting $\dot{V}o_2/f_R$ for normal subjects is 10–20 ml · breath$^{-1}$. Typically this increases to 80–100 ml · breath$^{-1}$ at maximum exercise. The pattern of increase is a rising exponential up to the region of $\dot{V}_E\theta$. Above $\dot{V}_E\theta$, when ventilation is completely uncoupled from metabolism and carotid body stimulation accelerates $f_R$, it is not unusual to observe a reduction in $\dot{V}o_2/f_R$ (Figure 4.34A).

### Abnormal responses (Figure 4.34B)

A submaximal exercise response will be associated with a submaximal $\dot{V}o_2/f_R$. Also, failure to observe a fall in $\dot{V}o_2/f_R$ towards end exercise most likely indicates a submaximal effort. Individuals with obstructive or restrictive pulmonary disease will exhibit a low maximum $\dot{V}o_2/f_R$. Both groups can exhibit a decrease in $\dot{V}o_2/f_R$ towards end exercise. Generally, $\dot{V}o_2/f_R$ is lower in restrictive compared with obstructive individuals.

## Ratio of inspiratory to expiratory time ($T_I/T_E$)

### Definition, derivation, and units of measurement

- The ratio of inspiratory to expiratory time, also called the *I/E* ratio, indicates what proportion of the time taken for each breath is devoted to inspiration versus expiration. Hence, $T_I/T_E$ is a measure of breathing pattern.
- The conventional method for measuring ventilation uses a flow transducer. Mixing chamber systems use unidirectional transducers, which summate exhaled breaths to derive exhaled minute ventilation. Breath-by-breath systems are more sophisticated, integrating exhaled flows with each breath to derive expired tidal volume or both expired and inspired tidal volume, depending on whether the flow transducer is unidirectional or bi-directional. Whole breath time ($T_{TOT}$) is used to calculate respiratory rate. Clearly, ($T_{TOT}$) is the sum of inspired time ($T_I$) and expired time ($T_E$) whereas $T_I/T_E$ is the ratio of these times.

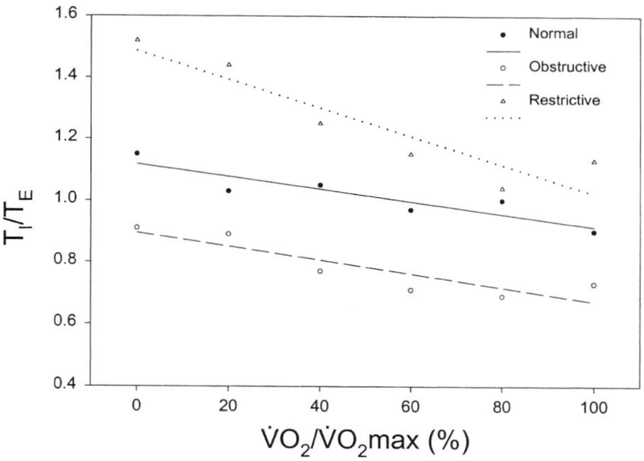


**Figure 4.35** Relationship between $T_I/T_E$ and percentage of $\dot{V}o_{2max}$ for normal subjects and patients with obstructive or restrictive disease. Mean data points and regression lines are shown. Generally, $T_I/T_E$ in obstructive patients is less than in normal subjects, whereas in restrictive patients it is higher.

$$f_R = \frac{60}{T_{TOT}} \quad (4.42)$$

$$T_{TOT} = T_I + T_E \quad (4.43)$$

$$I/E \text{ ratio} = \frac{T_I}{T_E} \quad (4.44)$$

Knowledge of $f_R$ or $T_{TOT}$, together with either $T_I$ or $T_E$, enables one to calculate the $T_I/T_E$.

- Being the ratio of two time intervals, $T_I/T_E$ has no units.

### Normal response (Figure 4.35)

Measured nonintrusively, $T_I/T_E$ is normally 0.8–1.0, both at rest and at maximum exercise. When a subject first breathes through a mouthpiece, $T_I/T_E$ might be disturbed by artificial prolongation of $T_I$. Hence, it is common throughout an incremental exercise test to see $T_I/T_E$ slowly decline (Figure 4.35).

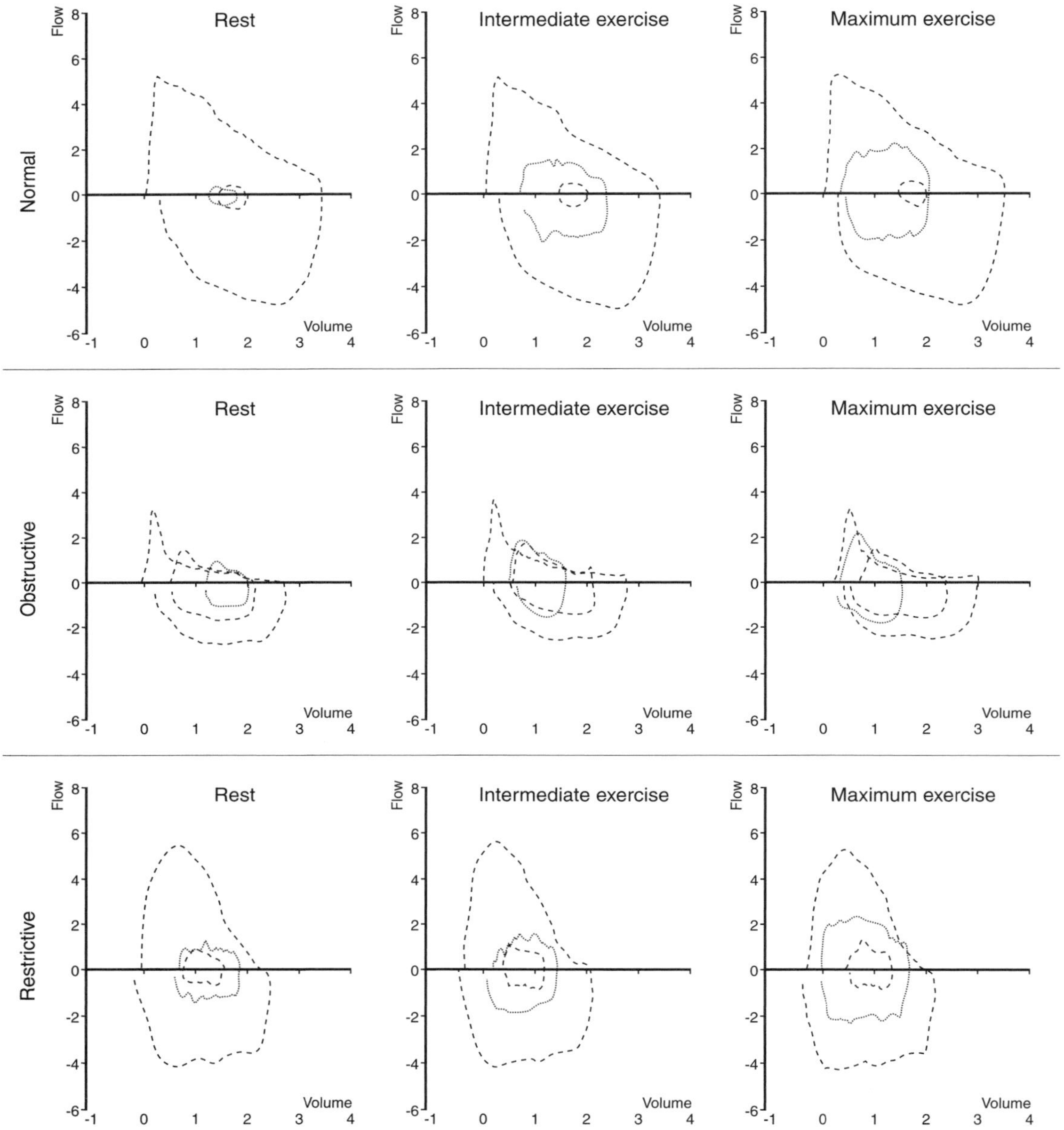


**Figure 4.36** Flow–volume loops for rest, intermediate exercise intensity, and maximum exercise in a normal subject (top row), a patient with obstructive disease due to chronic bronchitis (middle row), and a patient with restrictive disease due to pulmonary interstitial fibrosis (bottom row). In each panel the pretest maximal expiratory and inspiratory flow volume envelope is shown as the outer dashed line. The pretest resting loop is shown as the inner dashed line.

Given the various mechanical factors of the human respiratory system, including airway resistance and lung recoil, $T_I/T_E$ has an optimum value, rather like ventilation–perfusion ratio ($\dot{V}/\dot{Q}$). Coincidentally, this value appears to be approximately 0.8, the same as the ideal $\dot{V}/\dot{Q}$.

### Abnormal responses (Figure 4.35)

Acceptance of the concept of an ideal $T_I/T_E$ allows one to judge abnormalities of breathing pattern during exercise testing.

In obstructive pulmonary disease such as chronic bronchitis or asthma, expiratory flows are limited and there is an obligatory $T_E$ required to avoid dynamic hyperinflation as breath time shortens during exercise. Hence, a greater proportion of the breath time needs to be devoted to expiration compared with a normal subject. Thus, $T_I/T_E$ is less than 0.8 (Figure 4.35).

In restrictive pulmonary disease, such as pulmonary fibrosis or kyphoscoliosis, expiratory flow is facilitated by increased lung or chest wall recoil, whereas inspired flow is constrained by the same phenomenon. There is an obligatory $T_I$ required to avoid dynamic hypoinflation as breath time shortens towards maximum exercise. Hence, a greater proportion of the breath time needs to be devoted to inspiration compared with a normal subject. Thus, $T_I/T_E$ is greater than 0.8 (Figure 4.35).

## Inspiratory and expiratory flow: volume relationships ($\dot{V}_I$: $V$ and $\dot{V}_E$: $V$)

### Definition, derivation, and units of measurement

- Using a forced maneuver, it is possible to define the maximal inspiratory and expiratory flow capabilities for the respiratory system at various stages of lung volume. The typical maximal flow–volume plot shown in the top left-hand panel of Figure 4.36 illustrates that flow is critically dependent upon lung volume during the course of a single breath. This phenomenon is partly explained by changes in airway caliber with changes in lung volume.
- The maximal flow–volume loop is defined at rest using a forced single-breath maneuver. Then, inspiratory and expiratory flows can be observed at different stages of exercise for comparison with the theoretical maximal values to seek evidence of flow limitation. The method depends upon referencing flow to instantaneous lung volume, since absolute lung volume may change during exercise. This is accomplished at the time of recording tidal airflow by asking the subject to perform a maximal inspiration to total lung capacity (TLC). There is reasonable evidence that TLC does not change during exercise and so can be used as a reference point for absolute lung volume. Of course, this analytical approach is critically dependent on the subject being able to achieve TLC on command by performing inspiratory capacity maneuvers at various stages during exercise.
- The units of flow are $l \cdot s^{-1}$.

### Normal response

Typical inspiratory and expiratory flows during resting tidal breathing, an intermediate level of exercise intensity, and maximal exercise are shown in the top row of panels of Figure 4.36, superimposed on the normal maximal flow–volume plot. Although inspiratory and expiratory flows are measured in $l \cdot s^{-1}$, normal values are not clearly defined for a given individual. In fact, the flow–volume relationship is interpreted visually. Note the inspiratory maneuvers to TLC (shown as negative flows), which have been used to determine the position of each flow loop on the volume axis. It can be seen that the increase in tidal volume ($V_T$) with increasing exercise intensity is mainly due to an increase in the end-inspiratory lung volume (EILV). Normally, however, end-expiratory lung volume (EELV) simultaneously decreases during exercise and this change makes an important contribution to the increased tidal volume.

The tidal flow–volume loop is not expected to impinge upon the maximal flow–volume envelope with increasing exercise intensity in normal subjects. However, we now recognize that some degree of expiratory airflow limitation is normal, particularly in endurance-trained subjects at higher exercise intensities. The extent to which this phenomenon may influence maximal exercise capacity is not known.

### Abnormal responses

Clinical experience in the interpretation of flow–volume loops during exercise is still limited. Nevertheless, evidence of airflow obstruction during inspiration or expiration and volume restriction either in terms of tidal volume or encroachment on TLC can be identified.

Expiratory flow limitation, as seen in asthma or chronic bronchitis, imposes a concavity on the expiratory limb of the flow–volume curve. Early impingement of the tidal flow–volume loop on this envelope causes a shift to a higher operational lung volume. This phenomenon is called dynamic hyperinflation (see the middle row of Figure 4.36).

Restrictive pulmonary disease results in a reduced TLC, either as a result of reduced lung or chest wall compliance, or alternatively due to respiratory muscle weakness. The reduced TLC imposes a constraint on inspiratory capacity throughout exercise and can be identified as early encroachment of the tidal flow–volume loop on TLC (see the bottom row of Figure 4.36).

Finally, it should be appreciated that expiratory flow limitation (obstruction), by causing dynamic inflation, also results in a relative restrictive abnormality as the operational lung volume approaches TLC.

## Ventilatory equivalents ($\dot{V}_E/\dot{V}O_2$ and $\dot{V}_E/\dot{V}CO_2$)

### Definition, derivation, and units of measurement

- Ventilatory equivalents are measures of breathing efficiency, which relate instantaneous minute ventilation to the metabolic rate of oxygen uptake or carbon dioxide output.
- Ventilatory equivalents are secondary variables derived as the ratio of instantaneous minute ventilation to oxygen uptake ($\dot{V}_E/\dot{V}O_2$) or carbon dioxide output ($\dot{V}_E/\dot{V}CO_2$).
- Being ratios of two flows, ventilatory equivalents have no units.

### Normal response (Figure 4.37A)

Resting ventilatory equivalents are variable, but generally 30–60. The effect of breathing through a mouthpiece, particularly for the first time, can induce a degree of hyperventilation and result in higher resting ventilatory equivalents. During exercise a subject is more inclined to match ventilation appropriately to metabolic exchange of oxygen and carbon dioxide.

Ventilatory equivalents fall steadily during the early stage of incremental exercise. The explanation for this can be seen by geometrical consideration of graphs of ventilation versus $\dot{V}O_2$ or $\dot{V}CO_2$. Both plots have positive intercepts on the *y*-axis. Instantaneous values for $\dot{V}_E/\dot{V}O_2$ and $\dot{V}_E/\dot{V}CO_2$, represented by the slope of lines drawn from the origin, can be seen to fall, plateau, and then rise once ventilation becomes uncoupled from the parameter on the *x*-axis. The points of departure from the plateau values are different for $\dot{V}_E/\dot{V}O_2$ and $\dot{V}_E/\dot{V}CO_2$, based on different underlying physiological mechanisms. The $\dot{V}_E/\dot{V}O_2$ begins to increase when $\dot{V}_E$ becomes dissociated from $\dot{V}O_2$, i.e., when $\dot{V}_E$ responds to additional carbon dioxide generated by bicarbonate buffering of lactate. The inflection point for $\dot{V}_E/\dot{V}O_2$ can therefore be used to identify the metabolic threshold ($\dot{V}O_2\theta$). By contrast, $\dot{V}_E/\dot{V}CO_2$ does not begin to increase until $\dot{V}_E$ becomes dissociated from $\dot{V}CO_2$, i.e., when buffering mechanisms can no longer prevent a fall in blood pH and $\dot{V}_E$ responds to carotid body stimulation. The inflection point for $\dot{V}_E/\dot{V}CO_2$ can therefore be used to identify the ventilatory threshold or respiratory compensation point ($\dot{V}_E\theta$). Appreciation of the pattern of changes in $\dot{V}_E/\dot{V}O_2$ and $\dot{V}_E/\dot{V}CO_2$ is helpful in the interpretation of incremental XT. As long as the respiratory exchange ratio is less than 1.0, $\dot{V}_E/\dot{V}O_2$ will be less than $\dot{V}_E/\dot{V}CO_2$. Of particular importance are the plateau values that are on average 25 for $\dot{V}_E/\dot{V}O_2$ and 28 for

$\dot{V}_E/\dot{V}co_2$ for younger normal subjects (Figure 4.37). With advancing age, as the physiological dead space in the lung increases, the plateau values of the ventilatory equivalents are higher, e.g., 30 for $\dot{V}_E/\dot{V}o_2$ and 33 for $\dot{V}_E/\dot{V}co_2$.

### Abnormal responses (Figure 4.37B)

Abnormal ventilatory equivalents imply that the level of minute ventilation is inappropriate for the metabolic exchange of oxygen and carbon dioxide.

High ventilatory equivalents represent inefficient ventilation and have two common causes: hyperventilation and increased physiological dead space. Arterial blood sampling and determination of $Paco_2$ are essential to distinguish between these two causes. With hyperventilation, high ventilatory equivalents are associated with a low $Paco_2$, whereas with increased physiological dead space alone, $Paco_2$ is normal.

Acute hyperventilation occurring early during incremental exercise can be recognized by simultaneous increases in $\dot{V}_E/\dot{V}o_2$ and $\dot{V}_E/\dot{V}co_2$ as opposed to the separate inflection patterns that are expected (Figure 4.37).

An abnormal pattern of ventilatory equivalents is commonly seen in patients with chronic lung disease whereby both values are high at rest and do not fall with an expected pattern during incremental exercise. Hence the plateau values might be 40–60 depending on the severity of the underlying lung disease.

Low ventilatory equivalents are not expected and if observed should prompt a search for technical problems.

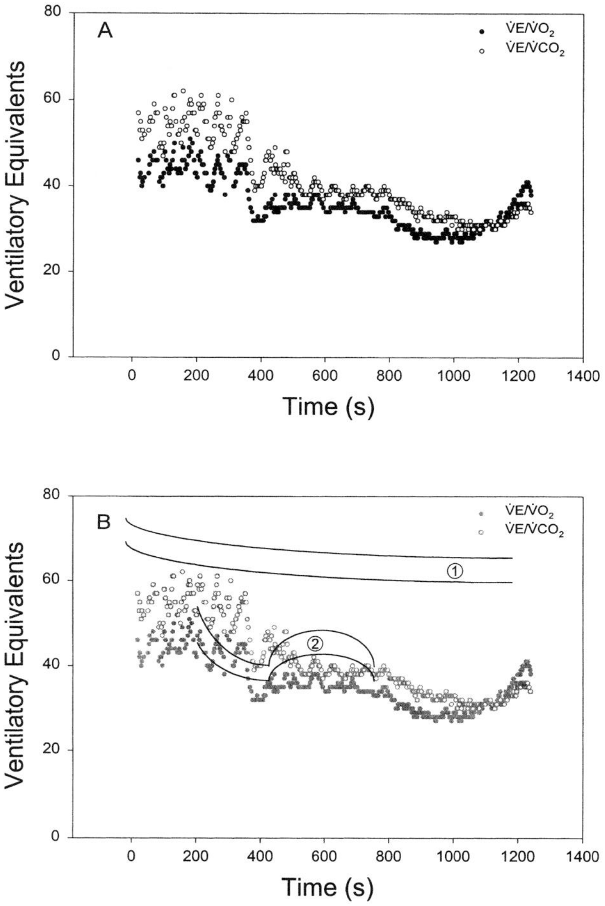


**Figure 4.37** Relationship between ventilatory equivalents and time during an incremental work rate XT. (A) Normal response. Note that while $R$ is less than 1.0, $\dot{V}_E/\dot{V}o_2$ is less than $\dot{V}_E/\dot{V}co_2$. $\dot{V}_E/\dot{V}o_2$ reaches a nadir about 25 and $\dot{V}_E/\dot{V}co_2$ reaches a nadir about 28. (B) Abnormal responses for ① chronic pulmonary disease resulting in high $V_D/V_T$ and ② acute hyperventilation causing simultaneous increases in both ventilatory equivalents.

## Arterial blood gas tensions ($Pao_2$ and $Paco_2$)

### Definition, derivation, and units of measurement

- Arterial blood gas tensions are the partial pressures of oxygen and carbon dioxide in the systemic arterial blood.
- Arterial blood for the measurement of $Pao_2$ and $Paco_2$ is usually sampled from the radial or brachial artery. Care must be taken to ensure that the samples are not contaminated with air bubbles. A small sample of blood is draw by automated pipette into a multipurpose gas analyzer which uses electrodes to determine pH, $Paco_2$, and $Pao_2$. Bicarbonate is typically calculated from pH and $Paco_2$ using the Henderson–Hasselbalch

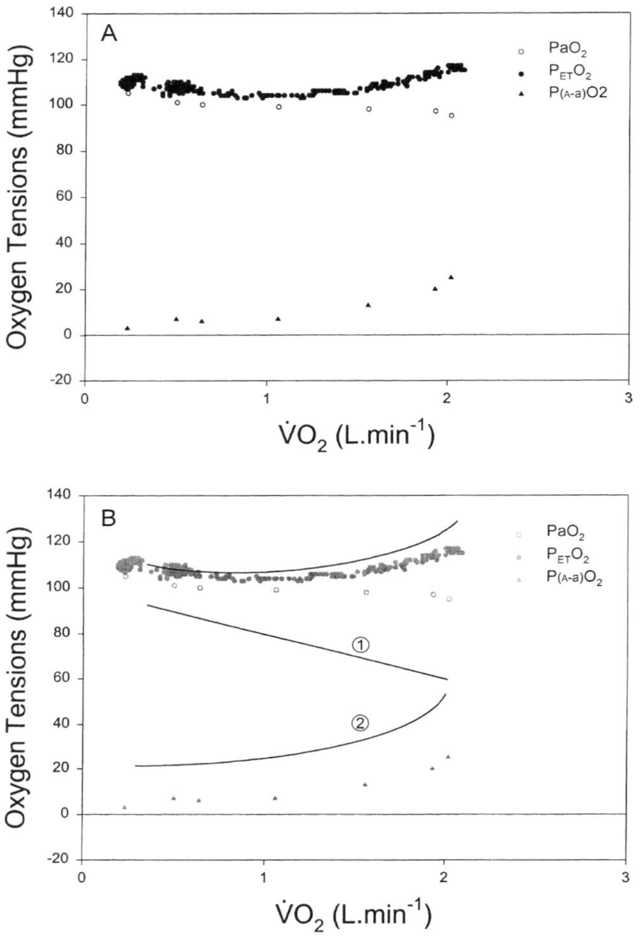


**Figure 4.38** Relationship between oxygen tensions and time during an incremental work rate XT. (A) Normal response. (B) Abnormal response with ① progressive fall in $Pa\text{O}_2$, and ② abnormally widened $P_{(A-a)}\text{O}_2$ gradient at maximum exercise.

equation (Equation 4.45), and oxyhemoglobin saturation is derived from $Pa\text{O}_2$ using a standard dissociation curve.

$$\text{pH} = \text{pK} + \log_{10}\frac{[\text{HCO}_3^-]}{\alpha \cdot Pa\text{CO}_2} \qquad (4.45)$$

where $\alpha$ is the solubility coefficient for carbon dioxide.

- The units of $Pa\text{O}_2$ and $Pa\text{CO}_2$ are millimeters of mercury (mmHg) in the USA and kiloPascals (kPa) in Europe, where:

$$\text{kPa} = \text{mmHg} \cdot 0.133 \qquad (4.46)$$

or:

$$\text{mmHg} = \text{kPa} \cdot 7.5 \qquad (4.47)$$

### Normal response (Figures 4.38A and 4.39A)

Arterial blood gas tensions are remarkably constant at rest and throughout a wide range of exercise intensities. This reflects the precision of the respiratory control mechanism, which matches alveolar ventilation to the changing metabolic demands for oxygen uptake and carbon dioxide output.

The accepted normal value for $Pa\text{O}_2$ declines with age owing to less efficient gas exchange with age-related alterations in lung structure. Resting $Pa\text{O}_2$, breathing room air, can be predicted by the equation:

$$Pa\text{O}_2 = 102 - (0.33 \cdot \text{age}) \qquad (4.48)$$

Normal $Pa\text{CO}_2$ is on average 40 mmHg, with a range from 36 to 44 mmHg. Small oscillations of $Pa\text{CO}_2$ are thought to occur and be involved in the fine control of ventilation. However, these oscillations are imperceptible in blood sampled from peripheral arteries and analyzed by typical laboratory gas analyzers.

Intense exercise, associated with lactic acidosis, can lead to additional stimulation of ventilation by the direct effect of acidemia on the carotid chemoreceptors. This compensatory component of the ventilatory response leads to increases in alveolar and arterial oxygen tensions along with decreases in alveolar and arterial carbon dioxide tensions. The magnitude of change in $Pa\text{O}_2$ and $Pa\text{CO}_2$ at intense exercise depends on the extent of the hyperventilation but an increase in $Pa\text{O}_2$ of 10 mmHg and fall in $Pa\text{CO}_2$ of 8 mmHg would be typical.

### Abnormal responses (Figures 4.38B and 4.39B)

Chronic lung disease and cardiovascular disease associated with abnormal right-to-left shunt result in abnormally low $Pao_2$ at rest and further reductions during exercise.

Early interstitial lung disease which slows oxygen diffusion in the lung can result in normal $Pao_2$ at rest but a progressive fall in $Pao_2$ during incremental exercise as cardiac output increases and pulmonary capillary transit time is decreased (Figure 4.38).

## End-tidal gas tensions ($P_{ET}o_2$ and $P_{ET}co_2$)

### Definition, derivation, and units of measurement

- End-tidal gas tensions are the partial pressures of oxygen and carbon dioxide observed at the end of each exhalation. The last gas exhaled from the lung is assumed to come from the alveolar compartment. Therefore, in the ideal lung, the end-tidal gas tensions would reflect the alveolar partial pressures of these gases.
- End-tidal gas tensions must be measured by continuously sampling the exhaled air stream using fast-responding gas analyzers. They can be displayed in real time by some metabolic measurement systems.
- The units of $P_{ET}o_2$ and $P_{ET}co_2$ are millimeters of mercury (mmHg) in the USA and kiloPascals (kPa) in Europe (see Equations 4.46 and 4.47).

### Normal response (Figures 4.38A and 4.39A)

The normal partial pressure profiles of exhaled oxygen and carbon dioxide are shown in Figure 4.40. The two profiles resemble "mirror images" of each other and the relative magnitudes of the changes they reflect depend on the respiratory exchange ratio ($R$). The end-tidal partial pressures are often described as plateaux but in reality they are slopes. Towards the end of exhalation, the oxygen tension actually continues to decrease slowly whereas the carbon dioxide tension increases slowly. These changes, which are subtle at rest, represent the continuing gas exchange between the blood and the alveolar gas. During exercise, as the metabolic rate increases, these alveolar slopes become steeper.

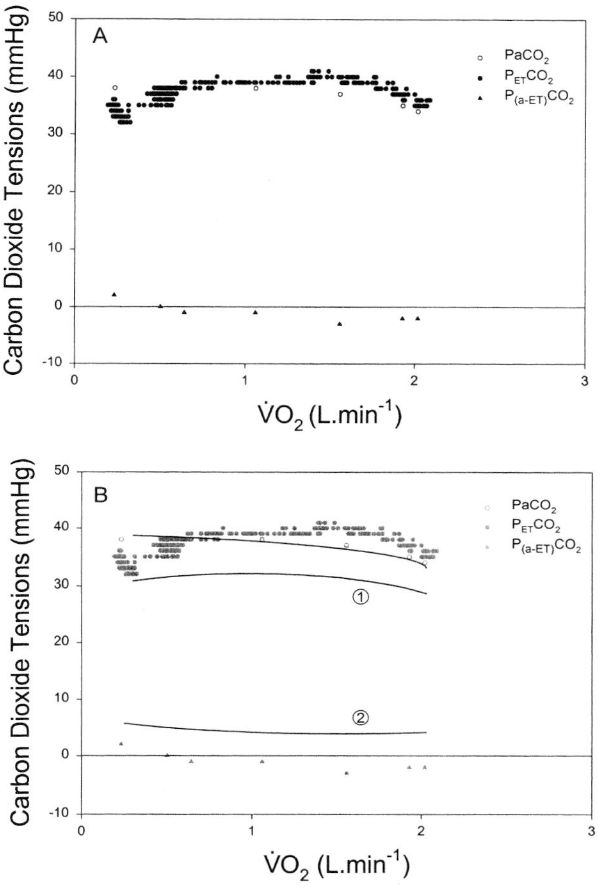


**Figure 4.39** Relationship between carbon dioxide tensions and time during an incremental work rate XT. (A) Normal response. (B) Abnormal response with ① persistently low $P_{ET}co_2$ and ② persistently positive $P_{(a-ET)}co_2$ throughout exercise.

### Abnormal responses (Figures 4.38B and 4.39B)

As illustrated by the "alveolar slope," end-tidal gas tensions are impacted by the rate of gas exchange in the lung. They are also affected by respiratory rate and breathing pattern in ways which are not so clearly defined.

An important influence on $P_{ET}o_2$ and $P_{ET}co_2$ is the magnitude of the physiological dead space,

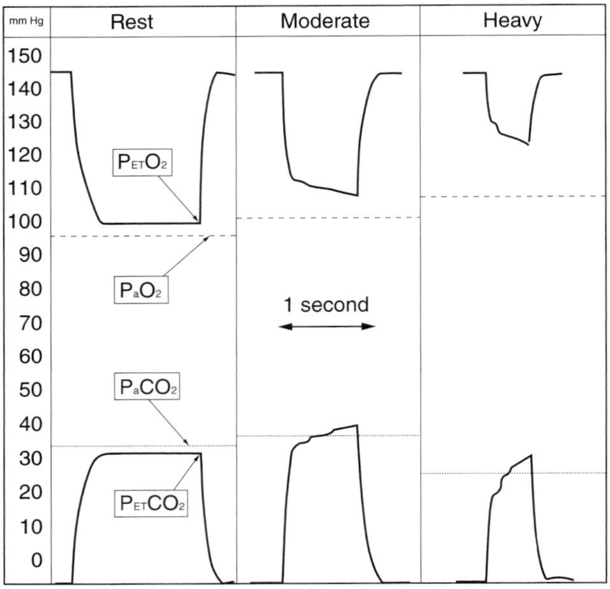


**Figure 4.40** Profiles of exhaled oxygen and carbon dioxide at rest and during moderate or high-intensity exercise. During exercise the "alveolar slope" for exhaled carbon dioxide steepens, so that $P_{ET}CO_2$ exceeds $PaCO_2$, resulting in a negative $P_{(a-ET)}CO_2$. During high-intensity exercise both $P_{ET}CO_2$ and $PaCO_2$ fall due to hyperventilation.

particularly the alveolar dead space. Figure 4.41 shows the simultaneous emptying of an ideal lung unit (on the left) and an unperfused lung unit representing alveolar dead space (on the right). Clearly, the relative amounts of air emptying from these two compartments determines to what extent end-tidal gas tensions differ from the gas tensions in the ideal lung unit, and consequently in the arterial blood. This concept will be explained more fully in the section on arterial–end-tidal carbon dioxide partial pressure difference (see below).

## Alveolar–arterial oxygen partial pressure difference ($P_{(A-a)}O_2$)

### Definition, derivation, and units of measurement

- $P_{(A-a)}O_2$ is the difference in partial pressure of oxygen between the arterial blood and the alveolar compartment of the lung. This represents the completeness or effectiveness of oxygen exchange in the lung. $P_{(A-a)}O_2$ is increased by diffusion impairment or admixture of inadequately oxygenated blood from areas of inappropriate ventilation–perfusion matching or shunt.
- $PaO_2$ is measured from an arterial blood sample whereas $P_AO_2$ is calculated using the simplified alveolar air equation:

$$P_AO_2 = P_IO_2 - \left(\frac{PaCO_2}{R}\right) \qquad (4.49)$$

where $P_IO_2$ is the inspired oxygen partial pressure and $R$ is the respiratory exchange ratio. Then:

$$P_{(A-a)}O_2 = P_AO_2 - PaO_2 \qquad (4.50)$$

- The units of $P_{(A-a)}O_2$ are millimeters of mercury (mmHg) in the USA and kiloPascals (kPa) in Europe (see Equations 4.46 and 4.47).

### Normal response (Figure 4.38A)

In a normal young adult, $P_{(A-a)}O_2$ is 5–10 mmHg. Most of this difference arises from venous admixture and normal anatomical shunt rather than from incomplete diffusion equilibration across the alveolar–capillary membrane. $P_{(A-a)}O_2$ increases with age, apparently due to reduced gas-exchanging efficiency associated with age-related alterations in the structure of the lung. $P_{(A-a)}O_2$ can be predicted by the following equation:

$$P_{(A-a)}O_2 = (0.33 \cdot \text{age}) - 2 \qquad (4.51)$$

where $P_{(A-a)}O_2$ is expressed in mmHg.

$P_{(A-a)}O_2$ increases during incremental exercise. The magnitude of this increase is about 20% for normal subjects around the predicted $\dot{V}O_{2max}$. Another estimate is that $P_{(A-a)}O_2$ increases by about 5.5 mmHg for every $1\,l \cdot min^{-1}$ increase in $\dot{V}O_2$. Again, diffusion limitation is unlikely to occur in normal subjects. However, three important factors influence oxygen diffusion across the alveolar–capillary membrane during exercise: (1) pulmonary capillary transit time (*Tpc*) is shortened; (2) mixed venous

**Table 4.6.** Reference values for oxygen partial pressure in arterial blood and alveolar–arterial difference

| Age (years) | $Pao_2$ (mmHg) | 95% CI (mmHg) | $P_{(A-a)}O_2$ (mmHg) | Upper 95% CI (mmHg) |
|---|---|---|---|---|
| 20 | 95 | 84–105 | 5 | 15 |
| 30 | 92 | 82–102 | 8 | 18 |
| 40 | 89 | 79–99 | 11 | 21 |
| 50 | 86 | 76–96 | 15 | 25 |
| 60 | 82 | 72–92 | 18 | 28 |
| 70 | 79 | 69–89 | 21 | 31 |
| 80 | 76 | 66–86 | 24 | 34 |

CI = Confidence interval.

oxygen partial pressure ($P\bar{v}O_2$) is reduced by increased peripheral oxygen extraction; and (3) alveolar oxygen partial pressure is increased by hyperventilation (Figure 4.42).
Elite athletes, with significantly elevated $\dot{V}O_{2max}$, can achieve widening of $P_{(A-a)}O_2$ to as much as 35 mmHg. All three of the factors mentioned above contribute to this phenomenon, but the most important is thought to be the substantial shortening of *Tpc* which accompanies the high cardiac output of the élite athlete.

Table 4.6 shows reference values for oxygen partial pressure in arterial blood and alveolar–arterial difference.

### Abnormal responses (Figure 4.38B)

Diffusion impairment increases $P_{(A-a)}O_2$ during incremental exercise as *Tpc* shortens (Figure 4.42). Both the slowed diffusion and shortened time for oxygen partial pressure equilibration contribute to this effect.

The response to incremental exercise in patients with interstitial lung disease is characterized by a progressive widening of $P_{(A-a)}O_2$ (Figure 4.38). Early interstitial lung disease may result in a normal $Pao_2$ and $P_{(A-a)}O_2$ at rest but an abnormal decrease in $Pao_2$ and increase in $P_{(A-a)}O_2$ during exercise. Hence, exercise testing may be the most sensitive means – indeed, the only means short of lung biopsy – of detecting such a condition. In severe interstitial lung disease $P_{(A-a)}O_2$ might be abnormal, even at rest.

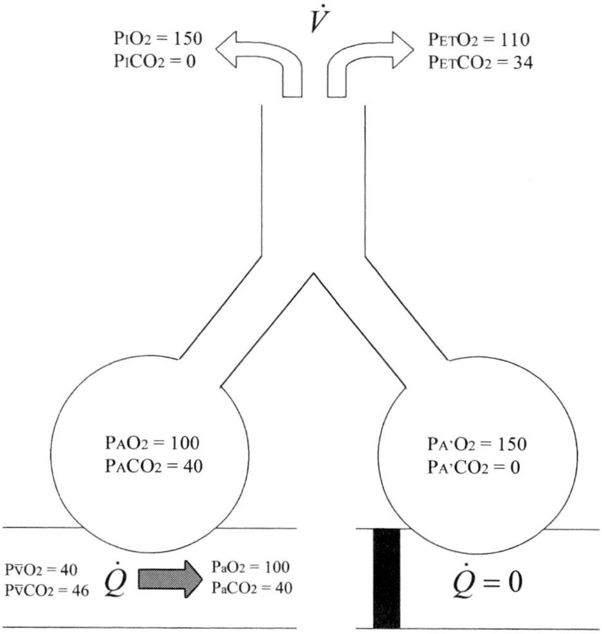


**Figure 4.41** Determinants of $P_{(a-ET)}CO_2$. (A) Ideal lung unit. (B) Alveolar dead space. Admixture of exhaled air from both units results in higher $P_{ET}O_2$ and lower $P_{ET}CO_2$ than ideal alveloar gas.

Increased physiological shunt also increases $P_{(A-a)}O_2$ – an effect that is likely to be exaggerated during incremental exercise. Examples of increased physiological shunt include lung consolidation, a lung tumor mass, the intrapulmonary vascular dilatations as seen in chronic liver disease, and cardiac septal defects. Rarely, in patients with pulmonary hypertension, the foramen ovale opens during incremental exercise, causing a sudden fall in $Pao_2$ and increase in $P_{(A-a)}O_2$.

Careful examination of $P_{(A-a)}O_2$ is helpful in assessing pulmonary gas exchange mechanisms during exercise. An abnormal $P_{(A-a)}O_2$ is indicative of diffusion impairment or inappropriately low $\dot{V}/\dot{Q}$, i.e., increased physiological shunt.

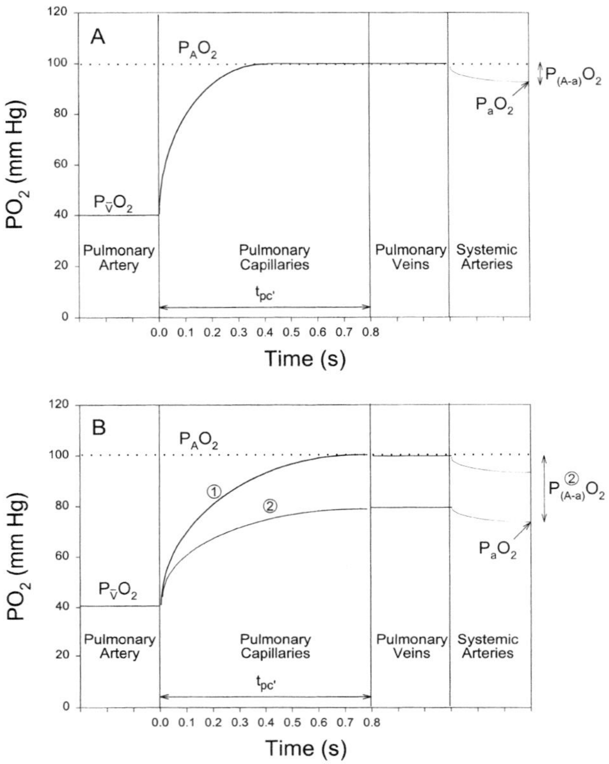


**Figure 4.42** Determinants of $P_{(A-a)}O_2$. (A) Normal diffusion equilibration for oxygen between pulmonary capillary blood and alveolar gas. Diffusion is typically complete within 0.4 s, or less than 50% of the pulmonary capillary transit time. (B) Profiles of slowed diffusion for ① early interstitial disease which would result in a widened $P_{(A-a)}O_2$ during exercise but not at rest and ② severe interstitial disease resulting in a widened $P_{(A-a)}O_2$ even at rest.

## Arterial–end-tidal carbon dioxide partial pressure difference ($P_{(a-ET)}CO_2$)

### Definition, derivation, and units of measurement

- $P_{(a-ET)}CO_2$ is the difference in carbon dioxide partial pressure between the arterial blood and the end-tidal gas. $PaCO_2$ is assumed to represent the $P_ACO_2$ in "ideal" gas-exchanging lung units. Therefore, $P_{(a-ET)}CO_2$ indicates the extent to which ideal alveolar gas has been diluted with gas from the physiological dead space.
- $PaCO_2$ is measured by arterial blood sampling. $P_{ET}CO_2$ is measured by sampling gas at the end of exhalation using a fast responding gas analyzer, then:

$$P_{(a-ET)}CO_2 = PaCO_2 - P_{ET}CO_2 \tag{4.52}$$

- The units of $P_{(a-ET)}CO_2$ are millimeters of mercury (mmHg) in the USA and kiloPascals (kPa) in Europe (see Equations 4.46 and 4.47).

### Normal response (Figure 4.39A)

We have already seen that, during exhalation in a normal individual at rest, the partial pressure of carbon dioxide rises exponentially from zero at the start of exhalation to reach the alveolar slope that represents the rate of metabolic carbon dioxide production. This fact is exemplified by the obvious increase in the "alveolar slope" during incremental exercise (Figure 4.40).

Assuming the lung was entirely composed of ideal lung units, $P_{ET}CO_2$ would represent ideal alveolar gas, and assuming complete equilibration of carbon dioxide partial pressures between the alveoli and the blood, $P_{ET}CO_2$ would equal $PaCO_2$. Actually, $P_{ET}CO_2$ is normally about 2 mmHg less than $PaCO_2$ due to admixture of gas from the alveolar dead space (Figure 4.41). Hence, the normal resting value for $P_{(a-ET)}CO_2$ is positive by about 2 mmHg.

During incremental exercise, an important change occurs. The alveolar slope becomes steeper due to increased metabolic carbon dioxide production. Meanwhile, $PaCO_2$ continues to represent the mean alveolar partial pressure of carbon dioxide ($P_ACO_2$) throughout the breath cycle. Consequently, $P_{ET}CO_2$ may actually exceed $PaCO_2$ (Figure 4.40). Hence, during exercise $P_{(a-ET)}CO_2$ becomes negative by about 2–4 mmHg in normal circumstances. During intense exercise, when acidemia causes compensatory hyperventilation, $P_ACO_2$ falls. Consequently, both $PaCO_2$ and $P_{ET}CO_2$ fall. They fall to approximately the same extent, so that $P_{(a-ET)}CO_2$ remains negative (Figure 4.39).

### Abnormal responses (Figure 4.39B)

Increases in physiological dead space result in proportional increases in $P_{(a-ET)}CO_2$. Certain types of lung disease, notably chronic obstructive pulmonary disease, emphysema, and pulmonary vascular disease, result in increased physiological dead space. Typically, these patients have abnormally increased $P_{(a-ET)}CO_2$ at rest, and may fail to demonstrate reversal of $P_{(a-ET)}CO_2$ from positive to negative during exercise (Figure 4.39).

Careful examination of $P_{(a-ET)}CO_2$ is helpful in assessing gas exchange mechanisms during exercise. An abnormal $P_{(a-ET)}CO_2$ is indicative of inappropriately high $\dot{V}/\dot{Q}$, i.e., increased physiological dead space.

## Dead space–tidal volume ratio ($V_D/V_T$)

### Definition, derivation, and units of measurement

- Since the respiratory system operates as a bidirectional pump, with each breath there is wasted ventilation or dead space. The physiological dead space ($V_{Dphysiol}$) comprises anatomical dead space ($V_{Danat}$) plus alveolar dead space ($V_{Dalv}$). $V_{Danat}$ represents the upper airway, trachea, and conducting bronchi and $V_{Dalv}$ represents nonperfused or underperfused areas of lung, hence:

$$V_{Dphysiol} = V_{Danat} + V_{Dalv} \tag{4.53}$$

- $V_D/V_T$ is calculated using the Bohr equation:

$$\frac{V_D}{V_T} = \frac{Paco_2 - P_{\bar{E}}co_2}{Paco_2} \tag{4.54}$$

Correct determination of $V_D/V_T$ necessitates arterial blood sampling for $Paco_2$. Some metabolic measurement systems erroneously purport to determine $V_D/V_T$ from noninvasive gas exchange measurements alone (i.e., without arterial blood sampling). Whilst this method might be approximately true in healthy young subjects, it is unreliable and potentially misleading in older subjects and patients with pulmonary disease. In Equation 4.54, $P_{\bar{E}}co_2$ is the mixed expired carbon dioxide partial pressure. This can be measured using a mixing chamber system but with a breath-by-breath system $P_{\bar{E}}co_2$ can be calculated from the instantaneous carbon dioxide output and ventilation.

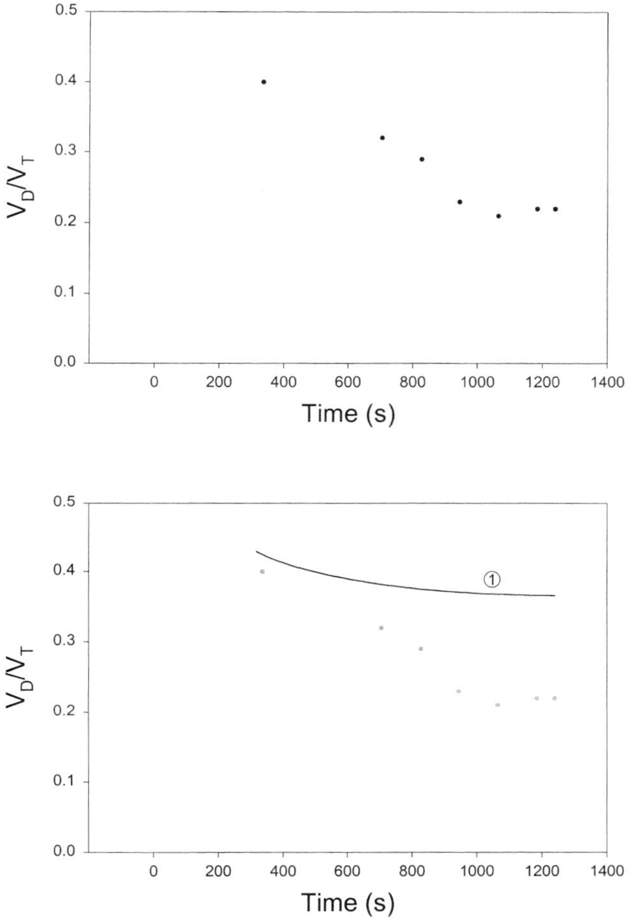


Figure 4.43 Relationship between $V_D/V_T$ and time during an incremental work rate XT. (A) Normal response. (B) Abnormal response for chronic obstructive pulmonary disease ①.

$$P_{\bar{E}}co_2 = (P_B - 47) \cdot \frac{\dot{V}co_2}{\dot{V}_E} \tag{4.55}$$

where $P_B$ is the barometric pressure and 47 represents the partial pressure of saturated water

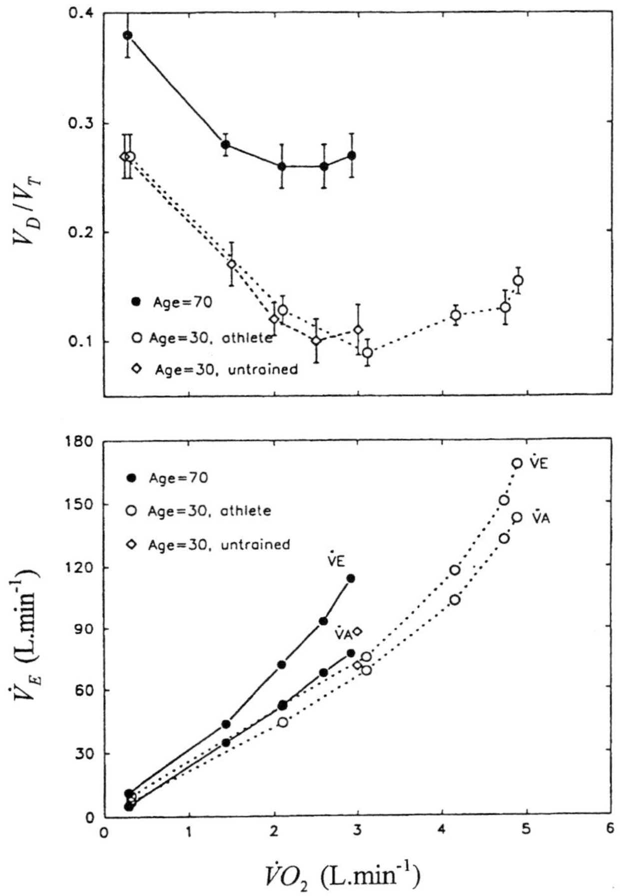


**Figure 4.44** Effect of increasing age on $V_D/V_T$ (top). The resulting steepening of the relationship between $\dot{V}_E$ and $\dot{V}O_2$ is shown below. Reproduced with permission from Johnson, B. D., Badr, M. S. & Dempsey, J. A. (1994). Impact of the aging pulmonary system on the response to exercise. *Clin. Chest Med.*, **15**, 229–46.

vapor at body temperature. During collection of exhaled gases, dead space is artificially increased by the additional mouthpiece and breathing valve. In these circumstances it becomes appropriate to correct $V_D/V_T$ for the added dead space ($Vds$).

$$\frac{V_D}{V_T} = \frac{Paco_2 - P_{\bar{E}}co_2}{Paco_2} - \frac{Vds}{V_T} \quad (4.56)$$

- $V_D/V_T$ is the fraction of each breath wasted. Being the ratio of two volumes, $V_D/V_T$ has no units. It is sometimes expressed as a percentage.

### Normal response

During resting breathing, $V_D$ constitutes about one-third of the tidal volume, i.e., $V_D/V_T$ approximately equals 33%. During incremental exercise, $V_D/V_T$ normally falls with an exponential pattern reaching lowest values of 15–20% (Figure 4.43).

The fall in $V_D/V_T$ with exercise is explained in two ways. Firstly, whilst tidal volume increases substantially during incremental exercise, changes in dead space are relatively small. Secondly, as pulmonary blood flow increases during exercise, ventilation and perfusion become better matched throughout the lungs, thus reducing alveolar dead space. The fall in $V_D/V_T$ with increasing exercise intensity serves to improve the efficiency of ventilation as the demand for gas exchange increases.

$V_D/V_T$ is higher in older subjects, reflecting less efficient ventilation. This observation is likely to be explained by the common finding of mild degrees of emphysema or abnormal lung architecture in autopsies of older individuals without actual recognized lung disease. These findings are presumed to represent a natural age-related deterioration of the lung.

It is advisable to take age into account when judging whether $V_D/V_T$ is normal or abnormal (Figure 4.44). At maximal exercise:

$$\frac{V_D}{V_T} = 0.4 \cdot \text{age} \quad (4.57)$$

### Abnormal responses (Figure 4.43B)

A normal $V_D/V_T$ depends upon appropriate matching of ventilation and perfusion in the lungs. Lung units that are ventilated but not perfused constitute alveolar dead space and increase $V_D/V_T$. Any lung disease which results in inequality of $\dot{V}/\dot{Q}$, such as chronic obstructive pulmonary disease or, particularly, pulmonary vascular disease, results in high

$V_D/V_T$ at rest and failure of $V_D/V_T$ to fall appropriately during incremental exercise (Figure 4.43).

## Lactate (La)

### Definition, derivation, and units of measurement

- Blood lactate (lactic acid) level during exercise is governed by several factors but primarily by the balance between its rate of accumulation or efflux from exercising muscles and its rate of disposal elsewhere in the body. The principal sites of lactate disposal are thought to be the liver, heart, brain, and nonexercising muscle.
- Blood lactate varies depending on whether an arterial or venous blood sample is obtained. In general, when blood is sampled from a nonexercising limb, arterial lactate is higher than venous lactate because of its uptake and metabolism by the tissues. Although an arterial sample might therefore be preferred, a venous sample might be more readily obtained and should suffice for a reasonably accurate estimation of circulating blood lactate.

  Blood lactate tends to increase for approximately 2 min after the termination of exercise. Therefore, if the maximum blood lactate level for an exhaustive exercise test is desired, then the sample should be obtained after approximately 2 min of recovery. It is good laboratory practice to standardize the timing of the sample so that staff can derive a better sense of what constitutes a normal and abnormal response.
- The units of measurement of lactate vary between laboratories. Some use milligrams per deciliter ($mg \cdot dl^{-1}$), whereas others use millimoles per liter ($mmol \cdot l^{-1}$). Conversion between these units is based on knowing that the molecular weight of lactic acid is 90, hence:

$$mg \cdot dl^{-1} = mmol \cdot l^{-1} \cdot 9 \qquad (4.58)$$

or:

$$mmol \cdot l^{-1} = mg \cdot dl^{-1} \cdot 0.111 \qquad (4.59)$$

### Normal response

The normal reference value for blood lactate at rest is 5–20 $mg \cdot dl^{-1}$ or 0.5–2.2 $mmol \cdot l^{-1}$. During a symptom-limited incremental exercise test the anticipated increase in lactate is governed by several factors, including subject motivation and degree of physical training.

Even during low-intensity exercise a small increase in blood lactate is seen. However, it is usual for the level to stabilize, reflecting a balance between lactate production from exercise muscle and lactate disposal by other tissues. This change has been called "early lactate."

As discussed in detail earlier in this chapter, the metabolic threshold, $\dot{V}o_2\theta$, represents the transition between two important physiological domains of exercise. According to our understanding of these domains, $\dot{V}o_2\theta$ also represents the onset of blood lactate accumulation, i.e., an imbalance between lactate production and disposal. The normal $\dot{V}o_2\theta$ occurs above 40% of the reference value for $\dot{V}o_{2max}$ and this should be equally true for the onset of blood lactate accumulation. Studies that have related serial arterial blood lactate measurements to the gas exchange indices used for the identification of $\dot{V}o_2\theta$ have demonstrated that $\dot{V}o_2\theta$ is the threshold above which lactate shows a sustained increase. Interpretation of the lactate threshold can be achieved using Table 4.4. Identification of the lactate threshold is facilitated by serial blood lactate measurements or at least by a specimen after 4 min of an incremental test that is calculated to terminate at about 10 min.

A well-motivated subject can be expected to achieve a lactate level of 40–100 $mg \cdot dl^{-1}$ (4.4–11.0 $mmol \cdot l^{-1}$). Greater motivation and tolerance of muscle fatigue result in higher end-exercise lactate levels.

### Abnormal responses

Failure to exhibit a significant increase in blood lactate during symptom-limited incremental exercise is abnormal. Possible explanations include lack of subject motivation, i.e., suboptimal effort, nonmetabolic causes of exercise limitation, and McArdle's disease. Note that a subject whose end-exercise blood lactate is 15–30 mg · dl$^{-1}$ (1.7–3.3 mmol · l$^{-1}$) could have just begun to accumulate lactate before termination of exercise. Some individuals with low tolerance of muscle fatigue exhibit this type of response.

A premature increase in blood lactate, i.e., before reaching 40% of the reference value for $\dot{V}O_{2max}$, is abnormal and should be accompanied by a low $\dot{V}O_2\theta$. A diagnostic approach to interpretation of a low $\dot{V}O_2\theta$ is described in Chapter 5.

Finally, an exaggerated increase in blood lactate with an unexpectedly high maximum value is abnormal and may reflect severe cardiovascular abnormalities or failure of cellular energy generation through restoration of ATP. Blood lactate values of 60–120 mg · dl (6.7–13.3 mmol · l$^{-1}$) are suspicious for these types of abnormality, especially when associated with a reduced $\dot{V}O_{2max}$. At present no clear-cut parameters exist for normal and abnormal blood lactate levels. Therefore, maximum lactate should be interpreted carefully with respect to the $\dot{V}O_{2max}$ achieved.

## Ammonia ($NH_3$)

### Definition, derivation, and units of measurement

- Blood ammonia increases with exercise, tending to reach a maximum with exhaustion.
- Ammonia is derived by the alternative pathway for ATP regeneration: firstly, two ADP molecules combine under the influence of the enzyme myokinase to form ATP and AMP. This reaction serves to restore a favorable ATP:ADP ratio.

$$2\text{ADP} \rightarrow \text{ATP} + \text{AMP} \quad (4.60)$$

Secondly, AMP is removed by the enzyme myoadenylate deaminase, generating inosine and ammonia.

$$\text{AMP} \rightarrow \text{Inosine} + \text{NH}_3 \quad (4.61)$$

This pathway appears to be activated when oxygen is in short supply and therefore ATP cannot be regenerated fast enough by oxidative phosphorylation alone.

- The units of measurement of ammonia vary between laboratories. Some use micrograms per deciliter (μg · dl$^{-1}$), whereas others use micromoles per liter (μmol · l$^{-1}$). Conversion between these units is based on knowing that the molecular weight of ammonia is 17, hence:

$$\mu g \cdot dl^{-1} = \mu mol \cdot l^{-1} \cdot 1.7 \quad (4.62)$$

or:

$$\mu mol \cdot l^{-1} = \mu g \cdot dl^{-1} \cdot 0.59 \quad (4.63)$$

### Normal response

Normal values for blood ammonia at rest are 5–70 μg · dl$^{-1}$ (3–40 μmol · l$^{-1}$). Normal values for ammonia at maximum exercise have not been well established. As with lactate, end-exercise ammonia levels undoubtedly relate in part to subject motivation and fitness level. A well-motivated normal subject typically achieves a maximum ammonia level of 120–200 μg · dl$^{-1}$ (70–120 μmol · l$^{-1}$).

### Abnormal responses

Failure to exhibit a significant increase in blood ammonia during symptom-limited incremental exercise is abnormal. Possible explanations include lack of subject motivation, i.e., suboptimal effort, nonmetabolic causes of exercise limitation, and the rare metabolic disorder, myoadenylate deaminase deficiency.

A premature increase in blood ammonia is abnormal and should be accompanied by a low $\dot{V}O_2\theta$. A diagnostic approach to interpretation of a low $\dot{V}O_2\theta$ is described in Chapter 5.

Finally, an exaggerated increase in blood ammonia with an unexpectedly high maximum value is abnormal and usually reflects failure of cellular energy generation through normal restoration of ATP via oxidative phosphorylation. This occurs in a variety of metabolic and other myopathies, notably the mitochondrial myopathies, which may include mitochondrial DNA mutations. A blood ammonia value greater than 200 $\mu g \cdot dl^{-1}$ (120 $\mu mol \cdot l^{-1}$) is suspicious for these types of abnormality. As with lactate, no clear-cut parameters exist for normal and abnormal blood ammonia levels. Therefore, maximum ammonia should be interpreted carefully with respect to the $\dot{V}o_{2max}$ achieved.

## Rating of perceived exertion (RPE)

### Definition, derivation, and units of measurement

- Rating of perceived exertion is a concept devised by Gunnar Borg, the Swedish psychophysicist. Borg appreciated that in human physiology the relationship between most applied stimuli (K) and their perception ($\psi$) followed Stevens' law of psychophysics. Hence, the relationship between these two variables could be represented by a power function:

$$\Psi = K^n \tag{4.64}$$

  In the case of many human physiological responses, e.g., perception of light intensity, the loudness of sound, and pain, the value of the exponent ($n$) is between 1 and 2. In the case of exercise the applied stimulus is exercise intensity and the perception of particular interest is exertion. Borg devised a series of psychometric scales to record $\psi$. The two most common representations of these scales are the RPE scale and the CR10 scale. These are category scales because they have graded labels. In addition, they have ratio properties that recognize the underlying power function and are intended to linearize the scale of response. Examples of these scales are included in Appendix D.
- The RPE scale is the most commonly used scale for rating of perceived exertion. The main advantage of the RPE scale is that the given ratings grow linearly with exercise intensity, $f_C$ and $\dot{V}o_2$ (Figure 4.45). RPE is then easy to compare with other physiological measurements of the exercise response. A disadvantage of the CR10 scale is that the number range is small. Also for ratings of perceived exertion the CR10 scale does not give the simple linear relationship to exercise intensity that the RPE scale does. In most situations it is preferable to use the RPE scale for perceived exertion and the CR10 scale for other sensations. The RPE is obtained by showing the scale to an exercising subject with appropriate written or verbal instructions. The instructions recommended by Borg are shown with the scales in Appendix D.
- These perceptions are integers selected from the particular scales.

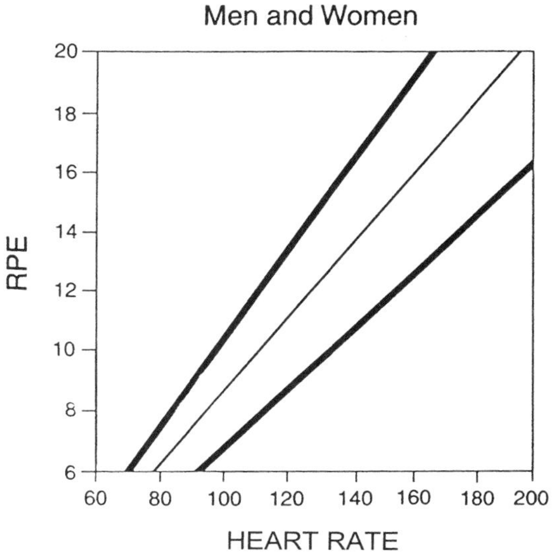


**Figure 4.45** Relationship between RPE and $f_C$ for men and women performing cycle ergometer exercise. Reproduced with permission from Borg, G. (1998). *Borg's Perceived Exertion and Pain Scales.* Champaign, IL: Human Kinetics.

### Normal response

There is sufficient experience using the 6–20 scale during incremental exercise to know that with a symptom-limited maximal effort RPE is expected to be 16–18. At the metabolic threshold RPE is expected to be 12–14. An RPE of 19 or 20 is rare.

Corresponding points on the 1–10 scale would be a maximum effort of 6–8 and a metabolic threshold at 3–5. Perceived exertion of 9 or 10 on this scale is rare.

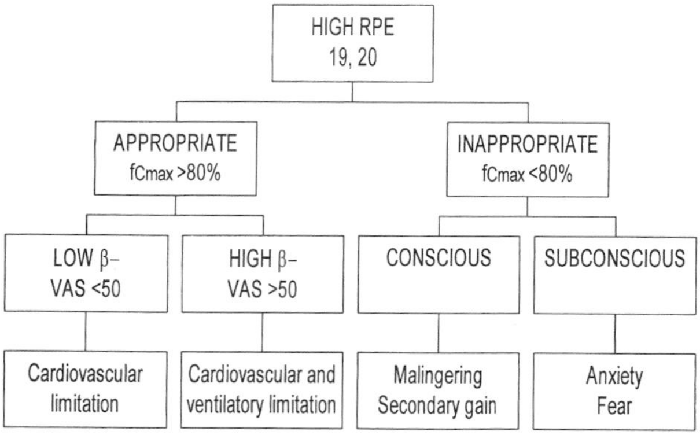


**Figure 4.46** Interpretation of high RPE. Firstly, the RPE is judged to be appropriate or inappropriate based on the cardiovascular response. An appropriately high RPE is then compared with the subject's perception of breathlessness (*β*–) on a visual analog scale (VAS). An inappropriately high RPE is examined for conscious or subconscious components.

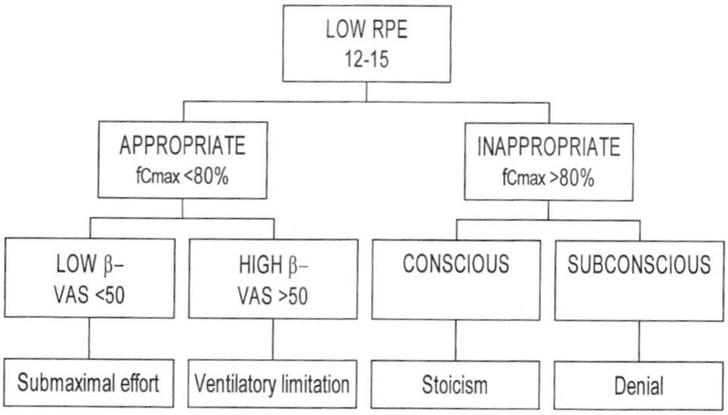


**Figure 4.47** Interpretation of low RPE. Firstly, the RPE is judged to be appropriate or inappropriate based on the cardiovascular response. An appropriately low RPE is then compared with the subject's perception of breathlessness (*β*–) on a visual analog scale (VAS). An inappropriately low RPE is examined for conscious or subconscious components.

### Abnormal responses

Knowledge of how RPE usually relates to exercise intensity in normal subjects allows identification of abnormal perceptual responses and can help explain exercise intolerance. The preferred approach is to determine whether RPE is inappropriately high or low compared with the cardiovascular response.

An inappropriately high RPE might include a rating of 19 or 20 at end exercise, particularly if $\dot{V}O_{2max}$ was reduced or low normal. Also an RPE greater than 14 would be considered inappropriately high when there is no accompanying evidence of a metabolic threshold having been achieved.

An inappropriately high RPE can be regarded as intentional (conscious) or unintentional (unconscious) based on an impression of whether the subject is intentionally rating perceived exertion high for secondary gain or whether it appears that there is truly a perceptual abnormality. This approach can be developed in conjunction with a separate evaluation of breathlessness to give further insight into abnormal symptom perception (Figures 4.46 and 4.47).

## Breathlessness (*β*–)

### Definition, derivation, and units of measurement

- The visual analog scale is a psychometric tool that can be used conveniently to quantify breathlessness (*β*–) during exercise. This scale offers a valuable alternative to the RPE scale, which is best reserved for rating perceived exertion and is not ideally suited to quantification of breathlessness. The usual scale is a 100-mm line representing the range of breathlessness from "not at all breathless" to "extremely breathless" or "the most breathless you have ever felt." An example of a visual analog scale for quantifying *β*– is included in Appendix D.
- The visual analog scale is shown to the subject immediately after the end of incremental exercise test and subjects are asked to mark the line at a point that indicates how breathless they felt at maximum exercise. The accuracy and therefore the value of a visual analog scale is dependent on the subject properly understanding the meaning of the scale and carefully marking it to represent the symptom being assessed.
- *β*– on the visual analog scale is usually expressed

without units. Alternatively it can be expressed as a percentage.

### Normal response

Visual analog scales for breathlessness have been shown to correlate reasonably well with minute ventilation during exercise. Hence, $\beta-$ can be compared with the ventilatory response to assess whether the symptom is appropriately matched to the physiological variables.

There is a loose correlation between $\beta-$ at maximum exercise and $\dot{V}_{E\max}$ expressed as a percentage of ventilatory capacity:

$$\beta- \approx \frac{\dot{V}_{E\max}}{\dot{V}_{E\mathrm{cap}}} \qquad (4.65)$$

At maximum exercise, a normal subject will score $\beta-$ at 50–90, corresponding to utilization of 60–100% of ventilatory capacity (Figure 4.48). Visual analog data are not as rigorous as many of the physiological parameters that have been discussed. However, with regular use, a sense of the appropriateness of symptom perception during exercise can be derived using this instrument. The score for $\beta-$ can then be used in conjunction with RPE, as shown in Figures 4.46 and 4.47.

### Abnormal responses

Patients with pulmonary disease may reach their ventilatory capacities during exercise and exhibit true ventilatory limitation. Given that such individuals utilize close to 100% of their ventilatory capacity, it is not unusual for them to score $\beta-$ between 90 and 100. $\beta-$ greater than 90 is unusual in the absence of ventilatory limitation and can be associated unconsciously with anxiety or consciously with malingering or a desire for secondary gain.

By contrast, $\beta-$ less than 50 is unusual with a true maximal effort. When $\beta-$ is low, the exercise practitioner should consider whether this is appropriate, due to submaximal effort, or whether it is inappropriate due to stoicism or denial.

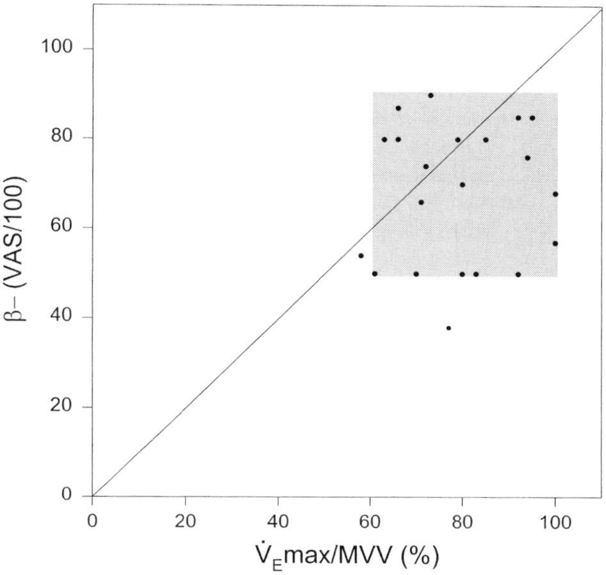


**Figure 4.48** Relationship between breathlessness ($\beta-$) and ventilation as a percentage of ventilatory capacity for 21 patients with a variety of diseases limiting exercise capacity but apparently normal symptom perception. The majority utilized 60–100% of ventilatory capacity at maximum exercise and recorded $\beta-$ scores between 50 and 90. VAS = Visual analog score; MVV = maximum voluntary ventilation.

A schema for the interpretation of $\beta-$ in conjunction with RPE is shown in Figures 4.46 and 4.47.

## FURTHER READING

American College of Sports Medicine (1995). *ACSM's Guidelines for Exercise Testing and Prescription*, 5th edn. Philadelphia: Williams & Wilkins.

Åstrand, P.-O. & Rodahl, K. (1986). *Textbook of Work Physiology. Physiological Bases of Exercise*, 3rd edn. New York: McGraw-Hill.

Åstrand, I., Åstrand P.-O., Hallbäck, I. & Kilbom, Å. (1973). Reduction in maximal oxygen uptake with age. *J. Appl. Physiol.*, **35**, 649–54.

Borg. G. (1998) *Borg's Perceived Exertion and Pain Scales.* Champaign, IL: Human Kinetics.

Chacko, K. A. (1995). American Heart Association Medical/Scientific Statement, 1994 revisions to the classification of functional capacity and objective assessment of patients with diseases of the heart. *Circulation*, **92**, 2003–5.

Cooper, C. B. (1995). Determining the role of exercise in chronic pulmonary diseases. *Med. Sci. Sports Exerc.*, **27**, 147–57.

Hansen, J. E., Sue, D. Y. & Wasserman, K. (1984). Predicted values for clinical exercise testing. *Am. Rev. Respir. Dis.*, **129** (suppl.), S49–55.

Hansen, J. E., Casaburi, R., Cooper, D. M. & Wasserman, K. (1988). Oxygen uptake as related to work rate increment during cycle ergometer exercise. *Eur. J. Appl. Physiol.*, **57**, 140–5.

Jones, N. L. & Campbell, E. J. M. (1982). *Clinical exercise Testing*, 2nd edn. Philadelphia: W. B. Saunders.

Lim, P. O., MacFayden, R. J., Clarkson, P. B. M. & MacDonald, T. M. (1996). Impaired exercise tolerance in hypertensive patients. *Ann. Intern. Med.*, **124**, 41–55.

Nunn, J. F. (1977). *Applied Respiratory Physiology*, 2nd edn. London: Butterworths.

Shvartz, E. & Reibold, R. C. (1990). Aerobic fitness norms for males and females aged 6 to 75 years: a review. *Aviat. Space Environ. Med.*, **61**, 3–11.

Spiro, S. G., Juniper, E., Bowman, P. & Edwards, R. H. T. (1974). An increasing work rate test for assessing the physiological strain of submaximal exercise. *Clin. Sci. Mol. Med.*, **46**, 191–206.

Stringer, W. W., Hansen, J. E., Wasserman, K. (1997). Cardiac output estimated noninvasively from oxygen uptake during exercise. *J. Appl. Physiol.*, **82**, 908–12.

Weber, K. T. & Janicki, J. S. (1985). Cardiopulmonary exercise testing for evaluation of chronic heart failure. *Am. J. Cardiol.*, **55**, 22A–31A.

Weber, K. T., Kinasewitz, G. T., Janicki, J. S. & Fishman, A. P. (1982). Oxygen utilization and ventilation during exercise in patients with chronic cardiac failure. *Circulation*, **65**, 1213–23.

Whipp, B. J., Davis, J. A., Torres, F. & Wasserman, K. (1981). A test to determine parameters of aerobic function during exercise. *J. Appl. Physiol. Respirat. Environ. Exerc. Physiol.*, **50**, 217–21.

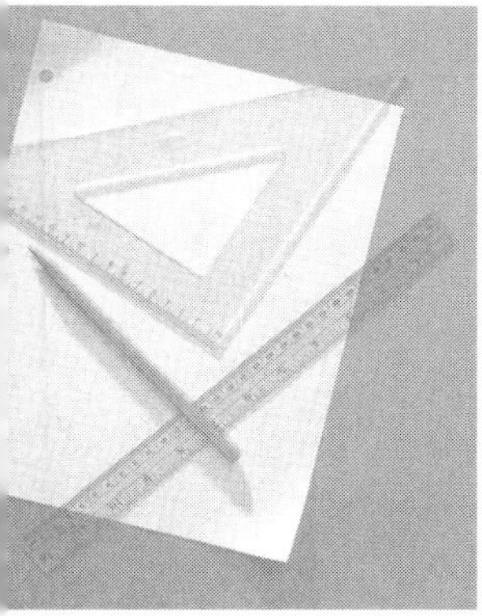

5

# Data integration and interpretation

## Introduction

Proper selection and use of well-calibrated instruments and an appropriate test protocol should produce one or more of the measured variables described in Chapter 4. These variables now require integration, one with another, and meaningful interpretation to complete the purpose of the exercise test.

Some tests, such as field tests, yield one specific measured variable. These variables are typically compared with reference values (so-called predicted normal values) or related to serial measurements for a given individual. They do not necessarily require integration with other results. The interpretation of individual variables has been thoroughly explained in Chapter 4. However, a brief consideration of the derivation and limitations of reference values will now be addressed.

Laboratory exercise tests, notably the maximal incremental work rate protocols, yield an impressive array of data. The results can be bewildering unless organized and interpreted in a systematic manner. This chapter describes how test data can be displayed, in graphical or tabular format, thus enabling the practitioner to evaluate these data systematically and arrive at conclusions that address the specific purpose of the test.

Based on logical data displays of multiple variables, a scheme for the recognition of specific response patterns can be developed. The scheme presented in this chapter acknowledges that clinical exercise testing is often limited in its ability to point to a specific diagnosis. However, for each abnormal response pattern, the implications are discussed and examples of clinical conditions giving rise to that pattern are given.

## Comparison of single variables with reference values

### Population sample means

Once a measurement is obtained in an exercising subject, the inclination is to ask what this value should be in normal circumstances. Reference values, often called predicted normal values, exist for many physiological variables. They are commonly obtained as mean values from the study of large samples of the supposedly normal human population.

In reality, all individuals do not have an identical value for a given physiological parameter. There is biological variability, which usually results in a normal distribution of values around the population mean. Hence, if we measure $\dot{V}O_{2max}$ in 1000 normal individuals of the same age, gender, and body weight, we will obtain a range of values with a bell-shaped distribution about the mean. The degree of variability is characterized statistically by the standard deviation of the mean (Figure 5.1).

When comparing measured values from an individual with reference values from a sample population, several factors must be taken into consideration: (1) Does the individual subject match

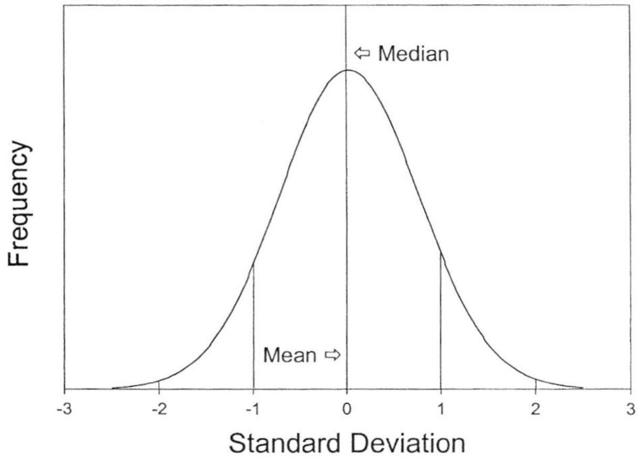


**Figure 5.1** Normal distribution of a hypothetical variable illustrating identical mean and median. The $x$-axis is represented in terms of standard deviation (SD), illustrating that 68% of the data lie within 1 SD either side of the mean, whereas 95% of data lie within 2 SD either side of the mean. The 95% confidence limits for the $x$-variable can also be appreciated from this graph.

the sample population? (2) Was the sample population representative of the normal condition? (3) What was the variability of the measurement in the sample population? The third question is important in determining whether a single measured value is sufficiently different from the population mean to be considered abnormal. Here, we rely upon statistical analysis to define normality.

Knowledge of the standard deviation of the mean or biological variability of the measurement enables one to predict that a percentage of all normal measurements will fall within a certain confidence interval based on the standard deviation. Thus, for a normally distributed variable approximately 95% of normal values will lie within 2 SD (actually 1.96 SD) of the population mean, as shown in Figure 5.1.

One can see that the biological variability of the measurement is crucial. The variability is small for measurements such as $\dot{V}O_{2max}$, $\dot{V}O_{2rest}$, $PaO_2$, $PaCO_2$, and RPE but substantial for measures such as $f_{Cmax}$, $\dot{V}_{Emax}$, $V_D/V_T$ and $\beta$– score. The most important ramification of these facts is in the prediction of maximum heart rate and the use of this estimate to derive $\dot{V}O_{2max}$ from submaximal exercise data. The standard deviation for $f_{Cmax}$ is 10 min$^{-1}$, meaning that 95% of normal individuals will exhibit $f_{Cmax}$ within 20 min$^{-1}$ above or below the predicted mean value. Such considerations clearly render estimates of $\dot{V}O_{2max}$ based on predicted $f_{Cmax}$ at best uncertain and often unreliable.

## Prediction equations

Several important measured variables of the exercise response are influenced by descriptive or anthropometric characteristics of the subject. It is important to keep this consideration in mind when comparing any measured variable with a reference value obtained from a prediction equation. The best example is $\dot{V}O_{2max}$, which is well known to be related to age, gender, and body mass. The influence of such characteristics can be assessed in population studies by regression analysis. The details of this approach are best researched in a text of biomedical statistics. However, many exercise variables are predicted by regression equations, which attempt to quantitate the relative influences of other major characteristics on the measurement in question. Examples of prediction equations for $\dot{V}O_{2max}$ are shown in Table C1 of Appendix C. By this approach it is possible to say that about 80% of the variability of $\dot{V}O_{2max}$ is accounted for by age, gender, and body mass. By similar considerations, it is also possible to state that only about 60% of the variability of $f_{Cmax}$ is accounted for by the age of the subject.

## Nomograms

A convenient method for prediction of normal values is the use of the nomogram. Usually, a nomogram consists of three parallel straight lines each graduated for a different variable, so that another straight line cutting across all three graduated lines intersects the related values of each variable. An example of a nomogram linking $f_C$, $\dot{W}$, and $\dot{V}O_{2max}$ (the Åstrand–Ryhming nomogram) is shown in Appendix C (Figure C5).

## Comparison of serial measurements for single variables

### Response to physical conditioning or rehabilitation

Repeated measurement of the same variable in the same individual gives greater statistical power to determine differences from normality and meaningful changes. In the realm of exercise testing this approach is most valuable in periodic assessment of physical fitness and progress monitoring with physical training or rehabilitation.

This can be achieved very effectively using field tests to measure physical performance in terms of running speed or distance (Figure 5.2). Alternatively, serial physiological assessments can be obtained using the more complex integrative exercise test to determine $\dot{V}o_{2max}$ and $\dot{V}o_2\theta$. Many athletes judge their level of physical conditioning by monitoring resting heart rate. Integrative exercise testing offers a more precise method of looking at submaximal heart rates in relation to metabolic rate through the slope of the cardiovascular response, $\delta f_C/\delta\dot{V}o_2$. Successful physical training should result in reduction of this slope as well as increased $\dot{V}o_{2max}$.

Comparison of serial measurements is best applied to single variables obtained from identical work rate protocols. For example, the performance of identical constant work rate XTs before and after successful physical training should result in reductions in $f_C$, $\dot{V}co_2$, $\dot{V}_E$ and most likely symptom scores at identical moments in the exercise protocol. Arguably these findings offer the most reliable evidence of a "true" physiological training response. When the work rate protocols are identical in relation to time, reductions in $f_C$, $\dot{V}o_2$, and $\dot{V}_E$ should be sought at identical times during each of the tests (so-called isotime analysis). Where the relationship between work rate and time is less certain, changes in single variables can be sought at the same work rate (so-called isowork analysis).

When the isotime or isowork approaches are used, special consideration should be given to the observation of reduced $\dot{V}o_2$ following physical train-



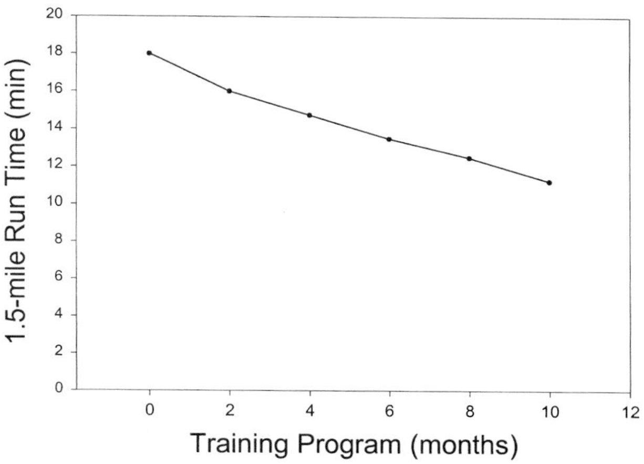

**Figure 5.2** Hypothetical graph of 1.5-mile running times for a 30-year-old female progressing from poor to superior fitness category during a 10-month training program.

ing or rehabilitation. Such a change implies improved biomechanical or work efficiency. Biomechanical efficiency is an important aspect of physical training but not strictly a manifestation of physiological improvement. Runners are familiar with the term "running economy," used to describe biomechanical efficiency for field XTs.

In the practice of rehabilitation for patients with chronic pulmonary disease, deliberate strategies are employed to reduce the ventilatory requirement or $\dot{V}_E$ for a given work rate. These strategies are based on an understanding of the determinants of the slope of the ventilatory response, $\delta\dot{V}_E/\delta\dot{V}o_2$, as discussed in Chapter 4. Hence avoidance of excessive carbohydrate ingestion just before exercise reduces $R$. Peripheral adaptations reduce lactic acidosis (i.e., they increase $\dot{V}o_2\theta$) and thereby reduce $\dot{V}co_2$ and also reduce $R$. Avoidance of rapid shallow breathing improves breathing efficiency and reduces $V_D/V_T$. Each of these changes in and of itself will contribute to reducing ventilatory requirement and hopefully increase functional capacity in these patients.

### Progression or regression of illness

In the realm of clinical assessment, serial measurement of specific exercise variables can be used to assess the progression or regression of certain disease processes.

Various walking tests are commonly used to assess the functional capacity of patients with cardiovascular and pulmonary diseases in terms of distance covered in a given time. Similarly, 1-mile walking tests and 12-min run or 1.5-mile run tests are often used with apparently healthy populations as field test measures of aerobic capacity. These tests can be designed to give additional information, such as the requirement for supplemental oxygen or symptom perception and rate of heart rate recovery.

Integrative exercise tests can be used to compare several more specific physiological measures. One or other of these measures might be directly relevant to the disease process in question.

For example, changes in $\dot{V}_{Emax}$ in patients with chronic pulmonary disease who have true ventilatory limitation might reflect a response to therapeutic intervention or alternatively reflect disease progression. Similarly, in patients with chronic pulmonary disease, alterations in exercise gas exchange, e.g., $P_{(A-a)}O_2$ and $P_{(a-ET)}CO_2$, can be indicators of a treatment response or alternatively of deterioration.

Whenever exercise capacity is deemed to be an important outcome in the clinical management of certain diseases, comparison of serial measurements can be used to assess the effectiveness of treatment. Thus, in chronic obstructive pulmonary disease $\dot{V}_{Emax}$ may increase with bronchodilator therapy. In fibrosing alveolitis $P_{(A-a)}O_2$ at maximum exercise should be reduced with effective corticosteroid or immunosuppressive treatment. In congestive heart failure $\dot{V}O_{2max}$ should be increased by successful pharmacotherapy whereas, unfortunately, too often drugs prescribed for cardiovascular disease actually impair the exercise response.

## Reduction and display of multiple data

### General approach

Multiple data need organization to assist interpretation. Two approaches are commonly used: tabular display, and graphical display. Both offer specific advantages and they can be usefully combined in developing an interpretation. Table 5.1 shows a systematic approach for the interpretation of multiple data.

#### Step 1: Reason for testing

One question remains of paramount importance in the conduct and analysis of an exercise test. This question is, of course, the reason for referral and testing. The entire approach to exercise testing should be geared to the specific purpose of answering this question. Hence, the selection of the test protocol should be appropriate and the method by which the results are collated and displayed should enable the practitioner to answer the questions posed by the referral.

A brief exercise or medical history is helpful in this regard. For example, a subject might have known pulmonary and cardiovascular disease but the reason for testing is to determine which of these problems limits exercise capacity. Alternatively, a subject may have no known medical problems and simply wish to know how $\dot{V}O_{2max}$ and $\dot{V}O_2\theta$ have responded to a physical training program. Also, the person referring the subject might have a predictable purpose in requesting exercise testing, e.g., a surgeon who is interested in preoperative risk assessment.

#### Step 2: Technical factors

An important requirement of every exercise test is to record any technical problems that may have occurred. These could include mouthpiece intolerance, leaking, poor-quality ECG, malfunction of the work rate controller, inability to draw blood samples, or any type of instrument failure. Such problems must obviously be taken into consideration when analyzing and interpreting the results.

Every test should be carefully scrutinized to ensure that the environmental conditions were accurately recorded and that all calibrations were satisfactory. Environmental conditions include

**Table 5.1.** Systematic approach for the analysis of multiple data from integrative exercise testing

| Step | Focus | Questions | Primary focus | Additional focus |
|---|---|---|---|---|
| 1 | Reason for testing | Why was the exercise test requested? | Known diagnoses<br>Specific question | Who referred |
| 2 | Technical factors | Was the test technically adequate? | $\dot{V}O_2/\dot{W}$<br>Test duration<br>Calibration | Technical problems<br>Medical problems |
| 3 | Parameters of aerobic performance | Was there normal aerobic capacity?<br>Was there normal work efficiency? | $\dot{V}O_{2max}$, $\delta\dot{V}O_2/\delta\dot{W}$, or $\eta^{-1}$, $\dot{V}O_2\theta$, $\tau\dot{V}O_2$ | $\dot{V}O_2$ warm-up (intercept) |
| 4 | Cardiovascular response | Was there cardiovascular limitation?<br>Was the cardiovascular response pattern normal? | $f_{Cmax}$, $\delta f_C/\delta\dot{V}O_2$, $\dot{V}O_2/f_C$ | $f_{Crest}$, ECG, systemic arterial pressure |
| 5 | Ventilatory response | Was there ventilatory limitation?<br>Was the ventilatory response pattern normal? | $\dot{V}_{Emax}$, MVV, $\dot{V}_{Ecap}$, $V_T$, $f_R$, $T_I/T_E$ | |
| 6 | Gas exchange | Were gas exchange mechanisms normal?<br>Was there evidence for wasted ventilation or wasted perfusion? | $Paco_2$, $V_D/V_T$, $Pao_2$, $P_{(A-a)}O_2$, $Spo_2$ | $P_{ET}CO_2$, $P_{(a-ET)}CO_2$, $P_{ET}O_2$, $\dot{V}_E/\dot{V}O_2$, $\dot{V}_E/\dot{V}CO_2$, $R$ |
| 7 | Muscle metabolism | Was there suggestion of myopathy? | Lactate, ammonia, creatine kinase | $\dot{V}O_2\theta$, $\delta\dot{V}O_2/\delta\dot{W}$ |
| 8 | Symptom perception | What symptoms limited exercise?<br>Was perceived exertion consistent with cardiovascular response?<br>Was breathlessness consistent with ventilatory response? | Reason for stopping RPE, $\beta$– | Subjective effort<br>Objective effort |
| 9 | Conclusion | What were the specific physiological limitations?<br>What was the answer to the question posed? | Steps 3–8<br>Pattern recognition | |

barometric pressure and ambient temperature. Gas exchange measurements at altitude, (e.g., in Denver at 1500 m or Cheyenne at 2300 m) must take into account the proportionately lower partial pressure of oxygen.

As described in Chapter 2, all instruments must be calibrated on a regular basis and, for gas exchange measurement, the flow transducer and gas analyzers should be calibrated before each test. Calibration data should be examined to ensure consistency, i.e., low variance, in calculated tidal volumes when using a standard calibration syringe. For the gas analyzers both accuracy and response characteristics are important. During breath-by-breath measurement, a common problem is prolongation of the phase delay of the gas analyzers due to problems with the sampling line. This problem alone can cause serious errors in calculated $\dot{V}O_2$ and $\dot{V}CO_2$, regardless of the accuracy of the instruments.

The best indicator of a successful incremental XT is found in the robustness of the $\dot{V}O_2$–$\dot{W}$ relationship and should be one of the first elements of the data set to be examined to ensure that there were no untoward technical problems during the test.

The tester should also examine the correlation of heart rate by ECG with the values recorded by the metabolic cart, throughout the test. Discrepancies can arise at higher exercise intensities due to electrical interference degrading the ECG signal.

Although not strictly technical factors, any medical problems which affect exercise performance should also be recorded.

### Step 3: Parameters of aerobic performance

Once the test purpose is clearly defined and technical problems have been assessed, the next fundamental step in data analysis is to examine the four parameters of aerobic capacity: $\dot{V}O_{2max}$, $\eta^{-1}$, $\dot{V}O_2\theta$ and $\tau\dot{V}O_2$ whenever or however they have been measured.

Using the convention described in Table 4.1, aerobic capacity or $\dot{V}O_{2max}$ can be stated to be normal (>80% and ≤120%), higher than predicted, or reduced to varying degrees. A normal $\dot{V}O_{2max}$ implies normal exercise capacity, although it is conceivable that $\dot{V}O_{2max}$ could be spuriously high due to technical problems, thus masking an underlying physiological abnormality. A low $\dot{V}O_{2max}$ demands explanation through further steps of the analysis.

A normal $\dot{V}O_2$–$\dot{W}$ relationship indicates a successful test and implies that technical problems were unlikely to have influenced this aspect of the results.

### Step 4: Cardiovascular response

With regard to the cardiovascular response, two questions are of fundamental importance:

1. Was there evidence of cardiovascular limitation?
2. Was the cardiovascular response pattern normal?

An approach to answering these questions is described later in this chapter.

Cardiovascular limitation with a normal response pattern is the normal physiological response, whereas cardiovascular limitation with an abnormal response pattern or absence of cardiovascular limitation is abnormal and demands further explanation.

### Step 5: Ventilatory response

With regard to the ventilatory response, two questions are of fundamental importance:

1. Was there evidence of ventilatory limitation?
2. Was the ventilatory response pattern normal?

An approach to answering these questions is described later in this chapter.

Ventilatory limitation is not expected in normal subjects. Therefore, evidence of ventilatory limitation or an abnormal ventilatory response pattern requires further explanation.

Ventilatory limitation must be judged in relation to a subject's actual ventilatory capacity rather than a normal predicted value. Hence, a person with obstructive pulmonary disease can be expected to have reduced ventilatory capacity but may or may not have ventilatory limitation.

### Step 6: Gas exchange

An integrative exercise test which yields measures of $\dot{V}_E$, $\dot{V}O_2$, $\dot{V}CO_2$, and end-tidal gas tensions can be interpreted to help determine whether any abnormality of gas exchange was present. However, arterial blood sampling is crucial for the calculation of $P_{(A-a)}O_2$, $P_{(a-ET)}CO_2$, and $V_D/V_T$ which are the definitive physiological measures of gas exchange efficiency. When normal patterns of change in ventilatory equivalents and end-tidal gas tensions are observed during an XT without arterial blood sampling, there are not likely to be severe or limiting gas exchange abnormalities. A single arterial blood sample obtained whilst gas exchange measurements are being made at rest allows a precise determination about resting gas exchange and can be used in conjunction with subsequent noninvasive data. However, an early or subtle gas exchange abnormality may only manifest itself at maximum exercise. When subtle gas exchange abnormalities are suspected, arterial blood sampling at maximum exercise is clearly desirable.

### Step 7: Muscle metabolism

A person with musculoskeletal disease, such as myopathy, is unlikely to exhibit normal responses for the parameters of aerobic performance. Abnormalities of the cardiovascular and ventilatory responses are also likely to occur. These findings *per se* are often nondiagnostic.

Examination of the physiological data together with measurements of blood lactate, ammonia, and creatine kinase are recommended to characterize the musculoskeletal response.

### Step 8: Symptom perception

An important requirement of any symptom-limited exercise test is a record of the specific symptoms or reasons that caused the subject to stop exercise. This information should be recorded immediately upon termination of the exercise test and will be helpful in the subsequent test interpretation. The subject should be allowed to describe in his or her own words the limiting symptoms or other reasons for stopping an exercise test. However, in order to obtain consistency in recording these data, a defined list can used from which to prompt the subject who has difficulty assigning or categorizing a limiting symptom. Table 5.2 shows the commonly described reasons subjects give for stopping an exercise test.

**Table 5.2.** Common symptoms or other reasons for stopping exercise

| Symptoms or other reasons for stopping exercise |
|---|
| Breathlessness |
| Leg fatigue |
| Breathlessness and leg fatigue |
| General fatigue |
| Chest pain |
| Palpitations |
| Dizziness |
| Dry mouth |
| Physical discomfort |

The use of psychometric scales, described in Chapter 4, enhances the symptomatic evaluation during an exercise test. The valuable correlation between rating of perceived exertion (RPE) and heart rate allows the observer to judge whether the subject's perception of effort was appropriate for the cardiovascular response. The approximate correspondence of breathlessness score on a 100-mm visual analog scale with the proportion of ventilatory capacity utilized ($\dot{V}_{E\max}/\dot{V}_{E\text{cap}}$) allows the observer to judge whether the subject's perception of breathlessness was appropriate for the ventilatory response. Symptoms that appear to be inappropriate compared with the physiological responses suggest conscious or subconscious nonphysiological or psychogenic components (see Chapter 4).

### Step 9: Conclusion

Once this stepwise process of interpretation is completed, it should be possible to define one or more specific physiological limitations to exercise in a given subject. In the case of clinical exercise testing, it may not be possible to attribute these limitations to a specific disease but usually a focused differential diagnosis can be suggested.

The final task in exercise interpretation is to address the question posed in referral of the subject. A systematic analysis, such as that outlined above, offers the best chance of being able to answer this question and thereby to satisfy the person requesting the exercise test.

## Tabular display

The systematic approach described above is helped considerably by the extraction and tabulation of key variables from the raw data obtained during an

**Table 5.3.** Tabular summary for multiple data from integrative exercise testing

| Name (last, first) | ID no. | Age (years) | Gender (M/F) | Date of study (m/d/y) |
|---|---|---|---|---|
| **Anthropometric** | | **Technical** | | **Diagnosis** |
| Height (in.) | | Barometer (mmHg) | | |
| Height (m) | | Ambient T (°C) | | |
| Weight (lb) | | $F_IO_2$ (%) | | |
| Weight (kg) | | Valve dead space (ml) | | |
| | | $\ddot{W}$ (W · min$^{-1}$) | | |
| Body mass index (kg · m$^{-2}$) | | $\dot{W}$ (W) | | |
| **Pulmonary function** | **Predicted** | **Observed** | **%Predicted** | **Comment** |
| FVC (l) | | | | |
| $FEV_1$ (l) | | | | |
| $FEV_1$/FEV (%) | | | | |
| MVV (l · min$^{-1}$) | | | | |
| **Aerobic capacity** | **Predicted** | **Observed** | **%pred$\dot{V}O_{2max}$** | **Comment** |
| $\dot{V}O_{2max}$ (l · min$^{-1}$) | | | | |
| $\dot{V}O_2\theta$ (l · min$^{-1}$) | | | | |
| $\delta\dot{V}O_2/\delta W$ (ml · min$^{-1}$ · W$^{-1}$) | 10.3 | | | |
| $\dot{V}O_{2unloaded}$ (l · min$^{-1}$) | | | | |
| **Cardiovascular response** | **Predicted** | **Observed** | **%Predicted** | **Comment** |
| $f_{Cmax}$ (min$^{-1}$) | | | | |
| Cardiac reserve (min$^{-1}$) | 0 | | | |
| $\dot{V}O_2/f_{Cmax}$ (ml) | | | | |
| $f_{Crest}$ (min$^{-1}$) | | | | |
| Resting ECG | | | | |
| Exercise ECG | | | | |
| | **Rest** | **Exercise (max.)** | **Recovery (2 min)** | |
| Systolic BP (mmHg) | | | | |
| Diastolic BP (mmHg) | | | | |
| **Ventilatory response** | **Predicted** | **Observed** | **%MVV** | **Comment** |
| $\dot{V}_{Emax}$ (l · min$^{-1}$) | | | | |
| Ventilatory reserve (l · min$^{-1}$) | $>15$ | | | |
| $V_{Tmax}$ (l) | | | | |
| $f_{Rmax}$ (min$^{-1}$) | $<50$ | | | |
| $T_I/T_E$ at end exercise | 0.8 | | | |

**Table 5.3.** *(cont.)*

| Gas exchange | Rest | Threshold | Maximum | Comment |
|---|---|---|---|---|
| $\dot{V}_E/\dot{V}O_2$ | | | | |
| $\dot{V}_E/\dot{V}CO_2$ | | | | |
| $P_{ET}O_2$ (mmHg) | | | | |
| $P_{ET}CO_2$ (mmHg) | | | | |
| $R$ | | | | |
| $SpO_2$ (%) | | | | |
| $PaO_2$ (mmHg) | | | | |
| $PaCO_2$ (mmHg) | | | | |
| $P_{(A-a)}O_2$ (mmHg) | | | | |
| $P_{(a-ET)}CO_2$ (mmHg) | | | | |
| $V_D/V_T$ (%) | | | | |
| **Muscle metabolism** | **Rest** | **Exercise (4 min)** | **Recovery (2 min)** | **Comment** |
| Lactate (mg · dl$^{-1}$) | | | | |
| Ammonia (μg · dl$^{-1}$) | | | | |
| Creatine kinase (U · l$^{-1}$) | | | | |
| | **Predicted** | **Observed** | | |
| $RQ_{mus}$ ($\delta\dot{V}CO_2/\delta\dot{V}O_2$) | 0.95 | | | |
| **Symptom perception** | **Rest** | **Exercise (max.)** | | **Comment** |
| Effort (observer impression) | | | | |
| Symptoms (subjective) | | | | |
| Perceived exertion (Borg scale/20) | | | | |
| Breathlessness (VAS scale/100) | | | | |

incremental exercise test. Condensing the data to a single page so that all elements of the test can be viewed simultaneously and interrelated is ideal.

Suggested elements of a tabular summary are shown in Table 5.3. This table combines identifying characteristics for the subject, known clinical diagnoses, anthropometric data, environmental conditions, protocol definition, aerobic capacity, cardiovascular response, ventilatory response, gas exchange, muscle metabolism, and symptom perception.

## Graphical display

Graphs are most valuable for studying the interrelationship of certain data and trending phenomena, either within a single test or with the passage of time to examine the progression of illness or the effects of physical training or rehabilitation.

Many investigators have found value in placing as many as nine graphs on a single page so that multiple relationships and trending phenomena can be viewed simultaneously.

### Nine-panel display

One such approach is the nine-panel display, popularized by Harbor-UCLA Medical Center. An example of a nine-panel display is shown in Figure 5.3 and the important elements of this display are listed in Table 5.4.

The nine-panel display has a logical layout.

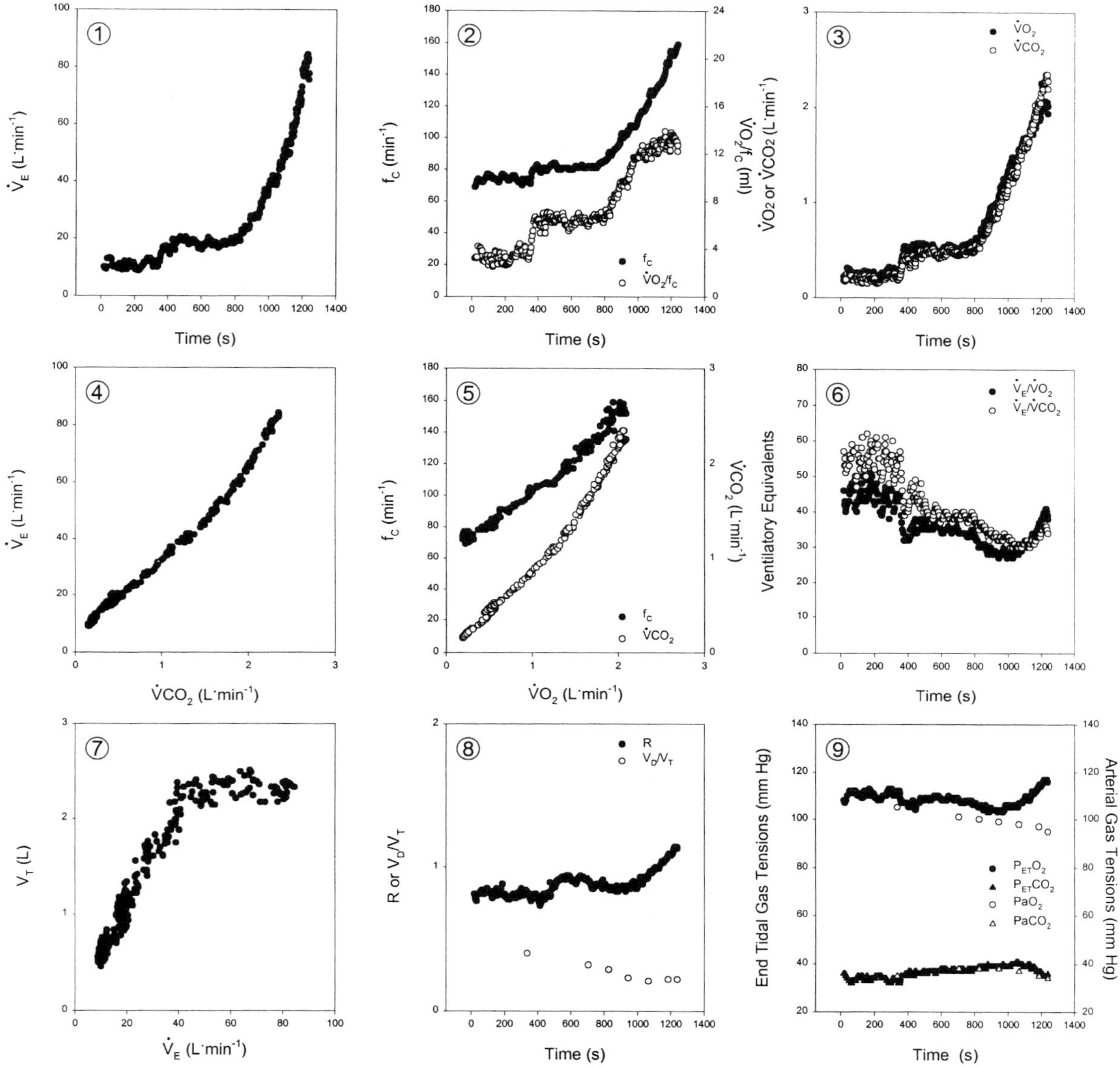


**Figure 5.3** Nine-panel display for a maximal incremental XT. Refer to Table 5.4 for a description of the individual graphs.

**Table 5.4.** Elements of a nine-panel display for multiple data from integrative exercise testing

| Graph | Variables | Relevance |
|---|---|---|
| 1 | $\dot{V}_E$ vs. time (or $\dot{W}$) | Ventilatory response |
| 2 | $f_C$ and $\dot{V}O_2/f_C$ vs. time (or $\dot{W}$) | Cardiovascular response |
| 3 | $\dot{V}O_2$ and $\dot{V}CO_2$ vs. time (or $\dot{W}$) | Metabolic response |
| 4 | $\dot{V}_E$ vs. $\dot{V}CO_2$ | Ventilatory threshold |
| 5 | $f_C$ vs. $\dot{V}O_2$ | Cardiovascular response |
| | $\dot{V}CO_2$ vs. $\dot{V}O_2$ | Metabolic threshold |
| 6 | $\dot{V}_E/\dot{V}O_2$ and $\dot{V}_E/\dot{V}CO_2$ vs. time (or $\dot{W}$) | Gas exchange |
| 7 | $V_T$ vs. $\dot{V}_E$ | Ventilatory response |
| 8 | $R$ and $V_D/V_T$ vs. time (or $\dot{W}$) | Gas exchange |
| 9 | $PaO_2$, $PaCO_2$, $P_{ET}O_2$, and $P_{ET}CO_2$ vs. time (or $\dot{W}$) | Gas exchange |

Graphs which depict the ventilatory response are arranged in the first column (panels 1, 4, and 7). Graphs which depict the cardiovascular response are together in the second column (panels 2 and 5). Graphs which depict the gas exchange responses are grouped at the bottom right (panels 5, 6, 8, and 9).

This arrangement also facilitates identification of other key response patterns. Graphs 6 and 9 can be used in conjunction to help identify the metabolic threshold. A vertical line through the inflection points for $\dot{V}_E/\dot{V}O_2$ and $P_{ET}O_2$ can be extrapolated on to graph 3 to read $\dot{V}O_2\theta$.

Most metabolic carts have adopted the nine-panel display as a graphical option and allow users to select and customize their own plots.

### Four-panel displays

An alternative approach to the graphical representation of data is to use a series of four four-panel displays to focus separately on aerobic performance, the cardiovascular response, the ventilatory response and gas exchange. Examples of these displays are shown in Figures 5.4–5.7 and their important elements are listed in Table 5.5.

These four displays can be used to analyze the important components of the exercise response. They should be studied in conjunction with each other but can also be used to focus on specific questions or concerns about an individual study.

*Aerobic performance (Figure 5.4)*

For an incremental work rate study, the four-panel display of aerobic performance allows three of the four important parameters of aerobic performance to be precisely studied ($\dot{V}O_{2max}$, $\eta^{-1}$, and $\dot{V}O_2\theta$).

Panel 1 shows the fundamental relationship between $\dot{V}O_2$ and $\dot{W}$, allowing the slope to be compared with its predicted normal value of $10.3\,ml \cdot min^{-1} \cdot W^{-1}$. Furthermore, this panel allows a comparison of $\dot{V}O_{2max}$ with its reference value.

Panel 2 shows the relationship between $f_C$ and $\dot{W}$. This panel allows $f_{Cmax}$ to be compared with its reference value. The slope of this relationship can also be assessed.

Panel 3 shows the relationship between $\dot{V}_E$ and $\dot{W}$. This panel allows $\dot{V}_{Emax}$ to be compared with the measured MVV or predicted $\dot{V}_{Ecap}$.

Panel 4 shows the relationship between $\dot{V}CO_2$ and $\dot{V}O_2$ and enables the metabolic threshold $\dot{V}O_2\theta$ to be determined.

The fourth parameter of aerobic performance, $\tau\dot{V}O_2$, is reflected in the phasic response of oxygen uptake shown in panel 1. However, there are methodological difficulties in determining $\tau\dot{V}O_2$ from the incremental test. For a constant work rate test, the four-panel display of aerobic performance would allow the determination of time constants for each of $\dot{V}O_2$, $\dot{V}CO_2$, $f_C$, and $\dot{V}_E$.

*Cardiovascular response (Figure 5.5)*

Panel 1 shows the relationship between $f_C$ and $\dot{W}$. Furthermore, this panel allows a comparison of $f_{Cmax}$ with its reference value.

Panel 2 shows the fundamental relationship between $f_C$ and $\dot{V}O_2$. This panel is most important in judging the pattern of the cardiovascular response and also allows a comparison of $f_{Cmax}$ with $\dot{V}O_{2max}$.

Panel 3 shows $\dot{V}O_2/f_C$ with increasing work rate.

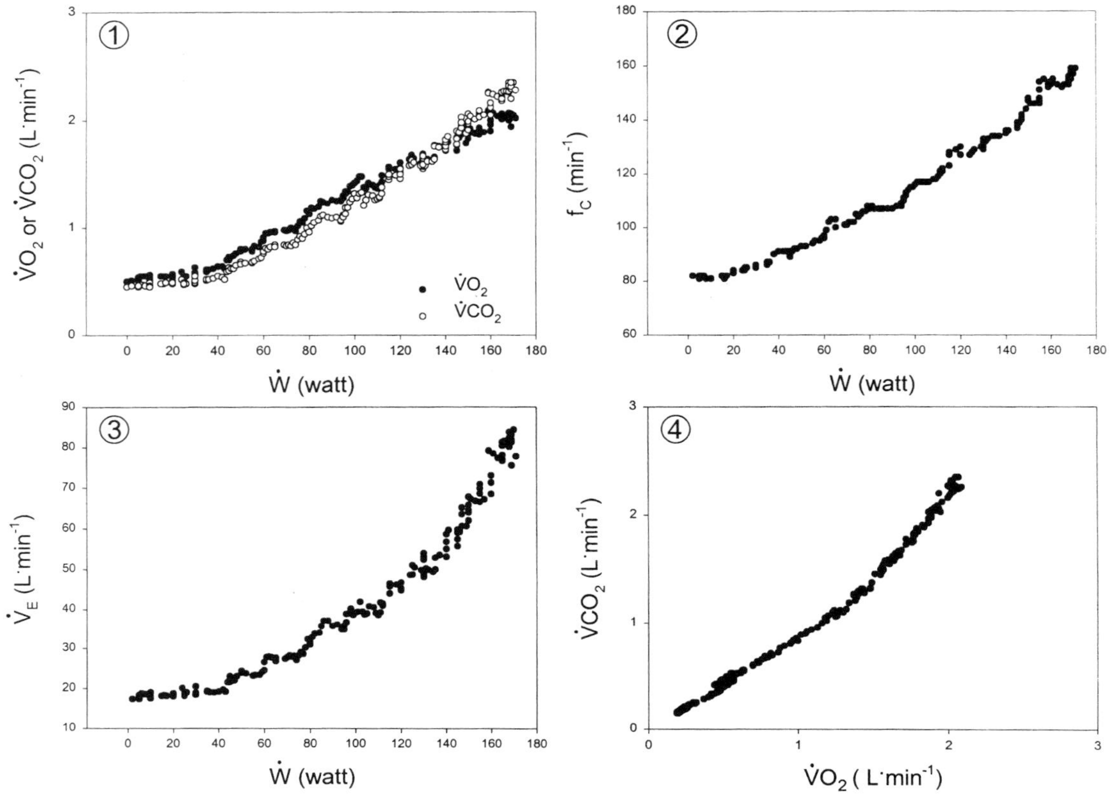


**Figure 5.4** Aerobic capacity: four-panel display. Refer to Table 5.5 for a description of the individual graphs.

Panel 4 shows the relationship between $\dot{V}o_2$ and $\dot{W}$, which is the important foundation upon which to judge the cardiovascular response.

*Ventilatory response (Figure 5.6)*
Panel 1 shows the relationship between $\dot{V}_E$ and $\dot{W}$. Furthermore, this panel allows a comparison of $\dot{V}_{Emax}$ with measured MVV or predicted $\dot{V}_{Ecap}$.

Panel 2 shows the fundamental relationship between $\dot{V}_E$ and $\dot{V}o_2$. This panel is important in judging the overall pattern of the ventilatory response.

Panel 3 is the inverse Hey plot of $V_T$ *versus* $\dot{V}_E$. This panel offers an approach for judging the pattern of the ventilatory response.

Panel 4 shows the relationship between $\dot{V}_E$ and $\dot{V}co_2$. This panel allows the ventilatory threshold $\dot{V}_E\theta$ to be identified. Identification of the value of $\dot{V}_E$ which corresponds to $\dot{V}_E\theta$ in panel 2 allows this threshold to be expressed in terms of $\dot{V}o_2$.

*Gas exchange (Figure 5.7)*
This plot is set out to facilitate the identification of the metabolic threshold.

Panel 1 displays the relationship between $\dot{V}co_2$ and $\dot{V}o_2$ and allows $\dot{V}o_2\theta$ to be determined by the pattern of its response. The $\dot{V}o_2\theta$ determined in this way has been shown to be the most accurate and reliable method for ascertaining the metabolic threshold from gas exchange measurements.

Panel 2 shows the relationships of $\dot{V}_E/\dot{V}o_2$ and

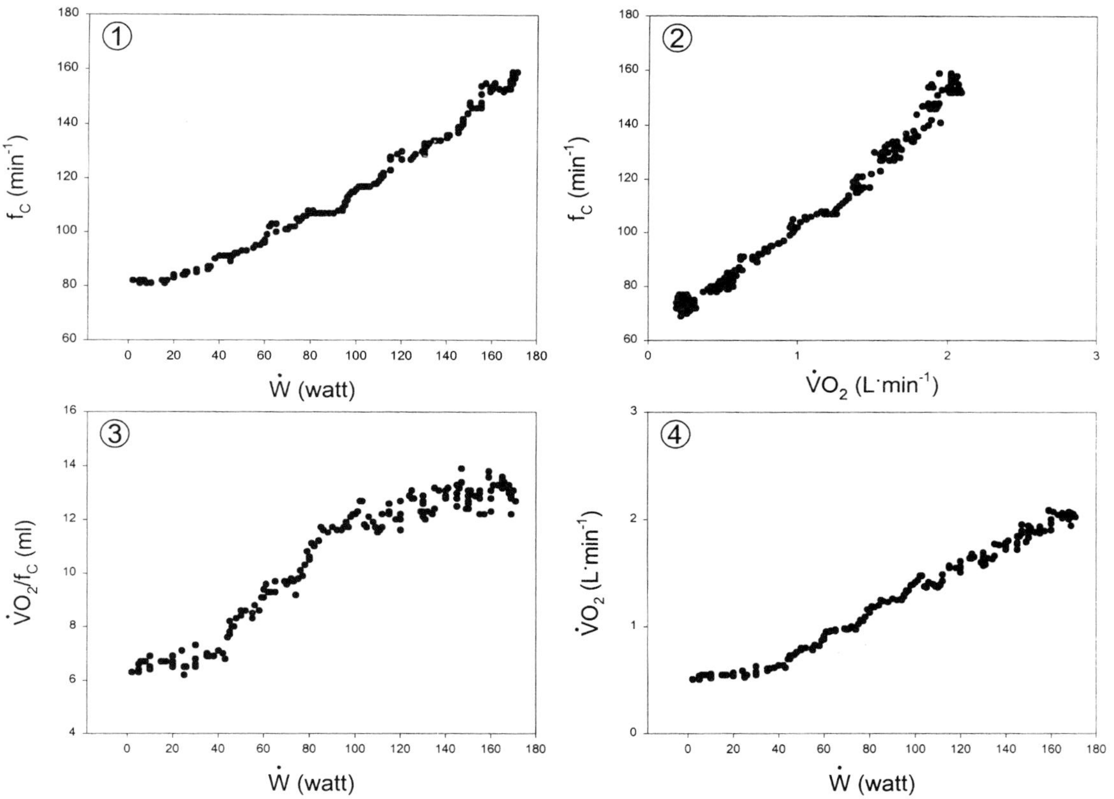


**Figure 5.5** Cardiovascular response: four-panel display. Refer to Table 5.5 for a description of the individual graphs.

$\dot{V}_E/\dot{V}co_2$ with increasing work rate. These plots illustrate the so-called dual criterion.

Panel 3 displays the relationship between $R$ and $\dot{W}$. Although complex and influenced by hyperventilation, this relationship often exhibits a threshold corresponding to $\dot{V}o_2\theta$.

Panel 4 shows the relationships of $P_{ET}o_2$ and $P_{ET}co_2$ with increasing work rate. Panels 2 and 4 can be used in conjunction to help identify the metabolic threshold. A vertical line is drawn through the inflection points for $\dot{V}_E/\dot{V}o_2$ and $P_{ET}o_2$ to determine the work rate at which the metabolic threshold occurred. Importantly, at the metabolic threshold, $\dot{V}_E/\dot{V}co_2$ and $P_{ET}co_2$ should not exhibit simultaneous upward or downward deflections respectively. This work rate must then be applied to a plot of $\dot{V}o_2$ versus $\dot{W}$ or to raw tabular data to determine the actual value for $\dot{V}o_2\theta$.

Values for $Pao_2$ and $Paco_2$ can also be added to panel 4, allowing for estimation of $P_{(A-a)}o_2$ and $P_{(a-ET)}co_2$.

## Sequential graphing to display trending phenomena

Certain variables derived from exercise testing are of such paramount importance that they stand alone and can be scrutinized in relation to predicted reference values or previously observed responses for an individual subject. In this context graphs can

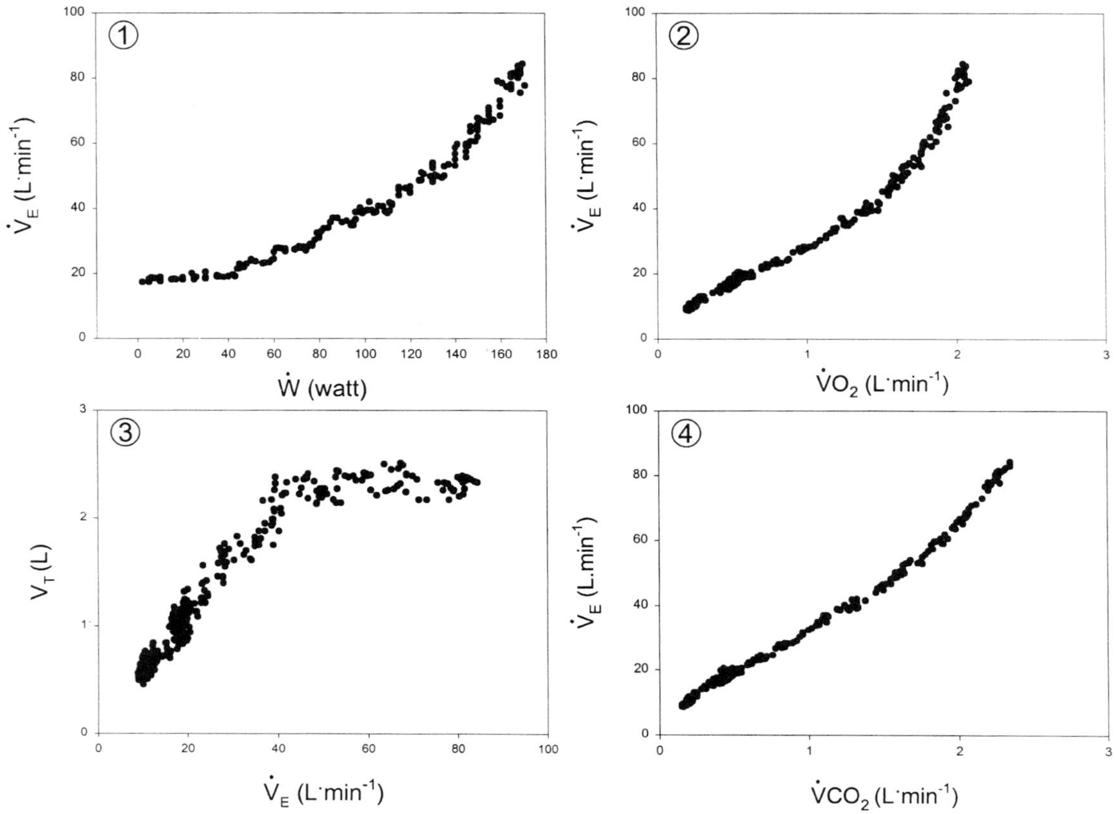


**Figure 5.6** Ventilatory response: four-panel display. Refer to Table 5.5 for a description of the individual graphs.

be helpful in displaying trending phenomena over time and between tests.

Variables relating to maximal performance which lend themselves to this type of display are walking or running time, $d_W$, $d_R$, $\dot{V}o_{2max}$, $\dot{V}o_2\theta$, $f_{Cmax}$, and $\dot{V}_{Emax}$. Variables that relate to submaximal performance can be displayed similarly to illustrate a physiological training effect. Most useful in this regard are $\dot{V}o_2$, $\dot{V}co_2$, $f_C$, $\dot{V}_E$, $f_R$, and lactate at a predetermined and fixed constant work rate. Figure 5.8 shows an example of the ventilatory response to four constant work rates before and after 8 weeks of cycle ergometer training in healthy subjects. The reduced levels of ventilation at higher work rates reflect reductions in blood lactate for the same exercise protocols after training.

## Diagnostic response patterns for multiple data

### Cardiovascular limitation

#### Definition and identification

Cardiovascular limitation is considered to occur when a subject achieves a value for $f_{Cmax}$ during incremental exercise that is within 2 SD of the reference value. This defining limit is conveniently calculated as being 20 min$^{-1}$ below predicted $f_{Cmax}$, estimated using one of the equations shown in Chapter 4. Importantly, the variance associated with estimation of $f_{Cmax}$ based on age is such that these estimates are often quite unreliable. Occasionally, during incremental exercise, a plateau value for $f_{Cmax}$ can be identified and this increases

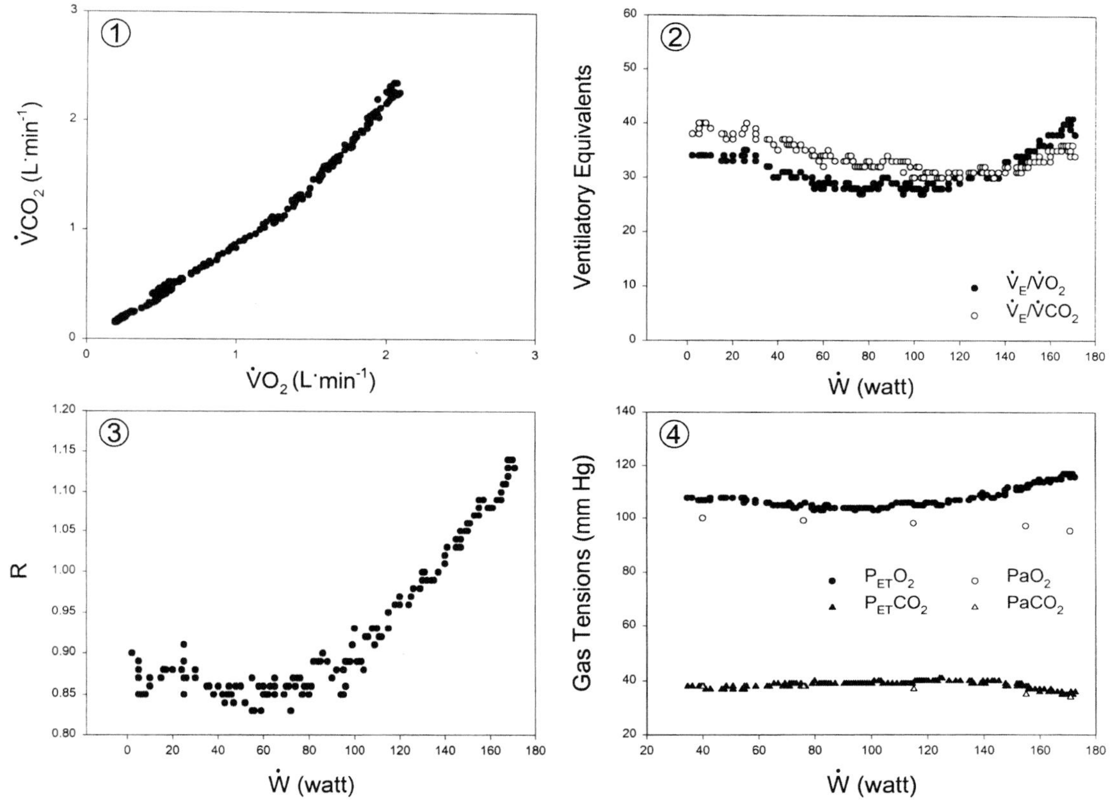


**Figure 5.7** Gas exchange: four-panel display. Refer to Table 5.5 for a description of the individual graphs.

the confidence with which cardiovascular limitation can be identified.

Cardiovascular limitation is to be expected in normal individuals. The main difficulty in identifying the normal cardiovascular response is the accuracy with which maximum heart rate for an individual can be predicted. Factors that are completely independent of the cardiovascular response, such as mechanical ventilatory limitations, abnormal symptom perception, or suboptimal effort for whatever reason, can cause termination of incremental exercise before predicted $f_{Cmax}$ is attained.

Cardiovascular limitation is best identified by examining tabular data for $f_{Cmax}$ and $\dot{V}o_2/f_{Cmax}$ (Table 5.6) in conjunction with panel 2 of a nine-panel display (Figure 5.3).

### Conditions exhibiting this response pattern

*Normal response*

Cardiovascular limitation is expected in normal individuals in conjunction with a normal or high $\dot{V}o_{2max}$.

*Athletic response*

Cardiovascular limitation is also expected in the physically trained or well-conditioned individual.

As a result of improved peripheral oxygen extraction by exercising muscle and increased cardiac stroke volume, the athlete requires a lower heart rate to attain the same cardiac output and $\dot{V}o_2$. In addition, there is a neural component by which the parasympathetic drive increases while

**Table 5.5.** Elements of the four-panel displays for multiple data from integrative exercise testing

| Four-panel display | Graph | Variables |
|---|---|---|
| Aerobic performance | 1 | $\dot{V}O_2$ and $\dot{V}CO_2$ vs. $\dot{W}$ |
| | 2 | $f_C$ vs. $\dot{W}$ |
| | 3 | $\dot{V}_E$ vs. $\dot{W}$ |
| | 4 | $\dot{V}CO_2$ vs. $\dot{V}O_2$ |
| Cardiovascular response | 1 | $f_C$ vs. $\dot{W}$ |
| | 2 | $f_C$ vs. $\dot{V}O_2$ |
| | 3 | $\dot{V}O_2/f_C$ vs. $\dot{W}$ |
| | 4 | $\dot{V}O_2$ vs. $\dot{W}$ |
| Ventilatory response | 1 | $\dot{V}_E$ vs. $\dot{W}$ |
| | 2 | $\dot{V}_E$ vs. $\dot{V}O_2$ |
| | 3 | $V_T$ vs. $\dot{V}_E$ |
| | 4 | $\dot{V}_E$ vs. $\dot{V}CO_2$ |
| Gas exchange | 1 | $\dot{V}CO_2$ vs. $\dot{V}O_2$ |
| | 2 | $\dot{V}_E/\dot{V}O_2$ and $\dot{V}_E/\dot{V}CO_2$ vs. $\dot{W}$ |
| | 3 | $R$ vs. $\dot{W}$ |
| | 4 | $P_{ET}O_2$ and $P_{ET}CO_2$ vs. $\dot{W}$ |

**Table 5.6.** Cardiovascular limitation

| |
|---|
| **Defining variables** |
| $f_{Cmax}$ |
| $\dot{V}O_2/f_{Cmax}$ |
| **Conditions exhibiting this response pattern** |
| Normal response |
| Athletic response |
| Cardiovascular disease |
| Medications (e.g., $\beta$-sympathomimetic antagonists, calcium channel antagonists) |

sympathetic tone decreases. Hence, an individual who is physically well conditioned will exhibit a low $f_{Crest}$, shallow $f_C$–$\dot{V}O_2$ slope and high $\dot{V}O_2/f_C$ at maximal exercise. $f_{Cmax}$ should still be achieved but at a higher $\dot{V}O_{2max}$. The athlete characteristically has a high $\dot{V}O_2\theta$, both as an absolute value and also as percentage of measured and predicted $\dot{V}O_{2max}$.

*Cardiovascular disease*

Cardiovascular disease can be subdivided into four categories: (1) coronary artery disease; (2) cardiomyopathy; (3) valvular heart disease; and (4) congenital heart disease. Each of these conditions is associated with cardiovascular limitation. However, attainment of $f_{Cmax}$ is typically associated with a low $\dot{V}O_{2max}$ (see below).

*Unusual conditions*

Certain drugs, notably $\beta$-sympathomimetic antagonists and calcium channel antagonists, constrain heart rate increases during exercise, thus preventing attainment of predicted $f_{Cmax}$. In these cases it is tempting to state that cardiovascular limitation did not occur. However, when the data are examined in conjuction with the $f_C$–$\dot{V}O_2$ slope, it appears that these subjects have a unique type of cardiovascular limitation.

## Abnormal cardiovascular response pattern

### Definition and identification

An abnormal cardiovascular response pattern is characterized primarily by abnormal form and slope of the $f_C$–$\dot{V}O_2$ relationship. Since the oxygen pulse represents instantaneous values of $\dot{V}O_2/f_C$ and the asymptotic oxygen pulse equates to the inverse of the $f_C$–$\dot{V}O_2$ slope, then an abnormal cardiovascular response pattern can also be exhibited by an abnormal maximal oxygen pulse. An abnormal cardiovascular response pattern is typically associated with a value for $\dot{V}O_{2max}$ that differs from the reference value. This is because the altered $f_C$–$\dot{V}O_2$ slope causes attainment of a different $\dot{V}O_{2max}$ at predicted $f_{Cmax}$.

An abnormal cardiovascular response pattern is best identified by examining panels 4 and 2 of a nine-panel display (Figure 5.3) in conjunction with tabular data for $f_{Cmax}$ and $\dot{V}O_2/f_{Cmax}$. An abnormal cardiovascular response pattern may also be associated with a resting bradycardia or tachycardia, abnormal blood pressure response, or ECG abnormalities (Table 5.7).

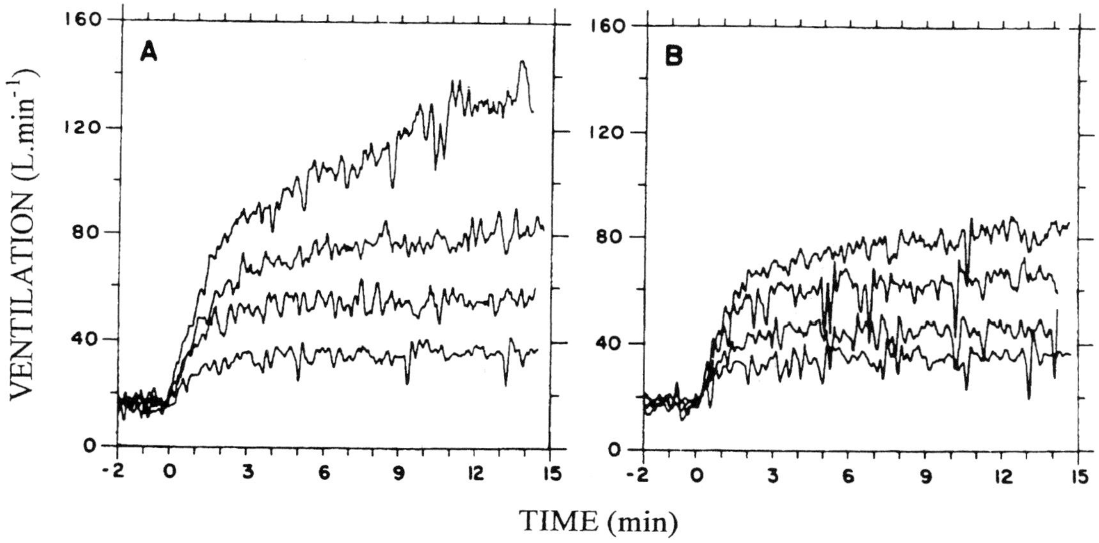


**Figure 5.8** Graphs showing ventilatory requirement for exercise at four different constant work rates (A) before and (B) after 8 weeks of strenuous cycle ergometer training in young health subjects. Reproduced with permission from Casaburi, R., Storer, T. W. & Wasserman, K. (1987). Mediation of reduced ventilatory response to exercise after endurance training. *J. Appl. Physiol.*, **63**, 1533–8.

**Table 5.7.** Abnormal cardiovascular response pattern

| |
|---|
| **Defining variables** |
| $f_{Crest}$ |
| $\delta f_C / \delta \dot{V}O_2$ |
| $\dot{V}O_2/f_C$ |
| Systemic arterial pressure |
| ECG |
| **Conditions exhibiting this response pattern** |
| Physical deconditioning |
| Cardiovascular disease (e.g., CAD, CM, VHD, CHD) |
| Systemic hypertension |
| Pulmonary vascular disease |
| Medications (see Table 5.8) |
| Chronotropic incompetence |
| Anxiety |
| Dysrhythmias |
| Thyrotoxicosis |

CAD = Coronary artery disease; CM = cardiomyopathy; VHD = valvular heart disease; CHD = congenital heart disease.

## Conditions exhibiting this response pattern

### *Physical deconditioning*

Physical deconditioning is essentially impairment in the ability of exercising skeletal muscle to extract and utilize oxygen from the blood. The physiological changes in muscle that signify deconditioning are opposite to those that distinguish the physically trained individual. Therefore, the deconditioned individual will have reduced muscle capillarity, reduced mitochondrial density, and reduced oxidative enzyme concentrations. Another distinction between physically trained and deconditioned individuals is seen in smaller cardiac stroke volume in deconditioned individuals. Together, these peripheral and central components result in an increased $f_{Crest}$, steeper $f_C$–$\dot{V}O_2$ slope, and reduced $\dot{V}O_2/f_C$ at maximum exercise. $\dot{V}O_{2max}$ is reduced and $\dot{V}O_2\theta$ is reduced both as an absolute value and also as a percentage of the reference value for $\dot{V}O_{2max}$. In deconditioned individuals $\dot{V}O_2\theta$ is typically between 40% and 50% of predicted $\dot{V}O_{2max}$.

*Cardiovascular disease*

Early cardiovascular disease is indistinguishable from physical deconditioning and it may be argued that the latter is a variant of the former. When an abnormal cardiovascular response pattern is identified, then other markers of cardiovascular disease should be sought. Preliminary physical examination can be used to identify signs of cardiomegaly, cardiac failure, valvular heart disease, or congenital heart disease. During exercise, the ECG should be scrutinized for evidence of myocardial ischemia and blood pressure monitored to detect exercise-induced hypertension. In the absence of such factors then it is reasonable to attribute an abnormal cardiovascular response pattern to deconditioning. Suspected cardiovascular disease warrants an echocardiogram. However, if no clinical evidence of cardiovascular disease can be found, then the ultimate way to distinguish early cardiovascular disease from deconditioning is to give the subject an exercise prescription over at least 6 weeks. Subjects with deconditioning are much more likely to show improvements in their exercise responses, perhaps even normalization of $\dot{V}O_{2max}$ and $\dot{V}O_2\theta$, which would distinguish this diagnosis.

*Systemic hypertension*

Systemic hypertension can develop during exercise, when it is not evident at rest. Essentially, hypertension increases cardiac afterload, myocardial work, and myocardial oxygen requirement. In these circumstances, increased cardiac output is usually achieved with relatively higher heart rate and smaller cardiac stroke volume. Such alterations are reflected in the cardiovascular response pattern as a steeper $f_C$–$\dot{V}O_2$ slope and lower $\dot{V}O_2/f_C$.

Exercise-induced hypertension appears to predict the development of significant resting systemic hypertension later in life. Thus, exercise serves as the physiological stimulus that reveals early alterations in systemic vascular conductance, presumably due to increased vascular tone or reduced vessel wall elasticity. A systolic blood pressure greater than 200 mmHg or a diastolic blood pressure greater than 100 mmHg during exercise along with pressures greater than 180/90 mmHg after 2 min of recovery warrant closer clinical scrutiny and regular checks for the development of resting hypertension.

*Pulmonary vascular disease*

Abnormal pulmonary vascular conductance, as seen in primary pulmonary hypertension, thromboembolic disease, and emphysema, diminishes stroke volume and thereby affects the cardiovascular response pattern during exercise. Increased $f_{Crest}$, steeper $f_C$–$\dot{V}O_2$ slope, and reduced $\dot{V}O_2/f_C$ at maximal exercise will be seen. Attributing these abnormalities to pulmonary vascular disease rather than any other form of cardiovascular impairment requires the identification of gas exchange abnormalities that accompany pulmonary vascular disease. Loss of portions of the pulmonary capillary bed results in both high and low $\dot{V}/\dot{Q}$ abnormalities. The high $\dot{V}/\dot{Q}$ abnormality (wasted ventilation) is manifest as increased $V_D/V_T$, increased ventilatory equivalents, and persistently positive $P_{(a-ET)}CO_2$ during incremental exercise. The low $\dot{V}/\dot{Q}$ abnormality is thought to be due to shortened pulmonary capillary transit time in nondiseased regions of the lung. This phenomenon (wasted perfusion) is manifest as an abnormal $P_{(A-a)}O_2$ gradient which widens progressively as cardiac output increases during incremental exercise.

Hence, an abnormal cardiovascular response pattern, in conjunction with evidence of the gas exchange abnormalities outlined above, and in the absence of cardiac or systemic vascular disease indicates the presence of pulmonary vascular disease.

*Medications*

The heart rate response to exercise is governed by sympathetic and parasympathetic mechanisms as well as the cardiac conduction pathways. Thus, medications which affect these control mechanisms can cause an abnormal cardiovascular response pattern. Drugs that affect the heart rate response are shown in Table 5.8. Drugs which decelerate heart rate or attenuate the heart rate response predictably cause a reduced $f_{Crest}$, shallower $f_C$–$\dot{V}O_2$ slope, and a

**Table 5.8.** Medications which affect the cardiovascular response pattern

| Drugs which decelerate $f_C$ | Drugs which accelerate $f_C$ |
|---|---|
| **$\beta$-sympathomimetic antagonists** | **Tricyclic antidepressants** |
| Propranolol, metoprolol, acebutolol | |
| **Calcium channel antagonists** | **Amphetamines** |
| Verapamil, diltiazem | |
| **Digoxin or other cardiac glycosides** | **Thyroxine** |
| | **$\beta$-sympathomimetic agonists** |
| | Albuterol (e.g., MDI), metaproterenol |
| | **Nicotine (recent smoking)** |
| | **Cocaine** |

MDI = Metered-dose inhaler.

spuriously high $\dot{V}O_2/f_C$. These changes may be mistaken for a physically trained response except that, when caused by medications, $\dot{V}O_{2max}$ and $\dot{V}O_2\theta$ are also reduced. Drugs that accelerate the heart rate response predictably cause increased $f_{Crest}$, steeper $f_C$–$\dot{V}O_2$ slope, and reduced $\dot{V}O_2/f_C$.

*Chronotropic incompetence*

Rarely, an abnormal cardiovascular response pattern is seen due to inherent dysfunction of the sinoatrial node. This has been called chronotropic incompetence and is thought usually to be due to ischemic heart disease. The manifestation of this condition is a failure to increase heart rate appropriately with increasing oxygen uptake. As with medications that slow the heart rate response, $\dot{V}O_2/f_C$ can be spuriously high. Diagnosis of chronotropic incompetence requires that the individual is not taking any medications that could impair sinoatrial node function.

*Anxiety*

Anxiety results in a heightened state of sympathetic activation. Thus, anxiety is associated with a familiar resting tachycardia and also higher heart rates during incremental exercise. The $f_C$–$\dot{V}O_2$ slope can be normal, although its intercept on the heart rate axis is increased and the subject may reach the predicted maximum heart rate prematurely. Anxiety can be distinguished from the anticipatory response which often precedes exercise. Anticipation results in a heart rate which is high at rest but which settles to an appropriate level once the exercise phase is underway.

*Unusual conditions*

Some individuals with significant coronary artery disease develop a critical imbalance between oxygen demand and supply during exercise. It is not unusual for this to occur at a relatively fixed heart rate or cardiac output. In these circumstances, whether or not the subject has angina pectoris, a distinct alteration can be seen in the pattern of the cardiovascular response during incremental exercise. The $f_C$–$\dot{V}O_2$ slope becomes steeper at the threshold for myocardial ischemia.

An abrupt alteration of the cardiovascular response pattern is also seen with the onset of a dysrhythmia during exercise, e.g., supraventricular tachycardia or atrial fibrillation.

Hyperthyroidism, due to excessive sympathetic stimulation, causes resting and exercise tachycardia and premature cardiovascular limitation. Furthermore, by the same mechanism, an exaggerated hypertensive response can occur. Hyperthyroidism is also sometimes characterized by the development of atrial fibrillation.

## Impaired oxygen delivery

### Definition and identification

Certain conditions potentially impair oxygen delivery to exercising muscles. Thus, oxygen delivery is reduced, either by decreased oxygen-carrying capacity of the blood or by reduced muscle blood flow. Oxygen-carrying capacity is affected by anemia or carboxyhemoglobinemia whilst muscle blood flow is impaired by peripheral vascular disease or cardiac disease. Each of these conditions is associated with impaired aerobic capacity and reduced $\dot{V}O_{2max}$.

When oxygen delivery to exercising muscle is impaired, the relationship between $\dot{V}O_2$ and external

**Table 5.9.** Impaired oxygen delivery

| |
|---|
| **Defining variables** |
| $\dot{V}o_{2max}$ |
| $\delta\dot{V}o_2/\delta\dot{W}$ or $\eta$ |
| $\dot{V}o_2\theta$ |
| **Conditions exhibiting this response pattern** |
| Carboxyhemoglobinemia |
| Anemia |
| Peripheral vascular disease |
| Cardiac disease |

work rate is abnormal. Hence, the $\dot{V}o_2$–$\dot{W}$ slope ($\eta^{-1}$) is reduced. This is particularly evident at higher work intensities when the demand for oxygen increases, thus presenting a greater challenge to the oxygen delivery mechanisms.

When muscle is deprived of sufficient oxygen for aerobic metabolism, premature reliance on anaerobic mechanisms can be anticipated. Therefore, $\dot{V}o_2\theta$ is reduced. As previously discussed, when $\dot{V}o_2\theta$ is less than 40% of predicted $\dot{V}o_{2max}$, definite pathology exists. However, when $\dot{V}o_2\theta$ lies in the 40–50% range it is difficult to distinguish between physical deconditioning and an early or mild disease process.

Impaired oxygen delivery can be identified by examining panels 3 and 5 of a nine-panel display (Figure 5.3) in conjunction with tabular data for $\dot{V}o_{2max}$ (Table 5.9). Panel 5 is used to determine $\dot{V}o_2\theta$.

## Conditions exhibiting this response pattern

*Carboxyhemoglobinemia*

The affinity of carbon monoxide for hemoglobin is over 200 times that of oxygen. Thus, the presence of carboxyhemoglobin (HbCO) in the blood denies hemoglobin the ability to transport oxygen. Consequently, significant levels of HbCO impair oxygen delivery to exercising muscle.

Increases in the level of HbCO cause proportional reductions in $\dot{V}o_{2max}$ and $\dot{V}o_2\theta$. However, discernible effects of HbCO on oxygen utilization and ventilation are not seen below $\dot{V}o_2\theta$.

Smokers can have HbCO levels up to 10% and occasionally higher. Experimentally an HbCO level of 10% was shown to reduce both $\dot{V}o_{2max}$ and $\dot{V}o_2\theta$ by 5–10%.

Incidentally, greater heart rate and blood pressure increases can be seen during exercise immediately after smoking, presumably due to the sympathomimetic effects of nicotine.

*Anemia*

Anemia, for whatever reason, represents a reduction in the hemoglobin concentration of the blood and therefore impacts oxygen-carrying capacity and oxygen delivery to exercising muscle. Thus, significant anemia reduces $\dot{V}o_{2max}$, $\dot{V}o_2\theta$ and the $\dot{V}o_2$–$\dot{W}$ slope ($\eta^{-1}$).

Anemia also reduces blood viscosity – an effect that might offset to some degree the reduced oxygen-carrying capacity by enhancing blood flow.

"Blood doping" (also called "blood boosting" or "blood packing") is a technique used by athletes to enhance physical performance. The effect occurs because of increased hemoglobin concentration, increased oxygen-carrying capacity, and increased oxygen delivery. One can easily appreciate that these physiological mechanisms are opposite to what occurs in anemia. Consequently, blood doping is expected to increase $\dot{V}o_{2max}$ and $\dot{V}o_2\theta$ but should have no influence on $\eta^{-1}$.

*Peripheral vascular disease*

In the case of peripheral vascular disease, the impaired oxygen delivery comes about because of poor systemic vascular conductance. This can be manifest in one leg and associated with symptoms of intermittent claudication or pain causing early exercise termination. Typically, $\dot{V}o_{2max}$ is reduced, but predicted $f_{Cmax}$ is not achieved. $\dot{V}o_2\theta$ may be low if lactic acid effluxes into the central circulation in sufficient quantity to produce discernible gas exchange alterations.

More generalized systemic atherosclerosis causes an exaggerated blood pressure response during exercise. Despite the reduced aerobic capacity, systolic blood pressure can be over 200 mmHg and diastolic blood pressure over 100 mmHg.

*Cardiovascular disease*
Clearly, cardiovascular disease itself impacts oxygen delivery when the ability to increase cardiac output or blood flow is impaired. As discussed above, cardiovascular diseases are important causes of reduced $\dot{V}O_{2max}$ and $\dot{V}O_2\theta$. They also impact the $\dot{V}O_2$–$\dot{W}$ slope ($\eta^{-1}$).

With coronary artery disease, the $\dot{V}O_2$–$\dot{W}$ slope may be initially normal but display a reduced slope at higher exercise intensity when myocardial ischemia causes ventricular dysfunction. Cardiomyopathy and valvular heart disease typically impact the $\dot{V}O_2$–$\dot{W}$ slope (and $\dot{V}O_2/f_C$) right from the onset of exercise.

## Ventilatory limitation

### Definition and identification

Ventilatory limitation is considered to occur when a subject reaches or approaches his or her ventilatory capacity ($\dot{V}_{Ecap}$) at maximum exercise. Arbitrarily, one can consider ventilatory limitation to occur when $\dot{V}_{Emax}$ is greater than 90% of $\dot{V}_{Ecap}$. Unlike $f_{Cmax}$ which is estimated, $\dot{V}_{Ecap}$ is usually measured as MVV or calculated from $FEV_1$. While it must be remembered that these approaches do not directly measure $\dot{V}_{Ecap}$ during conditions of exercise, they are none the less actual measurements and thereby likely to be more accurate than predicted $f_{Cmax}$. For this reason a tighter range can be used to define ventilatory limitation. It is not unusual for an individual with ventilatory limitation just to exceed $\dot{V}_{Ecap}$, for reasons expounded in Chapter 4.

Ventilatory limitation is not expected with the normal exercise response. Hence, ventilatory limitation is only likely to occur when ventilatory capacity is reduced. However, highly endurance-trained athletes, because they have successfully extended their cardiovascular response, use a significantly greater proportion of ventilatory capacity at maximum exercise and may approach ventilatory limitation even though their ventilatory capacity is normal.

Ventilatory limitation is best identified by examining tabular data for $\dot{V}_{Emax}$ and MVV (Table 5.10) in conjunction with panels 1, 4, and 7 of a nine-panel display (Figure 5.3). Panels 1 and 7 can be especially helpful in this regard if MVV or calculated $\dot{V}_{Ecap}$ is indicated on these graphs.

**Table 5.10.** Ventilatory limitation

| |
|---|
| **Defining variables** |
| $\dot{V}_{Emax}$ |
| $\dot{V}_{Ecap}$ or MVV |
| **Conditions exhibiting this response pattern** |
| Chronic pulmonary disease |
| Respiratory muscle weakness |
| Hyperventilation (rarely) |

### Conditions exhibiting this response pattern

*Chronic pulmonary disease*
In obstructive pulmonary disease, such as asthma or chronic bronchitis, ventilatory capacity is reduced and true ventilatory limitation is often identified. The breathlessness score is high, concomitant with the proportion of the ventilatory capacity utilized.

In restrictive pulmonary diseases, such as pulmonary fibrosis or kyphoscoliosis, ventilatory capacity is also reduced and true ventilatory limitation is often identified. Again, the breathlessness score is high, concomitant with the proportion of the ventilatory capacity utilized.

In many cases of chronic pulmonary disease, ventilatory limitation is precipitated by other factors that increase the ventilatory requirement for exercise. These factors include carbohydrate intake, inefficient breathing, increased $V_D/V_T$, and anxiety (see section on abnormal ventilatory response pattern, below).

*Respiratory muscle weakness*
Respiratory muscle weakness due to various forms of neuromuscular disease presents a specific form of restrictive ventilatory abnormality. Ventilatory capacity is reduced and therefore individuals with respiratory muscle weakness may be susceptible to true ventilatory limitation.

Sometimes, if a high intensity of exercise can be attained, an individual with respiratory muscle weakness may develop hypercapnic ventilatory failure (see below).

Individuals with respiratory muscle weakness typically experience severe breathlessness, even at rest. During exercise, the breathlessness score is high, concomitant with the proportion of the ventilatory capacity utilized.

*Extreme hyperventilation*

An individual with extreme hyperventilation due to psychological factors may conceivably exhibit ventilatory limitation. Other manifestations of hyperventilation would be apparent, including high ventilatory equivalents, high $P_{ET}O_2$, low $P_{ET}CO_2$, and low $PaCO_2$ (perhaps even $<20$ mm Hg).

## Abnormal ventilatory response pattern

### Definition and identification

The ventilatory response during exercise can be analyzed in two important ways. Firstly, consideration of the determinants of ventilatory requirement gives insight into the relationship between $\dot{V}_E$ and $\dot{V}O_2$, as described in Chapter 4. Secondly, breathing pattern can be assessed in terms of $V_T$, $f_R$, time components of the breath, and flow–volume relationships.

Ventilatory requirement and the related slope $\delta\dot{V}_E/\delta\dot{V}O_2$ are influenced by $R$, $PaCO_2$, and $V_D/V_T$. Hence, nutritional status that affects $R$, arterial $PaCO_2$ regulation and breathing efficiency can all alter ventilatory requirement.

Attempts to define the ventilatory response in terms of breathing pattern are handicapped by insufficient knowledge of factors regulating breathing pattern during incremental exercise. However, it seems intuitive that, given certain mechanical factors, there must be an optimum breathing pattern for an individual which would obtain the highest alveolar ventilation for a given minute ventilation ($\dot{V}_E$).

The traditional approach to breathing pattern analysis was described by Hey as the relationship between $V_T$ and $\dot{V}_E$. Unfortunately, this approach does not seem to discriminate between obstructive and restrictive pulmonary disease. Nevertheless, there is a tendency, shown by the Hey plot, for individuals with restrictive disease to achieve their $V_{T\max}$ at lower exercise intensity and thereafter rely almost entirely on an increase in $f_R$ to achieve a higher $\dot{V}_E$.

Considering breathing pattern in terms of the time components of the breath, two factors are of primary importance. They are total breath time ($T_{TOT}$) and $T_I/T_E$ ratio. From $T_{TOT}$ derives breathing frequency ($f_R$) and from $T_I/T_E$ derives $T_I$ and $T_E$. $V_T$ derives from $T_I$ and $T_E$ after taking into account mechanical factors such as respiratory muscle force, lung compliance, and airway resistance. In normal circumstances, $T_{TOT}$ should not be less than 1.2 s ($f_R < 50\ \text{min}^{-1}$) and $T_I/T_E$ should be approximately 0.8.

Finally, the flow–volume loop, which can be recorded with reasonable accuracy during exercise, allows an interpretation of two factors: encroachment on total lung capacity (restriction), and encroachment on the volume-related maximal expiratory flow (obstruction).

An abnormal ventilatory response pattern is best identified by examining tabular data for $\dot{V}_E$, $V_T$, $f_R$, $\dot{V}O_2/f_R$, and $T_I/T_E$ (Table 5.11) in conjunction with panels 1, 4, and 7 of a nine-panel display (Figure 5.3). Panel 7 is particularly useful in this regard if MVV and vital capacity are also displayed on the graph.

### Conditions exhibiting this response pattern

*Obstructive pulmonary disease*

In general, individuals with obstructive disease have reduced $V_T$ and achieve their $V_{T\max}$ at moderate-intensity exercise. The obligatory prolongation of expiratory time results in $f_{R\max}$ being within the normal range ($<50\ \text{min}^{-1}$).

Given that the nature of an obstructive ventilatory abnormality is difficulty with expiration, $T_E$ is typically prolonged or occupies a larger proportion of $T_{TOT}$. Therefore, the $T_I/T_E$ is less than 0.8.

**Table 5.11.** Abnormal ventilatory response pattern

| |
|---|
| **Defining variables** |
| $\dot{V}_E$ |
| $V_T$ |
| $f_R$ |
| $\dot{V}O_2/f_R$ |
| $T_I/T_E$ |
| **Conditions exhibiting this response pattern** |
| Obstructive pulmonary disease |
| Restrictive pulmonary disease |
| Neuromuscular disease |
| Nutritional factors |

The flow–volume loop shows compromised maximal expiratory flows and typically the expiratory flows during exercise encroach upon this envelope, indicating expiratory flow limitation. Furthermore, because of the expiratory flow limitation, the tidal flow–volume loop is typically shifted towards higher lung volumes (dynamic hyperinflation). Individuals with a primary obstructive ventilatory abnormality may therefore encroach upon total lung capacity and exhibit a secondary restrictive abnormality.

*Restrictive pulmonary disease*

Individuals with restrictive disease have reduced $V_T$ and achieve their $V_{T\max}$ at lower-intensity exercise. The primary restriction of $V_T$ means that increases in $\dot{V}_E$ are more dependent on $f_R$. Indeed, $f_{R\max}$ is often $>50\ \text{min}^{-1}$ at maximum exercise.

Given that the nature of a restrictive ventilatory abnormality is difficulty with inspiration, $T_I$ is typically prolonged or occupies a larger proportion of $T_{TOT}$. Therefore, the $T_I/T_E$ is greater than 0.8. Furthermore, with reduced lung compliance, as seen in pulmonary fibrosis, the increased elastic recoil enhances expiratory flow and shortens $T_E$, contributing to the increased $T_I/T_E$.

The flow–volume loop shows encroachment of tidal volume on total lung capacity early during incremental exercise. The coexistence of expiratory flow limitation at lower lung volumes has also been described in some cases of pulmonary fibrosis. This phenomenon, if present, appears to be secondary to the restriction, which prevents the bulk of expiratory flow being achieved at higher lung volumes.

Respiratory muscle weakness due to various forms of neuromuscular disease presents a specific form of restrictive ventilatory abnormality. Even in the presence of normal lung compliance, reduced inspiratory force results in slower inspiratory flow and generally smaller $V_T$ *with a higher* $f_R$. These findings may be evident at rest and worsen during incremental exercise.

Any of the breathing pattern abnormalities described above can be seen with respiratory muscle weakness.

*Nutritional status*

Carbohydrate ingestion just prior to exercise increases $\dot{V}CO_2$ and thereby increases ventilatory requirement. Measurable changes in $\dot{V}CO_2$ and $\dot{V}_E$ occur. Although advocated in chronic pulmonary disease, lower-carbohydrate (higher-fat) diets do not produce measurable reductions in ventilatory requirement in these patients.

## Abnormal ventilatory control

### Definition and identification

During exercise, alveolar ventilation should increase appropriately with the increased efflux of carbon dioxide. There are several important sources of exhaled $CO_2$ during incremental exercise. At low exercise intensity, exhaled $CO_2$ comes from aerobic metabolism. Above the metabolic threshold, additional exhaled $CO_2$ comes from bicarbonate buffering of accumulating lactate. Normally, during both of these phases, ventilation is precisely matched to $\dot{V}CO_2$ so that $P_ACO_2$ and $PaCO_2$ remain remarkably constant despite manifold increases in $\dot{V}CO_2$. Only during intense exercise, when a decrease in pH can no longer be prevented by buffering, does carotid body stimulation cause $\dot{V}_E$ to increase over and above that required for $CO_2$ elimination. This is an expected phase of true hyperventilation when both ventilatory equivalents show a sustained increase,

$P_{ET}CO_2$ falls, $P_{ET}O_2$ increases, and $PaCO_2$ also falls. Abnormal ventilatory control can result in inappropriately high or low levels of $\dot{V}_E$ during these various stages of the exercise response.

Inappropriately high $\dot{V}_E$ will be associated with increased $\dot{V}_E/\dot{V}O_2$, increased $\dot{V}_E/\dot{V}CO_2$, increased $P_{ET}O_2$, reduced $P_{ET}CO_2$, and reduced $PaCO_2$. This pattern is called hyperventilation. It can occur acutely during exercise or be associated with a chronic disturbance.

Inappropriately low $\dot{V}_E$ will be associated with reduced $\dot{V}_E/\dot{V}O_2$, reduced $\dot{V}_E/\dot{V}CO_2$, reduced $P_{ET}O_2$, increased $P_{ET}CO_2$ and increased $PaCO_2$. This pattern is called hypoventilation or ventilatory failure.

Sometimes abnormalities of ventilatory control are manifest as irregularities of ventilatory pattern, e.g., rapid shallow breathing or cyclical ventilation. The former may be due to subconscious influences of the higher central nervous system. The latter is typically due to degradation of the fine tuning of the biofeedback mechanism which determines the appropriate level of ventilation.

Abnormal ventilatory control is best identified by examining tabular data for $PaO_2$, $PaCO_2$, and $P_{(A-a)}O_2$ (Table 5.12) in conjunction with panels 2, 4, 6, and 9 of a nine-panel display (Figure 5.3). Panel 1 shows irregularities in $\dot{V}_E$; panel 4 allows identification of $\dot{V}_E\theta$; panels 6 and 9 show irregularities in ventilatory equivalents, end-tidal gas tensions, and arterial gas tensions.

**Table 5.12.** Abnormal ventilatory control

| |
|---|
| **Defining variables** |
| $\dot{V}_E$ |
| $\dot{V}_E/\dot{V}O_2$ |
| $\dot{V}_E/\dot{V}CO_2$ |
| $P_{ET}O_2$ |
| $P_{ET}CO_2$ |
| $PaO_2$ |
| $PaCO_2$ |
| **Conditions exhibiting this response pattern** |
| Acute hyperventilation |
| Chronic hyperventilation syndrome |
| Ventilatory failure (hypoventilation) |
| Rapid shallow breathing |
| Oscillating ventilation |

## Conditions exhibiting this response pattern

*Acute hyperventilation*

Hyperventilation implies inappropriately high $\dot{V}_E$, therefore high ventilatory equivalents and low $PaCO_2$. When hyperventilation occurs acutely during an exercise test protocol a sudden increase in $\dot{V}CO_2$ is expected. In addition, there is often a spurious and concomitant increase in $\dot{V}O_2$. The increase in $\dot{V}O_2$ is a technical problem but should be recognized in this context.

Acute hyperventilation is seen most frequently at rest or with the onset of unloaded pedaling on a cycle. Later, when the exercise stimulus is of greater intensity, ventilation often becomes better matched to metabolic rate and ventilatory equivalents fall appropriately.

The respiratory alkalosis, which results from significant acute hyperventilation, may cause symptoms such as lightheadedness, and paresthesia involving the hands and face.

*Chronic hyperventilation syndrome*

Some individuals, an example being those with chronic anxiety, can exhibit chronic hyperventilation. The abnormalities that accompany acute hyperventilation are likely to be present throughout the exercise study. In addition, the compensatory depletion of plasma bicarbonate may compromise the ability to buffer lactate, resulting in a shorter isocapnic buffering period during incremental exercise.

*Ventilatory failure (hypoventilation)*

True ventilatory failure implies inadequate alveolar ventilation and is associated with hypercapnia and hypoxia. Although $PaO_2$ is reduced, $P_{(A-a)}O_2$ is normal in pure hypoventilation. This is a relatively unusual finding during incremental exercise. Ventilatory failure occurs when mechanical factors severely limit the ventilatory response or, rarely, due to primary abnormalities of ventilatory control similar to the syndrome of primary alveolar hypoventilation seen in obese subjects.

*Rapid shallow breathing*

Rapid shallow breathing is an inefficient mode of ventilation, which results in increased $V_D/V_T$, i.e., significant wasted ventilation. This pattern of ventilatory abnormality is seen most commonly as a feature of acute or chronic hyperventilation. Commonly, it is associated with anxiety. It can occur in obstructive pulmonary disease when the resulting compromise of alveolar ventilation leads to oxyhemoglobin desaturation. Individuals with restrictive pulmonary disease exhibit rapid shallow breathing by virtue of their limited ability to increase tidal volume, as described above.

*Oscillating ventilation*

Oscillations in $\dot{V}_E$ are sometimes noted in cases of severe cardiac failure. This phenomenon is thought to represent a degrading of the ventilatory control mechanism, equivalent to Cheyne–Stokes breathing. In effect, the sluggish blood flow between the pulmonary capillary bed and the carotid body chemoreceptors prolongs the response time of the biofeedback mechanism which normally regulates $\dot{V}_E$ according to the chemical composition of the systemic arterial blood. The oscillations represent alternating undercorrection and overcorrection of $\dot{V}_E$ in response to afferent neural input to the central nervous system from the carotid body chemoreptors.

## Impaired gas exchange

### Definition and identification

In physiological terms, there are two types of gas exchange abnormality. These are increased physiological dead space, corresponding to high ventilation–perfusion abnormality, and increased physiological shunt, corresponding to low ventilation–perfusion inequality.

The high $\dot{V}/\dot{Q}$ abnormality, or increased dead space, produces high ventilatory equivalents in the presence of a relatively normal or high $Pa\text{CO}_2$. In addition, $P_{ET}\text{O}_2$ is high, $P_{ET}\text{CO}_2$ is low, and $P_{(a-ET)}\text{CO}_2$ is widened or persistently positive during incremental exercise. This pattern of abnormalities is confirmed by an increase in the calculated $V_D/V_T$.

The low $\dot{V}/\dot{Q}$ abnormality, or increased shunt, is characterized by reduced oxyhemoglobin saturation as determined by pulse oximetry ($Sp\text{O}_2$, reduced $Pa\text{O}_2$ and abnormally increased $P_{(A-a)}\text{O}_2$. Importantly, it is the low $\dot{V}/\dot{Q}$ abnormality which, if sufficiently severe, produces critical hypoxemia and true gas exchange failure.

The hallmark of gas exchange failure is inability to maintain adequate oxygenation of arterial blood during incremental exercise. Oxyhemoglobin desaturation can be detected by pulse oximetry, taking care to exclude any technical errors (Chapter 2). When arterial blood is available for analysis, a critical fall in $Pa\text{O}_2$ can be seen along with widening of the alveolar–arterial oxygen gradient. Only in the unusual setting of exercise under conditions of environmental hypoxia (e.g., extreme altitude) would desaturation be accompanied by a relatively normal $P_{(A-a)}\text{O}_2$.

When $\text{PaO}_2$ falls below 60 mmHg, carotid body responsiveness causes intense stimulation of ventilation. Thus, the onset of gas exchange failure is commonly accompanied by an exaggeration of the ventilatory response just prior to exercise termination.

Impaired gas exchange is best identified by examining tabular data for $Pa\text{O}_2$, $Sp\text{O}_2$, $P_{(A-a)}\text{O}_2$, $Pa\text{CO}_2$, $P_{(a-ET)}\text{CO}_2$, and $V_D/V_T$ (Table 5.13) in conjunction with panels 6, 8, and 9 of a nine-panel display (Figure 5.3).

### Conditions exhibiting this response pattern

*Emphysema*

Emphysema is destruction of the lung parenchyma by loss of the supporting connective tissue. The collapse of unsupported airways results in a mechanical impairment that is usually categorized as a form of obstructive pulmonary disease. Air spaces distal to the terminal bronchioles (1 mm diameter)

**Table 5.13.** Impaired gas exchange

| |
|---|
| **Defining variables** |
| $Pa\text{O}_2$ |
| $Sp\text{O}_2$ |
| $P_{(A-a)}\text{O}_2$ |
| $P_{(a-ET)}\text{CO}_2$ |
| $V_D/V_T$ |
| **Conditions exhibiting this response pattern** |
| Emphysema |
| Interstitial lung disease |
| Pulmonary vascular disease |
| Intracardiac shunt |

are enlarged. However, the lung destruction also specifically obliterates pulmonary capillaries, resulting in loss of pulmonary capillary bed. The obvious consequence of this process is an increased $V_D/V_T$ (high $\dot{V}/\dot{Q}$ abnormality). Individuals with emphysema exhibit increased $V_D/V_T$ at rest and a failure of $V_D/V_T$ to fall with a normal pattern during exercise.

The loss of pulmonary capillary bed produces a more complex gas exchange problem due to reduced vascular conductance in certain regions of the lung. Since the stimulus of incremental exercise demands an ever-increasing cardiac output, perfusion must be diverted to other nonemphysematous regions of the lung or, alternatively, blood flow needs to be accelerated through regions of diseased capillary bed. Both effects, particularly the latter, result in shunt (low $\dot{V}/\dot{Q}$ abnormality) with reduced $Pa\text{O}_2$ and increased $P_{(A-a)}\text{O}_2$. The ability to divert perfusion to less diseased regions of the lung may avert desaturation until higher exercise intensity. However, one can envisage a critical cardiac output or pulmonary blood flow above which desaturation is inevitable.

### *Interstitial lung disease*

Interstitial lung disease (ILD) is characterized by inflammation and fibrosis of the interstitial spaces, which separate the alveolar epithelium and capillary endothelium. Hence, ILD disrupts the pathway for pulmonary gas exchange. Furthermore, the disease process is often homogeneous, i.e., diffusely involving a large area of the lungs.

Disruption of the gas exchange pathway predictably impacts oxygen diffusion rather than carbon dioxide diffusion, for reasons explained in Chapter 4. As a result there is a widening of the $P_{(A-a)}\text{O}_2$ gradient and reduced $Pa\text{O}_2$. If $Pa\text{O}_2$ is reduced below 60 mmHg, significant oxyhemoglobin desaturation can be detected by pulse oximetry.

In its early stages, ILD may be insufficient to produce measurable gas exchange abnormalities at rest. However, the exercise stimulus, by virtue of the shortened pulmonary capillary transit time and reduced $P\bar{v}\text{O}_2$, offers the best method for challenging the physiological mechanisms of oxygen diffusion and revealing a subtle gas exchange abnormality. Exercise testing is the most sensitive and reliable method available for detecting the subtle gas exchange abnormalities that result from early ILD.

A characteristic pattern of gas exchange abnormality is associated with ILD. The $P_{(A-a)}\text{O}_2$ gradient widens progressively as cardiac output increases. Clearly this phenomenon relates to the steadily increasing pulmonary blood flow and shortened pulmonary capillary transit time. Whilst the shortened pulmonary capillary transit time challenges diffusion mechanisms, the increased pulmonary blood flow, particularly through regions of the lung with compromised ventilation, equates to shunt (low $\dot{V}/\dot{Q}$ abnormality). Both effects contribute to the progressive reduction in $Pa\text{O}_2$ seen during incremental exercise in ILD.

### *Pulmonary vascular disease*

The key to the diagnosis of pulmonary vascular disease is the demonstration of abnormal gas exchange, particularly increased $V_D/V_T$ (high $\dot{V}/\dot{Q}$ abnormality), accompanied by an abnormal cardiovascular response to exercise. In some cases the abnormal gas exchange can be explained by chronic pulmonary disease with resulting effects on the ventilatory response to exercise. When pulmonary function tests are normal, gas exchange abnormalities are likely to be caused by very early interstitial or obstructive disease or pulmonary vascular disease. The absence of demonstrable cardiac or peripheral vascular disease indicates that the abnormality of the cardiovascular response arises in the pulmonary circulation.

Pulmonary vascular diseases include primary pulmonary hypertension and secondary pulmonary hypertension, e.g., as a result of chronic thromboembolic disease. The physiological consequences are reduced pulmonary vascular conductance and pulmonary hypertension, which is exaggerated during exercise. The cardiovascular response during exercise is characterized by a steeper $f_C$–$\dot{V}O_2$ relationship or reduced $\dot{V}O_2/f_C$, leading to cardiovascular limitation at a low $\dot{V}O_{2max}$.

*Intracardiac shunt*

An extrapulmonary, right-to-left shunt results in a widened $P_{(A-a)}O_2$ gradient and reduced $PaO_2$. If the shunt flow is substantial, e.g. 10% of the cardiac output, this will cause significant hypoxemia, which reduces the oxygen-carrying capacity of the arterial blood and potentially affects the cardiovascular response to exercise by steepening the $f_C/\dot{V}O_2$ relationship. In turn, a steeper $f_C/\dot{V}O_2$ relationship leads to cardiovascular limitation at a low $\dot{V}O_{2max}$.

The commonest examples of these shunts are long-standing defects of the atrial or ventricular cardiac septum, which begin as left-to-right shunts but reverse their flow when pressures in the right side of the heart become persistently elevated above systemic or left-sided pressures.

There is an unusual example of a right-to-left shunt, which develops suddenly during exercise. This occurs if the foramen ovale, which is not fully sealed, opens abruptly as right atrial pressure increases. The sudden development of right-to-left shunt is detected by a marked fall in $PaO_2$, possibly accompanied by a steepening of the slope of the $f_C$–$\dot{V}O_2$ relationship.

## Abnormal muscle metabolism

### Definition and identification

Muscle metabolism is the primary determinant of oxygen uptake during exercise. Therefore, abnormal muscle metabolism is usually but not inevitably associated with a reduced $\dot{V}O_{2max}$. However, reduced aerobic capacity is not a specific finding.

**Table 5.14.** Abnormal muscle metabolism

| |
|---|
| **Defining variables** |
| $\dot{V}O_{2max}$ |
| $\dot{V}O_2\theta$ |
| Lactate |
| Ammonia |
| Creatine kinase |
| |
| **Conditions exhibiting this response pattern** |
| McArdle's syndrome |
| Myoadenylate deficiency |
| Carnitine palmitoyl transferase deficiency |
| Mitochondrial myopathy |
| Chronic fatigue syndrome |

Abnormal muscle metabolism typically results in a markedly reduced $\dot{V}O_2\theta$ (<40% of predicted $\dot{V}O_{2max}$) in the absence of demonstrable cardiovascular disease. Milder forms of myopathy will be associated with lesser reductions in $\dot{V}O_2\theta$ and will be difficult to distinguish from physical deconditioning.

The diagnosis of abnormal muscle metabolism must be aided by blood analysis; different types of myopathy are associated with specific profiles of abnormality.

Impaired muscle metabolism is best identified by examining tabular data for $\dot{V}O_2$, lactate, ammonia, and creatine kinase (Table 5.14) in conjunction with panels 3 and 5 of a nine-panel display (Figure 5.3). Panel 3 depicts $\dot{V}O_{2max}$ and panel 5 enables determination of $\dot{V}O_2\theta$.

### Conditions exhibiting this response pattern

*McArdle's syndrome*

McArdle's syndrome is an inherited lack of muscle phosporylase, which denies an individual the ability to utilize muscle glycogen for glycolysis. Individuals with this condition develop muscle cramping and fatigue at moderate exercise intensity.

In McArdle's syndrome, $\dot{V}O_{2max}$ is typically less than 50% of the reference value. Impairment of glycolysis means that an increase in blood lactate does not occur in McArdle's syndrome. Interestingly, false gas exchange thresholds have been described but these are likely to be due to hyperventilation associated with muscle pain, which characteristically develops when these individuals perform moderate-intensity exercise. Careful scrutiny of the ventilatory equivalents and end-tidal gas tensions should distinguish this phenomenon.

The cardiovascular response to incremental exercise is also abnormal in that predicted $f_{Cmax}$ will be attained at a considerably reduced $\dot{V}O_{2max}$. This has been interpreted as an attempt to increase delivery of oxidative substrate to contracting muscle, mediated through muscle sympathetic nervous system activation by muscle metabolites.

Reliance on the alternative metabolic pathway for ATP regeneration by deamination of ADP results in exaggerated increases in ammonia – as much as four times normal. Thus, measurement of lactate and ammonia during incremental exercise can help establish the diagnosis of McArdle's syndrome.

*Myoadenylate deaminase deficiency*

Myoadenylate deaminase deficiency was first described in 1978. The enzyme participates in the alternative pathway for ATP regeneration from ADP and its main role is thought to be the maintenance of high ATP : ADP ratios during strenuous muscular activity. Individuals with this condition complain of muscle cramps on exercise. Since myoadenylate deaminase is the major enzyme catalyzing the production of ammonia by contracting muscle, when it is deficient, increases in the blood ammonia level are not seen. On the other hand, reliance purely on anaerobic glycolysis for ATP regeneration causes premature and exaggerated increases in blood lactate. Creatine kinase levels can be mildly elevated. The EMG is nonspecifically abnormal.

Myoadenylate deaminase deficiency can be demonstrated by histochemical analysis of a muscle biopsy.

*Carnitine palmitoyl transferase deficiency*

Carnitine palmitoyl transferase (CPT) is an essential enzyme in fatty acid oxidation. Individuals with this condition complain of muscle pain, especially on prolonged exercise and particularly after fasting or taking a high-fat diet. Since there is little, if any, reliance on fatty acid oxidation to regenerate ATP during short-duration incremental exercise testing, it is not unusual to find that $\dot{V}O_{2max}$ is normal or only mildly reduced. $\dot{V}O_2\theta$ is typically reduced, e.g., 40–50% of predicted $\dot{V}O_{2max}$. Therefore, it is difficult to know to what extent this is due to physical deconditioning. Creatine kinase levels can be grossly elevated in this condition.

Muscle biopsy can be normal or show accumulation of lipid droplets between myofibrils. Histochemical analysis is necessary to confirm the diagnosis.

*Mitochondrial myopathy*

There exists a group of myopathic disorders where the abnormalities lie within the mitochondria. These include a variety of mitochondrial DNA abnormalities either inherited or acquired by point mutation, a phenomenon that seems surprisingly common. Another group of disorders affects the enzymes of the respiratory chain and thus prevents production of ATP by oxidative phosphorylation.

Individuals with mitochondrial myopathy have muscle pain on exercise and striking reductions in $\dot{V}O_{2max}$. Reliance on cytoplasmic pathways for the regeneration of ATP causes premature and exaggerated increases in lactate and ammonia during incremental exercise. Therefore $\dot{V}O_2\theta$ is also markedly reduced.

Muscle biopsy can show abnormal morphology either with red-ragged fibers or subsarcolemmal accumulations of abnormal mitochondria. These appearances are more convincing on electron microscopy.

*Chronic fatigue syndrome*

Chronic fatigue syndrome is a term used in the USA to describe a condition characterized by severe persistent debilitating fatigue which does not appear to have any identifiable medical or psychological basis. The condition may be due to an abnormal perception of effort. However, the symptoms are commonly indistinguishable from individuals with myopathy.

During incremental exercise testing, $\dot{V}O_{2max}$ and $\dot{V}O_2\theta$ are mildly reduced and a premature increase in blood lactate has been demonstrated. A resting tachycardia is often seen in conjunction with a steeper $f_C$–$\dot{V}O_2$ response. These individuals have increased perception of effort compared with normal subjects. Unfortunately, it is not known whether these effects are due to the disease or the physical deconditioning which results from inactivity.

In chronic fatigue syndrome exercise testing is requested to rule out cardiovascular disease or other reasons for exercise limitation and for designing an individualized exercise program.

**Table 5.15.** Abnormal symptom perception

| |
|---|
| **Defining variables** |
| RPE in conjunction with $f_C/f_{Cmax}$ |
| $\beta$– in conjunction with $\dot{V}_{Emax}/\dot{V}_{Ecap}$ |
| Objective impression of effort |
| Subjective reason(s) for exercise termination |
| Musculoskeletal discomfort |
| Other discomfort |
| **Conditions exhibiting this response pattern** |
| Chronic pulmonary disease |
| Malingering |
| Desire for secondary gain |
| Stoicism |
| Denial |
| Anxiety |
| Fear |
| Psychological disturbances |
| Arthritis |

## Abnormal symptom perception

### Definition and identification

When psychometric scales are skillfully used during exercise testing, the symptomatic response can be compared with the accompanying physiological responses. In this regard RPE should correlate with variables of the cardiovascular response, whereas a breathlessness score should loosely correlate with the proportion of ventilatory capacity utilized. Thus, it is possible to draw conclusions as to whether the symptomatic responses are inappropriately high or low compared with these physiological parameters. Symptom scores that are disproportionate to the underlying physiological responses constitute a unique diagnostic response pattern, which necessitates further explanation. A systematic approach to symptom evaluation has been described in Chapter 4.

Some individuals exhibit pure symptom limitation without evidence of simultaneous physiological limitation. Extreme scores on the psychometric scales, which are used to rate perceived exertion and breathlessness, can help identify pure symptomatic limitation. RPE of 18 or higher is sufficient to account for exercise cessation. Alternatively, a breathlessness score close to or greater than 90 on a scale of 100 implies that the subject feels close to ventilatory capacity. These sensations can be recorded without simultaneous physiological evidence of cardiovascular limitation, ventilatory limitation, or gas exchange failure, in which case they represent pure symptom limitation.

Abnormal symptom perception is best identified by examining tabular data for RPE, $f_{Cmax}$(%), $\beta$– and $\dot{V}_{Emax}/\dot{V}_{Ecap}$ (Table 5.15) and also comparing the objective impression of effort noted by the exercise practitioner with the reasons given for exercise termination by the subject. Occasionally, other symptoms that do not have a physiological basis cause exercise cessation. These symptoms are elicited by questioning the subject at the end of the exercise test. They may include discomfort from the mouthpiece, cycle saddle, or musculoskeletal system.

### Conditions exhibiting this response pattern

*Chronic pulmonary disease*

Chronic obstructive and restrictive pulmonary diseases are often associated with extreme breathlessness, which becomes reinforced by chronic fear and anxiety. In some of these individuals their symptoms have increased out of proportion to any underlying physiological abnormalities and become the sole limiting factor during maximal exercise.

*Malingering and desire for secondary gain (disproportionately high symptoms)*

Some individuals deliberately score symptoms high on psychometric scales. A reason in terms of secondary gain from doing so may be obvious or subtle. Examples may include claim for disability payments, a desire to retire from work, or for other purposes of financial compensation or litigation. Some individuals score disproportionately high symptoms for no other reason than that they desire ongoing medical attention and investigation. This behavior is described as malingering.

*Stoicism and denial (disproportionately low symptoms)*

There are two common reasons for disproportionately low symptom scores: stoicism and denial. A subject can intentionally underrate perceived exertion and underscore breathlessness through being stoical. Thus, stoicism is a conscious process, often exhibited for reasons of bravado. Determined athletes exhibit stoicism; also some patients exhibit stoicism despite having a definite disease process.

Denial is notably different from stoicism, implying unintentional or subconscious underrating or underscoring of symptoms. Denial is seen in athletes as they get older and are unwilling to accept the inevitable decline in maximal exercise performance. Denial is also seen in patients who subconsciously refuse to accept the existence of their disease process.

Clearly, distinguishing between stoicism and denial becomes a subtle judgment call on the part of the exercise professional.

*Psychological disturbances*

Various psychological disturbances, including anxiety neurosis, can precipitate exercise limitation without physiological limitation. Other features of anxiety may be evident from the submaximal physiological measurements, e.g., resting tachycardia or hyperventilation at any stage during the study.

Psychological disturbances are often unpredictable in the way they influence perception of effort and other exercise symptoms such as breathlessness. Disproportionately high or low symptoms that do not have any obvious explanation can be due to an obscure psychological disturbance.

Fear and anxiety most commonly lead to disproportionately high symptom scores, which can sometimes even limit the exercise response.

*Musculoskeletal disease*

Arthritis or other musculoskeletal disease can cause exercise cessation without physiological limitation. It would be unusual to require an incremental exercise test to reach the conclusion that musculoskeletal disease was the reason for exercise limitation. However, there may be circumstances where it is desired to measure physiological performance within the constraints of known musculoskeletal disease.

## Suboptimal effort

### Definition and identification

Suboptimal effort results in submaximal physiological values for the incremental exercise test. Hence, aerobic capacity is reduced and predicted maximum heart rate is not attained. In the absence of any identifiable physiological limitations or abnormal response patterns, $\dot{V}O_{2max} < 80\%$ of predicted together with $f_{Cmax}$ also $<80\%$ of predicted suggests suboptimal effort. Given that the underlying exercise response is otherwise normal, the reductions in $\dot{V}O_{2max}$ and $f_{Cmax}$ are usually proportional. The detection of $\dot{V}O_2\theta$ within the normal range further substantiates the diagnosis of a suboptimal effort, assuming all other aspects of the exercise response are normal. However, $\dot{V}O_2\theta$ may also be within the range of deconditioning, i.e., 40–50% of predicted

**Table 5.16.** Suboptimal effort

| |
|---|
| **Defining variables** |
| $\dot{V}O_{2max}$ |
| $f_{Cmax}$ |
| $\dot{V}_{Emax}$ |
| $\dot{V}O_2\theta$ |
| Lactate |
| RPE |
| $R$ |
| **Conditions exhibiting this response pattern** |
| Poor motivation |
| Psychological disturbances |
| Desire for secondary gain |
| Malingering |

$\dot{V}O_{2max}$ in the presence of suboptimal effort.

The expected increase in blood lactate that accompanies a true maximal effort is diminished or absent. End-exercise blood lactate should be at least 30 mg · dl$^{-1}$ to indicate a true maximal effort, in the absence of other confounding factors.

A true maximal effort is reliably associated with a rating of perceived exertion of 16–18 on the Borg scale. Thus an RPE < 16, in the absence of other confounding factors, is also consistent with suboptimal effort.

The respiratory exchange ratio, $R$, is often advocated as an indicator of maximum effort. An $R$ value less than 1.10 is unlikely to be observed with true maximal effort in the absence of other confounding factors. However, $R$ for a true maximum effort is extremely variable between individuals and attainment of an $R$ value of 1.10 should never be taken as an indication to terminate a maximal exercise test.

Suboptimal effort is best identified by examining tabular data for $\dot{V}O_{2max}$, $f_{Cmax}$, $\dot{V}_{Emax}$, $\dot{V}O_2$ lactate, RPE, and $R$ (Table 5.16) in conjunction with panels 1, 2, 3, 5, and 8 of a nine-panel display (Figure 5.3). Panel 5 shows a normal $f_C$–$\dot{V}O_2$ response pattern which ends prematurely before $f_{Cmax}$ and $\dot{V}O_{2max}$ have been achieved. The same panel allows determination of $\dot{V}O_2\theta$ from the $\dot{V}CO_2$–$\dot{V}O_2$ plot.

### Conditions exhibiting this response pattern

*Subconscious (unintentional) suboptimal effort*
Some individuals are simply poorly motivated for a maximal exercise test and consequently do not push themselves to give a true maximal effort. Their physiological measures fail to indicate any specific physiological limitations but nevertheless their perception of effort (RPE) may be relatively high. In these circumstances the inability to give a true maximal effort is unintentional. Furthermore, if successful measures can be implemented to improve motivation then a higher aerobic capacity should be elicited in a subsequent test.

Inability to give a true maximal effort is a feature of certain psychological disturbances. Therefore, the results of an exercise test in a person with established psychiatric diagnosis should be interpreted accordingly. Beware not to prejudge an individual because of suspected psychological factors which could mask an underlying somatic illness.

*Conscious (intentional) suboptimal effort*
Some individuals deliberately give a suboptimal effort to give the impression of reduced exercise capacity for reasons of secondary gain. These reasons may be obvious, such as a claim for disability payments, a desire to retire from work, or for other purposes of financial compensation or litigation. Sometimes the secondary gain is less obvious and requires subtle inquiry to reveal its nature.

Some individuals give a suboptimal effort for no other reason than they desire ongoing medical attention and investigation. This behavior is often described as malingering.

## FURTHER READING

Ben-Dov, I., Sietsema, K. E., Casaburi, R. & Wasserman, K. (1992). Evidence that circulatory oscillations accompany ventilatory oscillations during exercise in patients with heart failure. *Am. Rev. Respir. Dis.*, **145**, 776–81.

Burden, J. G. W., Killian, K. J. & Jones, N. L. (1983). Pattern of breathing during exercise in patients with interstitial lung disease. *Thorax*, **38**, 778–84.

Carroll, J. E., Hagberg, J. M., Brooke, M. H. & Shumate, J. B.

(1979). Bicycle ergometry and gas exchange measurements in neuromuscular diseases. *Arch. Neurol.*, **36**, 457–61.

Glantz, S. A. (1987). *Primer of Biostatistics*, 2nd edn. New York: McGraw Hill.

Hey, E. N., Lloyd, B. B., Cunningham, D. J., Jukes, M. G. & Bolton, D. P. (1966). Effects of various respiratory stimuli on the depth and frequency of breathing in man. *Respir. Physiol.*, **1**, 193–205.

Koike, A., Wasserman, K., Armon, Y. & Weiler-Ravell, D. (1991). The work-rate dependent effect of carbon monoxide on ventilatory control during exercise. *Respir. Physiol.*, **85**, 169–83.

Lauer, M. S., Francis, G. S., Okin, P. M., Pashkow, F. J., Snader, C. E. & Marwick, T. H. (1999). Impaired chronotropic response to exercise stress testing as a predictor of mortality. *J.A.M.A.*, **281**, 524–9.

Lim, P. O., MacFayden, R. J., Clarkson, P. B. M. & MacDonald, T. M. (1996). Impaired exercise tolerance in hypertensive patients. *Ann. Intern. Med.*, **124**, 41–55.

Loveridge, B., West, P., Anthonisen, N. R. & Kryger, M. H. (1984). Breathing patterns in patients with chronic obstructive pulmonary disease. *Am. Rev. Respir. Dis.*, **130**, 730–3.

Riley, M. S., O'Brien, C. J., McCluskey, D.R. & Nicholls, D. P. (1990). Aerobic work capacity in patients with chronic fatigue syndrome. *Br. Med. J.*, **301**, 953–6.

Weber, K. T. & Janicki, J. S. (1985). Cardiopulmonary exercise testing for evaluation of chronic cardiac failure. *Am. J. Cardiol.*, **55**, 22A–31A.

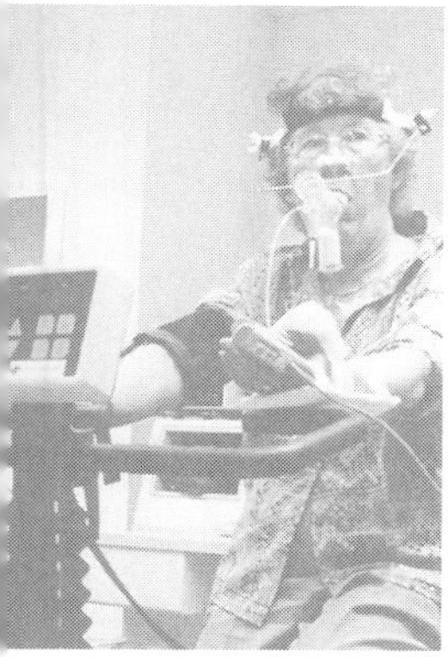

# 6

# Illustrative cases and reports

## Introduction

This chapter provides six carefully selected cases which are used to integrate the concepts of test purpose, instrumentation, testing methods, physiological responses, and interpretation of test results that have been developed in Chapters 1–5. These examples are not meant to represent an exhaustive examination of every set of responses that may be seen in clinical or performance exercise testing. Rather, these commonly encountered cases allow the reader to envisage the process of exercise testing leading to its natural conclusion – an interpretation of exercise performance based upon a systematic process of carefully applied methodologies and accurate collection of key response variables. Each case concludes with a brief statement about the outcome following exercise testing.

## Case 1: Declining exercise capacity with a history of asthma (CXT: diagnostic)

### Purpose

This 51-year-old male complained of declining exercise capacity. He had a history of asthma but normal pulmonary function tests. He used a salmeterol metered-dose inhaler (MDI: 2 puffs twice daily) and fluticasone MDI (2 puffs twice daily). He had never smoked. He was accustomed to running 2–3 miles, 4–5 days per week. A clinical exercise test (CXT) was requested to define his exercise limitations.

### Method

A diagnostic exercise test was chosen utilizing a ramp work rate protocol on a cycle ergometer. Based on the initial physical assessment and reported exercise habits, a ramp rate of $30\,W \cdot min^{-1}$ was chosen. Expired ventilation was measured using a two-way breathing valve and hot wire flow transducer. Therefore, flow–volume loops could not be obtained. The metabolic measuring system was set in breath-by-breath mode. Peripheral measurements included ECG, systemic arterial pressure, pulse oximetry, and serial arterial blood sampling.

After a period of equilibration at rest, he performed unloaded pedaling for 3 min followed by the ramp increase in work rate. He gave an excellent effort, achieving a maximum work rate of 300 W. He stopped exercise complaining of leg fatigue. There were no technical problems and no medical complications during the study.

### Results

#### Tabular data

See Table 6.1.

#### Graphical data

See Figure 6.1.

#### Aerobic capacity

$\dot{V}O_{2max}$ was $3.53\,l \cdot min^{-1}$ or $37\,ml \cdot kg^{-1} \cdot min^{-1}$ (138%

**Table 6.1.** Case 1: tabular data

| | | | |
|---|---|---|---|
| **Identification** | **ID no.** | **Age (years)** | **Gender (M/F)** |
| Illustrative case | 1 | 51 | M |
| **Anthropometric** | | **Technical** | |
| Height (in.) | 69 | Barometer (mmHg) | 757 |
| Height (m) | 1.75 | Ambient temperature (°C) | 22 |
| Weight (lb) | 209 | $F_IO_2$ (%) | 21% |
| Weight (kg) | 95 | Valve dead space (ml) | 80 |
| | | $\ddot{W}$ (W · min$^{-1}$) | 30 |
| Body mass index (kg · m$^{-2}$) | 31 | $\dot{W}_{max}$ (W) | 300 |
| **Pulmonary function** | **Predicted** | **Observed** | **%Predicted** |
| FVC (l) | 4.70 | 4.50 | 96% |
| $FEV_1$ (l) | 3.46 | 3.22 | 93% |
| $FEV_1$/FVC (%) | 74% | 72% | |
| MVV (l · min$^{-1}$) | 89 | 160 | 179% |
| **Aerobic capacity** | **Predicted** | **Observed** | **%pred$\dot{V}o_{2max}$** |
| $\dot{V}o_{2max}$ (l · min$^{-1}$) | 2.57 | 3.53 | 137% |
| $\dot{V}o_2\theta$ (l · min$^{-1}$) | 1.03 | 1.60 | 62% |
| $\delta\dot{V}o_2/\delta W$ (ml · min$^{-1}$ · W$^{-1}$) | 10.3 | 10.0 | |
| $\dot{V}o_{2unloaded}$ (l · min$^{-1}$) | | 0.80 | |
| **Cardiovascular response** | **Predicted** | **Observed** | **%Predicted** |
| $f_{Cmax}$ (min$^{-1}$) | 169 | 149 | 88% |
| Cardiac reserve (min$^{-1}$) | 0 | 20 | |
| $\dot{V}o_2/f_{Cmax}$ (ml) | 15.2 | 23.7 | 156% |
| $f_{Crest}$ (min$^{-1}$) | | 67 | |
| Resting ECG | SR 70/min, axis + 60, P-QRS-T configuration normal | | |
| Exercise ECG | No dysrhythmia and no evidence of myocardial ischemia | | |
| | **Rest** | **Exercise (max.)** | **Recovery (2 min)** |
| Systolic BP (mmHg) | 138 | 154 | 140 |
| Diastolic BP (mmHg) | 98 | 94 | 90 |
| **Ventilatory response** | **Predicted** | **Observed** | **%MVV** |
| $\dot{V}_{Emax}$ (l · min$^{-1}$) | 160 | 117 | 73% |
| Ventilatory reserve (l · min$^{-1}$) | >15 | 43 | |
| $V_{Tmax}$ (l) | 2.25 | 2.93 | |
| $f_{Rmax}$ (min$^{-1}$) | <50 | 41 | |
| $T_I/T_E$ at end exercise | 0.8 | 0.9 | |

**Table 6.1.** *(cont.)*

| Gas exchange | Rest | Threshold | Maximum |
|---|---|---|---|
| $\dot{V}_E/\dot{V}O_2$ | 35 | 26 | 33 |
| $\dot{V}_E/\dot{V}CO_2$ | 40 | 26 | 27 |
| $P_{ET}O_2$ (mmHg) | 103 | 104 | 115 |
| $P_{ET}CO_2$ (mmHg) | 39 | 42 | 38 |
| $R$ | 0.88 | 0.98 | 1.23 |
| $SpO_2$ (%) | 97 | 96 | 93 |
| $PaO_2$ (mmHg) | 90 | 99 | 88 |
| $PaCO_2$ (mmHg) | 44 | 43 | 39 |
| $P_{(A-a)}O_2$ (mmHg) | 9 | 6 | 29 |
| $P_{(a-ET)}CO_2$ (mmHg) | 5 | 1 | 1 |
| $V_D/V_T$ (%) | 36% | 18% | 16% |
| **Muscle metabolism** | **Rest** | **Exercise (4 min)** | **Recovery (2 min)** |
| Lactate ($mg \cdot dl^{-1}$) | | | 94 |
| Ammonia ($\mu g \cdot dl^{-1}$) | | | |
| Creatine kinase ($U \cdot l^{-1}$) | | | |
| | **Predicted** | **Observed** | |
| $RQ_{mus}$ ($\delta\dot{V}CO_2/\delta\dot{V}O_2$) | 0.95 | 1.00 | |
| **Symptom perception** | **Rest** | **Exercise (max.)** | |
| Effort (observer impression) | | Excellent | |
| Symptoms (subjective) | | Leg fatigue | |
| Perceived exertion (Borg scale/20) | | 10 | |
| Breathlessness (VAS scale/100) | | 21 | |

of reference). $\dot{V}O_2\theta$ was confidently detected at an oxygen uptake of $1.60 \, l \cdot min^{-1}$ or $17 \, ml \cdot kg^{-1} \cdot min^{-1}$ (62% of reference $\dot{V}O_{2max}$). Both of these measurements exceed the reference values. Work efficiency was normal, as judged by the relationship between $\dot{V}O_2$ and $\dot{W}$. $\dot{V}O_2$ for unloaded pedaling was increased commensurate with increased body weight.

## Cardiovascular response

$f_{Cmax}$ was $149 \, min^{-1}$ (88% of reference). He approached cardiovascular limitation. $\dot{V}O_2/f_{Cmax}$ was 23.7 ml (156% of reference) and $\delta f_C/\delta\dot{V}O_2$ was reduced consistent with physical conditioning. The ECG showed no dysrhythmia and no evidence of myocardial ischemia. Systemic arterial pressures were normal at rest, during exercise, and during recovery.

## Ventilatory response

$\dot{V}_{Emax}$ was $117 \, l \cdot min^{-1}$ (73% of measured MVV). He did not exhibit ventilatory limitation. $\delta\dot{V}_E/\delta\dot{V}O_2$ was normal. $V_{Tmax}$ and $f_{Rmax}$ were both within their expected ranges. $T_I/T_E$ was normal, indicating a normal ventilatory response pattern.

## Gas exchange

Ventilatory equivalents and end-tidal gas tensions showed normal response patterns. $V_D/V_T$ was 36% at rest and 16% at maximum exercise, which was normal. $P_{(A-a)}O_2$ was 9 mmHg at rest and 29 mmHg at maximum exercise, which was also normal. Oxygenation was normal throughout the study, as judged by pulse oximetry.

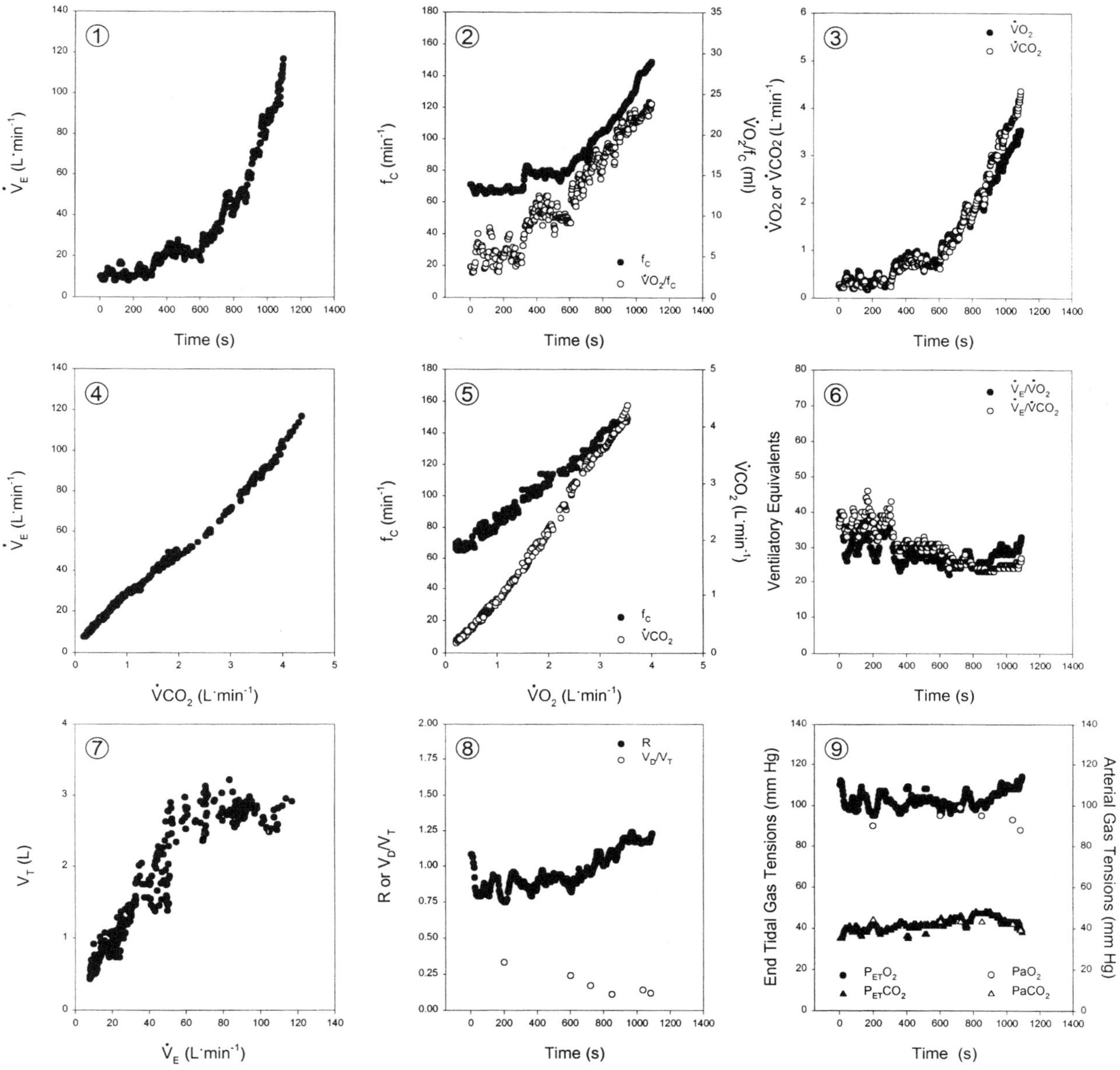


**Figure 6.1** Case 1. Nine-panel display. The data were obtained for a period of equilibration at rest then 3 min of unloaded pedaling followed by a ramp increase in work rate of 30 W · min$^{-1}$ to symptom-limited maximum.

### Muscle metabolism

$RQ_{mus}$ was normal, as judged by the lower slope of the $\dot{V}co_2$–$\dot{V}o_2$ relationship. He exhibited a normal increase in blood lactate.

### Symptom perception

His RPE was 10/20, which was inappropriately low compared with the cardiovascular response. His $\beta$–score was 21/100, which was inappropriately low compared with the proportion of his ventilatory capacity utilized.

## Interpretation

Increased aerobic capacity and increased metabolic threshold consistent with a physically well-conditioned subject. The cardiovascular response was also consistent with physical fitness. There was no evidence of ventilatory limitation. Gas exchange mechanisms and muscle metabolism appeared normal. Symptom perception was inappropriately reduced, consistent with stoicism.

### Addendum

The subject was reassured that he maintained an excellent level of fitness and that no physiological abnormalities existed to account for exercise limitation.

# Case 2: A sedentary young female preparing for exercise (PXT: fitness assessment)

## Purpose

This 26-year-old female wished to begin a regular exercise program for the purpose of weight management and cardiovascular risk reduction. She has a strong family history of coronary artery disease, diabetes, and obesity. Although not diabetic, she was 12 kg overweight. She was apparently in good health, having normal blood pressure and blood lipids. She was taking no medications and did not smoke. She had not exercised regularly for 8 years, but would prefer to walk or jog as her choice of activities.

## Method

After obtaining a Physical Activity Readiness Questionnaire (PAR-Q) and informed consent, a performance exercise test was conducted in the field using a Rockport 1-mile walk test. The purposes of the test were to assess her current level of cardiopulmonary fitness, to acquire physiological and perceptual responses during the test, and to establish a baseline for exercise prescription and progress monitoring. The test was administered on a measured outdoor track. A heart rate monitor was used to measure and record $f_C$ throughout the test. Ratings of perceived exertion were acquired every 440 yd. The subject was instructed to walk as fast as possible for the entire mile without running. After light stretching and a short walk to become familiar with the course, the subject began walking on a verbal signal to start that coincided with starting the stopwatch. Ambient air temperature was 24 °C; humidity was 55%. Body weight was measured before the test at 84 kg. Resting $f_C$ was 78 min$^{-1}$. The subject gave a good effort, did not exhibit any symptoms, and reported no ill effects from the exercise.

## Results

### Tabular data

See Table 6.2.

### Graphical data

See Figure 6.2.

### Predicted aerobic capacity

The 26-year-old subject's endurance time for the 1-mile walk was 18:59 (min:s). Her heart rate during the last 2 min of the walk averaged 171 min$^{-1}$, determined from the heart rate meter. These data, along with her body weight of 84 kg, were entered into the Rockport walking test equation for

**Table 6.2.** Case 2: tabular data for the Rockport 1-mile walk test

| Time (min) | $f_C$ (min$^{-1}$) | Lap time (min) | Distance (yd) | $\dot{V}O_2$ (ml · kg$^{-1}$ · min$^{-1}$) | RPE |
|---|---|---|---|---|---|
| 1 | 123 | | | | |
| 2 | 138 | | | | |
| 3 | 150 | | | | |
| 4 | 156 | | | | |
| 5 | 158 | 4:38 | 440 | 12.2 | 11 |
| 6 | 159 | | | | |
| 7 | 160 | | | | |
| 8 | 162 | | | | |
| 9 | 165 | 9:06 | 880 | 12.3 | 12 |
| 10 | 166 | | | | |
| 11 | 168 | | | | |
| 12 | 169 | | | | |
| 13 | 168 | | | | |
| 14 | 170 | 13:38 | 1320 | 12.4 | 13 |
| 15 | 171 | | | | |
| 16 | 170 | | | | |
| 17 | 171 | | | | |
| 18 | 170 | | | | |
| 19 | 171 | 18:59 | 1760 | 11.8 | 14 |

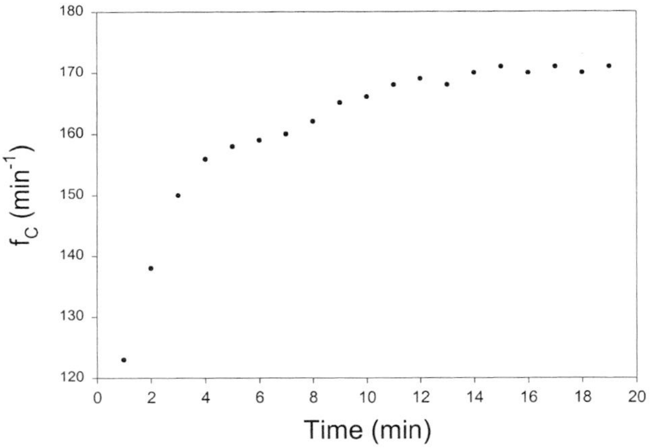


**Figure 6.2** Case 2. Relationship between $f_C$ and time for the Rockport 1-mile walk test.

prediction of $\dot{V}O_{2max}$, yielding a value of 27.0 ml · kg$^{-1}$ · min$^{-1}$. The test was performed at a relatively even pace with 440-yd lap times of 4:38, 4:28, 4:32, and 5:21 (min:s). These times suggest an average walking velocity of 19 min · mile$^{-1}$ (85 m · min$^{-1}$) and a corresponding $\dot{V}O_2$ of 12 ml · kg$^{-1}$ · min$^{-1}$ at this speed. No adverse symptoms were reported.

### Cardiovascular response

Her $f_C$ was 123 min$^{-1}$ after the first minute and 158 min$^{-1}$ at the end of the first 440 yd. From the end of the 11th minute of walking through the end of the test at 18:59, $f_C$ did not vary by more than 3 min$^{-1}$, reaching a peak value of 171 min$^{-1}$ during the last minute of the test. This steady-state $f_C$ represents 88% of the subject's maximal heart rate or 79% of the heart rate reserve (estimated $f_{Cmax}$–$f_{Crest}$).

### Symptom perception

Ratings of perceived exertion (RPE) increased slightly from 11 to 14 at each quarter-mile interval throughout the test (Table 6.2). Relative to the cardiovascular response, RPE was somewhat low.

## Interpretation

The predicted $\dot{V}O_{2max}$ of 27 ml · kg$^{-1}$ · min$^{-1}$ represents a below-average level of aerobic fitness for women aged 20–29 compared to the reference value of 36 ml · kg$^{-1}$ · min$^{-1}$ for this gender and age group. Thus, the predicted $\dot{V}O_{2max}$ represents 75% of the reference value and is suggestive of deconditioning. The cardiovascular response, as determined by $f_C$ alone, is higher than expected for the work rate which is also consistent with deconditioning. Symptom perception is inappropriately low, suggesting denial or stoicism.

### Addendum

After review of the test results and the development of a progressive walking, walk/jog program, the subject embarked on fulfilling this prescription 5 days per week. She exercised regularly for the next 9 weeks, averaging 0.36 kg per week weight loss.

## Case 3: An apparently healthy male complaining of exertional breathlessness and muscle fatigue (CXT: diagnostic)

### Purpose

This 44-year-old male complained of exertional breathlessness and muscle fatigue. He had no known medical problems and took no medications. He was completely sedentary, having stopped any regular exercise 8 months previously. He had a 10 pack-year smoking history but quit 1 month before his exercise evaluation. Resting pulmonary function tests were normal.

### Method

A diagnostic exercise test was chosen utilizing a ramp work rate protocol on a cycle ergometer. Based on initial physical assessment and reported exercise habits, a ramp rate of $15\,W \cdot min^{-1}$ was chosen. Ventilation was measured using a bi-directional flow transducer. The metabolic measuring system was set in breath-by-breath mode. Peripheral measurements included ECG, systemic arterial pressure, and pulse oximetry. A cannula was inserted in the right radial artery and sequential samples of arterial blood were obtained for the measurement of blood gases, lactate, ammonia, and creatine kinase.

After a period of equilibration at rest, he performed unloaded pedaling for 3 min followed by the ramp increase in work rate. He gave an excellent effort, achieving a maximum work rate of 197 W. He stopped exercise complaining of breathlessness. There were no technical problems and no medical complications during the study.

### Results

#### Tabular data

See Table 6.3.

#### Graphical data

See Figure 6.3.

#### Aerobic capacity

$\dot{V}O_{2max}$ was $2.06\,l \cdot min^{-1}$ (74% of reference). This was mildly reduced. $\dot{V}O_2\theta$ was confidently detected by gas exchange measurements at an oxygen uptake of $1.30\,l \cdot min^{-1}$ (47% of reference $\dot{V}O_{2max}$). This was normal. Work efficiency was abnormal, as judged by the relationship between $\dot{V}O_2$ and $\dot{W}$ which had a slope of $8.2\,ml \cdot min^{-1} \cdot W^{-1}$ compared with the reference value of $10.3\,ml \cdot min^{-1} \cdot W^{-1}$. $\dot{V}O_2$ for unloaded pedaling was within normal limits.

#### Cardiovascular response

$f_{Cmax}$ was $161\,min^{-1}$ (91% of reference). Hence he exhibited cardiovascular limitation. $\dot{V}O_2/f_{Cmax}$ was 12.9 ml (81% of reference) and $\delta f_C/\delta\dot{V}O_2$ was normal, consistent with a normal cardiovascular response pattern. The ECG showed no dysrhythmia and no evidence of myocardial ischemia. Systemic arterial pressures were normal throughout the study.

#### Ventilatory response

$\dot{V}_{Emax}$ was $83\,l \cdot min^{-1}$ (70% of measured MVV). Hence he did not exhibit ventilatory limitation. $\delta\dot{V}_E/\delta\dot{V}O_2$ was normal. $f_{Rmax}$ was within the expected range. $V_{Tmax}$ was lower than expected. There was a definite period of hyperventilation at moderate exercise intensity (see panels 1, 6, 8, and 9 of Figure 6.3).

#### Gas exchange

Gas exchange mechanisms were normal. $V_D/V_T$ was 18% at rest and 15% at maximum exercise. $P_{(A-a)}O_2$

**Table 6.3.** Case 3: tabular data

| **Identification** | **ID no.** | **Age (years)** | **Gender (M/F)** |
|---|---|---|---|
| Illustrative case | 3 | 44 | M |
| **Anthropometric** | | **Technical** | |
| Height (in.) | 66 | Barometer (mmHg) | 755 |
| Height (m) | 1.68 | Ambient temperature (°C) | 23 |
| Weight (lb) | 143 | $F_IO_2$ (%) | 21% |
| Weight (kg) | 95 | Valve dead space (ml) | 80 |
| | | $\ddot{W}$ (W · min$^{-1}$) | 15 |
| Body mass index (kg · m$^{-2}$) | 23 | $\dot{W}_{max}$ (W) | 197 |
| **Pulmonary function** | **Predicted** | **Observed** | **%Predicted** |
| FVC (l) | 4.09 | 4.73 | 116% |
| $FEV_1$ (l) | 3.37 | 3.85 | 114% |
| $FEV_1$/FVC (%) | 82% | 81% | |
| MVV (l · min$^{-1}$) | 87 | 119 | 136% |
| **Aerobic capacity** | **Predicted** | **Observed** | **%pred$\dot{V}o_{2max}$** |
| $\dot{V}o_{2max}$ (l · min$^{-1}$) | 2.79 | 2.06 | 74% |
| $\dot{V}o_2\theta$ (l · min$^{-1}$) | 1.12 | 1.30 | 47% |
| $\delta\dot{V}o_2/\delta W$ (ml · min$^{-1}$ · W$^{-1}$) | 10.3 | 8.2 | |
| $\dot{V}o_{2unloaded}$ (l · min$^{-1}$) | | 0.50 | |
| **Cardiovascular response** | **Predicted** | **Observed** | **%Predicted** |
| $f_{Cmax}$ (min$^{-1}$) | 176 | 161 | 91% |
| Cardiac reserve (min$^{-1}$) | 0 | 15 | |
| $\dot{V}o_2/f_{Cmax}$ (ml) | 15.9 | 12.9 | 81% |
| $f_{Crest}$ (min$^{-1}$) | | 74 | |
| Resting ECG | SR 76/min, rad + 100, LVH by voltage criteria, ST normal | | |
| Exercise ECG | No dysrhythmia and no evidence of myocardial ischemia | | |
| | **Rest** | **Exercise (max.)** | **Recovery (2 min)** |
| Systolic BP (mmHg) | 116 | 158 | 132 |
| Diastolic BP (mmHg) | 76 | 86 | 70 |
| **Ventilatory response** | **Predicted** | **Observed** | **%MVV** |
| $\dot{V}_{Emax}$ (l · min$^{-1}$) | 119 | 83 | 70% |
| Ventilatory reserve (l · min$^{-1}$) | >15 | 36 | |
| $V_{Tmax}$ (l) | 2.37 | 2.22 | |
| $f_{Rmax}$ (min$^{-1}$) | <50 | 40 | |
| $T_I/T_E$ at end exercise | 0.8 | 0.9 | |

**Table 6.3.** *(cont.)*

| Gas exchange | Rest | Threshold | Maximum |
|---|---|---|---|
| $\dot{V}_E/\dot{V}O_2$ | 25 | 24 | 38 |
| $\dot{V}_E/\dot{V}CO_2$ | 33 | 30 | 31 |
| $P_{ET}O_2$ (mmHg) | 105 | 107 | 120 |
| $P_{ET}CO_2$ (mmHg) | 36 | 36 | 35 |
| $R$ | 0.77 | 0.82 | 1.23 |
| $SpO_2$ (%) | 99 | 100 | 98 |
| $PaO_2$ (mmHg) | 97 | | 101 |
| $PaCO_2$ (mmHg) | 39 | | 34 |
| $P_{(A-a)}O_2$ (mmHg) | 1 | | 20 |
| $P_{(a-ET)}CO_2$ (mmHg) | 3 | | −1 |
| $V_D/V_T$ (%) | 18% | | 15% |
| **Muscle metabolism** | **Rest** | **Exercise (4 min)** | **Recovery (2 min)** |
| Lactate ($mg \cdot dl^{-1}$) | 11 | 12 | 59 |
| Ammonia ($\mu g \cdot dl^{-1}$) | 90 | 70 | 186 |
| Creatine kinase ($U \cdot l^{-1}$) | 96 | 96 | 109 |
| | **Predicted** | **Observed** | |
| $RQ_{mus}$ ($\delta\dot{V}CO_2/\delta\dot{V}O_2$) | 0.95 | 1.00 | |
| **Symptom perception** | **Rest** | **Exercise (max.)** | |
| Effort (observer impression) | | Excellent | |
| Symptoms (subjective) | | Dyspnea, leg fatigue | |
| Perceived exertion (Borg scale/20) | | 18 | |
| Breathlessness (VAS scale/100) | | 77 | |

was 1 mmHg at rest and 20 mmHg at end exercise, both of which were normal. Oxygenation was normal throughout the study, as judged by pulse oximetry.

### Muscle metabolism

$RQ_{mus}$ was normal, as judged by the lower slope of the $\dot{V}CO_2$–$\dot{V}O_2$ relationship. He displayed normal increases in lactate and ammonia levels during exercise. Creatine kinase levels were normal.

### Symptom perception

His RPE was 18/20, which was appropriate compared with the cardiovascular response. His $\beta$-score was 77/100, which was appropriate compared with the proportion of his ventilatory capacity utilized.

## Interpretation

Mildly reduced aerobic capacity with a normal metabolic threshold. He exhibited cardiovascular limitation with a normal cardiovascular response pattern. There was a period of hyperventilation but no evidence of ventilatory limitation. Gas exchange mechanisms were normal. Muscle metabolism was normal, although the ammonia increase was exaggerated. Symptom perception was appropriate. In conclusion, he showed minor nonspecific abnormalities and no evidence of cardiovascular or pulmonary disease to account for his breathlessness. The identification of hyperventilation during the exercise phase suggests a component of anxiety.

### Addendum

The subject was reassured that his breathlessness was normal and that he had no physiological

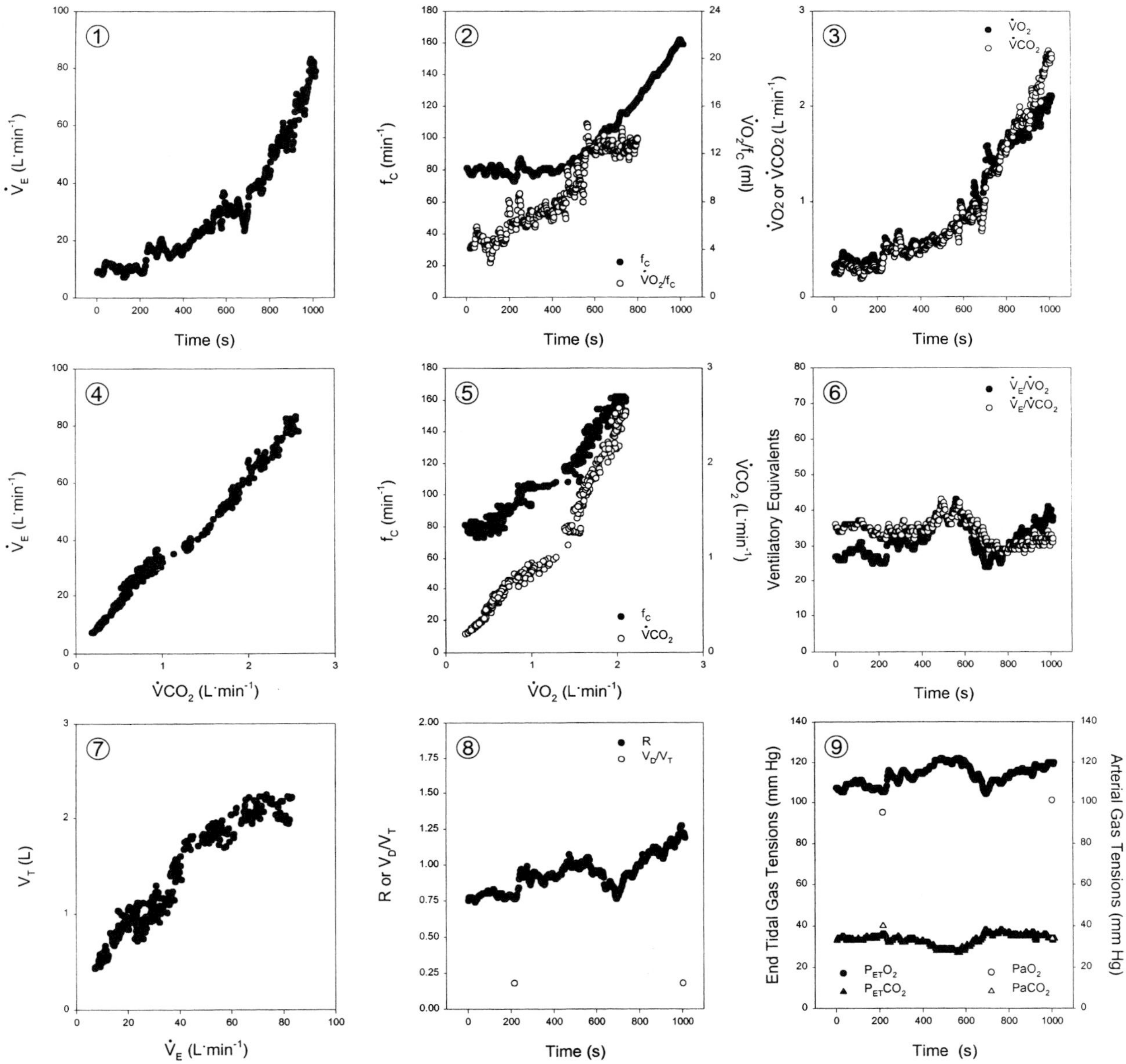


**Figure 6.3** Case 3. Nine-panel display. The data were obtained for a period of equilibration at rest then 3 min of unloaded pedaling followed by a ramp increase in work rate of 15 W · min⁻¹ to symptom-limited maximum.

abnormalities. Aerobic exercise training was recommended three times per week, for 30 min, with a target heart rate range of 100–120 beat·min$^{-1}$. He was encouraged to focus on slower, deeper breathing whenever troubled by breathlessness.

## Case 4: Initial evaluation for pulmonary rehabilitation (CXT: diagnostic)

### Purpose

This 71-year-old male wished to participate in a pulmonary rehabilitation program that consisted of structured exercise training. He was known to have chronic obstructive pulmonary disease with components of asthma and emphysema. Also, he had had coronary artery bypass surgery. His medications were diltiazem 180 mg daily, quinidine 324 mg daily, isosorbide mononitrate 60 mg daily, and simvastatin 10 mg daily. He had a 100 pack-year smoking history. He was able to hit golf balls for about 20 min three times a week but any greater physical activity was limited by breathlessness.

### Method

A diagnostic exercise test utilizing a ramp work rate protocol on a cycle ergometer was chosen in order to define his physiological limitations and to enable a safe and effective exercise prescription. Based on the initial physical assessment and reported exercise habits, a ramp rate of 10 W·min$^{-1}$ was chosen. Ventilation was measured using a two-way breathing valve and hot wire flow transducer. Therefore, flow–volume loops could not be obtained. The metabolic measuring system was set in breath-by-breath mode. Peripheral measurements included ECG, systemic arterial pressure, and pulse oximetry. A single arterial blood sample was obtained at rest for blood gases and a single venous blood sample was obtained after 2 min of recovery for lactate.

After a period of equilibration at rest, he performed unloaded pedaling for 3 min followed by the ramp increase in work rate. He gave an excellent effort, achieving a maximum work rate of 104 W. He stopped exercise complaining of breathlessness and leg fatigue. There were no technical problems and no medical complications during the study.

### Results

#### Tabular data

See Table 6.4.

#### Graphical data

See Figure 6.4.

#### Aerobic capacity

$\dot{V}O_{2max}$ was 1.55 l·min$^{-1}$ (80% of reference). Hence, aerobic capacity was low normal. $\dot{V}O_2\theta$ was confidently detected at an oxygen uptake of 0.95 l·min$^{-1}$ (49% of reference $\dot{V}O_{2max}$). This was within the expected range. Work efficiency was normal, as judged by the relationship between $\dot{V}O_2$ and $\dot{W}$. $\dot{V}O_2$ for unloaded pedaling was also normal.

#### Cardiovascular response

$f_{Cmax}$ was 120 min$^{-1}$ (81% of reference). He approached but did not truly exhibit cardiovascular limitation. $\dot{V}O_2/f_{Cmax}$ was 13.0 ml (100% of reference). $\delta f_C/\delta\dot{V}O_2$ was reduced due to the constraining effects of diltiazem on heart rate increase, thus resulting in a spuriously high oxygen pulse but a submaximal heart rate. The ECG showed rare premature ventricular contractions during the exercise phase but no ST or repolarization changes suggestive of myocardial ischemia. Systemic arterial pressures were normal at rest, during exercise, and during recovery.

#### Ventilatory response

$\dot{V}_{Emax}$ was 53 l·min$^{-1}$ (96% of measured MVV). He exhibited ventilatory limitation. $\delta\dot{V}_E/\delta\dot{V}O_2$ was normal. $V_{Tmax}$ and $f_{Rmax}$ were both within their expected

**Table 6.4.** Case 4: tabular data

| | | | |
|---|---|---|---|
| **Identification** | **ID no.** | **Age (years)** | **Gender (M/F)** |
| Illustrative case | 4 | 71 | M |
| **Anthropometric** | | **Technical** | |
| Height (in.) | 67 | Barometer (mmHg) | 749 |
| Height (m) | 1.70 | Ambient temperature (°C) | 24 |
| Weight (lb) | 145 | $F_{I}O_2$ (%) | 21% |
| Weight (kg) | 66 | Valve dead space (ml) | 80 |
| | | $\ddot{W}$ (W · min$^{-1}$) | 10 |
| Body mass index (kg · m$^{-2}$) | 23 | $\dot{W}_{max}$ (W) | 104 |
| **Pulmonary function** | **Predicted** | **Observed** | **%Predicted** |
| FVC (l) | 3.90 | 2.36 | 61% |
| $FEV_1$ (l) | 2.63 | 1.19 | 45% |
| $FEV_1$/FVC (%) | 67% | 50% | |
| MVV (l · min$^{-1}$) | 73 | 55 | 76% |
| **Aerobic capacity** | **Predicted** | **Observed** | **%pred$\dot{V}o_{2max}$** |
| $\dot{V}o_{2max}$ (l · min$^{-1}$) | 1.93 | 1.55 | 80% |
| $\dot{V}o_2\theta$ (l · min$^{-1}$) | 0.77 | 0.95 | 49% |
| $\delta\dot{V}o_2/\delta W$ (ml · min$^{-1}$ · W$^{-1}$) | 10.3 | 10.9 | |
| $\dot{V}o_{2unloaded}$ (l · min$^{-1}$) | | 0.58 | |
| **Cardiovascular response** | **Predicted** | **Observed** | **%Predicted** |
| $f_{Cmax}$ (min$^{-1}$) | 149 | 120 | 81% |
| Cardiac reserve (min$^{-1}$) | 0 | 29 | |
| $\dot{V}o_2/f_{Cmax}$ (ml) | 13.0 | 13.0 | 100% |
| $f_{Crest}$ (min$^{-1}$) | | 80 | |
| Resting ECG | SR 70/min, borderline widened QRS, normal ST, T | | |
| Exercise ECG | Rare PVCs during exercise, normal ST and repolarization | | |
| | **Rest** | **Exercise (max.)** | **Recovery (2 min)** |
| Systolic BP (mmHg) | 140 | 180 | 170 |
| Diastolic BP (mmHg) | 80 | 90 | 80 |
| **Ventilatory response** | **Predicted** | **Observed** | **%MVV** |
| $\dot{V}_{Emax}$ (l · min$^{-1}$) | 55 | 53 | 96% |
| Ventilatory reserve (l · min$^{-1}$) | >15 | 2 | |
| $V_{Tmax}$ (l) | 1.18 | 1.36 | |
| $f_{Rmax}$ (min$^{-1}$) | <50 | 41 | |
| $T_I/T_E$ at end exercise | 0.8 | 0.6 | |

**Table 6.4.** *(cont.)*

| Gas exchange | Rest | Threshold | Maximum |
|---|---|---|---|
| $\dot{V}_E/\dot{V}O_2$ | 41 | 31 | 34 |
| $\dot{V}_E/\dot{V}CO_2$ | 46 | 33 | 33 |
| $P_{ET}O_2$ (mmHg) | 106 | 104 | 107 |
| $P_{ET}CO_2$ (mmHg) | 39 | 43 | 43 |
| $R$ | 0.87 | 0.97 | 1.05 |
| $SpO_2$ (%) | 97 | 97 | 95 |
| $PaO_2$ (mmHg) | 74 | | |
| $PaCO_2$ (mmHg) | 45 | | |
| $P_{(A-a)}O_2$ (mmHg) | 22 | | |
| $P_{(a-ET)}CO_2$ (mmHg) | 6 | | |
| $V_D/V_T$ (%) | 46% | | |
| **Muscle metabolism** | **Rest** | **Exercise (4 min)** | **Recovery (2 min)** |
| **Lactate (mg · dl⁻¹)** | | | 35 |
| Ammonia (μg · dl⁻¹) | | | |
| Creatine kinase (U · l⁻¹) | | | |
| | **Predicted** | **Observed** | |
| $RQ_{mus}$ ($\delta\dot{V}CO_2/\delta\dot{V}O_2$) | 0.95 | 1.00 | |
| **Symptom perception** | **Rest** | **Exercise (max.)** | |
| Effort (observer impression) | | Good | |
| Symptoms (subjective) | | Dyspnea, leg fatigue | |
| Perceived exertion (Borg scale/20) | | 19 | |
| Breathlessness (VAS scale/100) | | 84 | |

ranges. However, $T_I/T_E$ was reduced consistent with an obstructive response pattern.

### Gas exchange

Ventilatory equivalents and end-tidal gas tensions showed normal response patterns. $V_D/V_T$ was 46% at rest which was marginally increased. $P_{(A-a)}O_2$ was 22 mmHg at rest, which is normal. Resting $PaO_2$ was 74 mmHg, whereas $PaCO_2$ was 45 mmHg, indicating a mild degree of alveolar hypoventilation. Oxygenation was normal throughout the study as judged by pulse oximetry.

### Muscle metabolism

$RQ_{mus}$ was normal, as judged by the lower slope of the relationship between $\dot{V}CO_2$ and $\dot{V}O_2$. He exhibited a normal increase in blood lactate.

### Symptom perception

His RPE was 19/20, which was inappropriately high compared with the cardiovascular response. His $\beta$–score was 84/100, which was appropriate compared with the proportion of his ventilatory capacity utilized.

## Interpretation

Low normal aerobic capacity with normal metabolic threshold. He exhibited ventilatory limitation with abnormal gas exchange characterized by mildly increased physiological dead space. The cardiovascular response was influenced by diltiazem but was not strictly limiting and significant evidence of myocardial ischemia was not identified. Muscle metabolism appeared normal. His perception of exertion was probably also influenced by diltiazem. This study indicated that his rehabilitation should

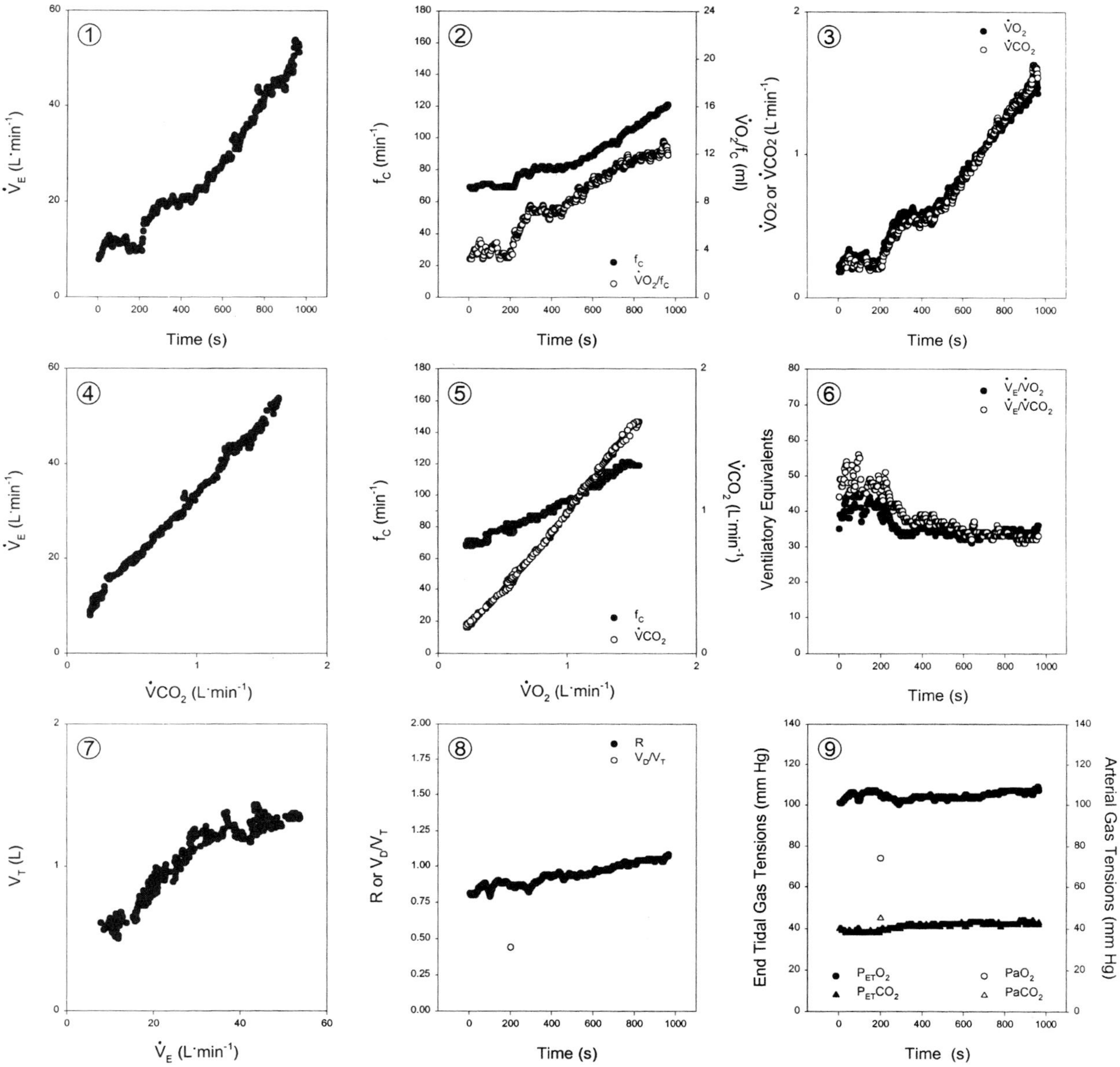


**Figure 6.4** Case 4. Nine-panel display. The data were obtained for a period of equilibration at rest then 3 min of unloaded pedaling followed by a ramp increase in work rate of 10 W · min$^{-1}$ to symptom-limited maximum.

focus on optimizing bronchodilator therapy to improve ventilatory mechanics and emphasize slower breathing to improve ventilatory efficiency. He had potential for physical reconditioning to reduce his ventilatory requirement for exercise.

### Addendum

The subject participated in a 6-week intensive rehabilitation program. Three months after the intensive phase he maintained a vigorous exercise program and was able to walk briskly on the treadmill for 60 min at 3 m.p.h. and 4% grade.

## Case 5: A history of occupational exposure (CXT: diagnostic)

### Purpose

This 58-year-old male complained of exertional breathlessness and decline in his exercise capacity. He used to walk 2 miles each day until 12 months prior to testing but was now sedentary. He gave a 12-year history of exposure to solvents during his work. He took nifedipine 60 mg daily for hypertension. He smoked in the past but quit 13 years prior to testing. A CXT was requested to assist with diagnosis.

### Method

A diagnostic exercise test was chosen utilizing a ramp work rate protocol on a cycle ergometer. Based on initial physical assessment and reported exercise habits, a ramp rate of $15\,W \cdot min^{-1}$ was chosen. Ventilation was measured using a bi-directional flow transducer. The metabolic measuring system was set in breath-by-breath mode. Peripheral measurements included ECG, systemic arterial pressure, and pulse oximetry. An arterial sample was obtained at rest for blood gases and venous sample obtained after 2 min of recovery for lactate.

After a period of equilibration at rest, he performed unloaded pedaling for 3 min followed by the ramp increase in work rate. He gave an excellent effort, achieving a maximum work rate of 131 W. He stopped exercise complaining of breathlessness. There were no technical problems and no medical complications during the study.

### Results

#### Tabular data

See Table 6.5.

#### Graphical data

See Figure 6.5.

#### Aerobic capacity

$\dot{V}O_{2max}$ was $1.61\,l \cdot min^{-1}$ (69% of reference). $\dot{V}O_2\theta$ was confidently detected at an oxygen uptake of $0.95\,l \cdot min^{-1}$ (41% of reference $\dot{V}O_{2max}$). Both of these values were reduced. Work efficiency was normal, as judged by the relationship between $\dot{V}O_2$ and $\dot{W}$. $\dot{V}O_2$ for unloaded pedaling was marginally increased commensurate with increased body weight.

#### Cardiovascular response

$f_{Cmax}$ was $166\,min^{-1}$ (102% of reference). He exhibited cardiovascular limitation. $\dot{V}O_2/f_{Cmax}$ was 9.7 ml (67% of reference) and $\delta f_C/\delta\dot{V}O_2$ was increased, consistent with attainment of maximum heart rate at low maximum oxygen uptake. The ECG showed no dysrhythmia and no evidence of myocardial ischemia. Systemic arterial pressures were marginally high at rest and at maximum exercise.

#### Ventilatory response

$\dot{V}_{Emax}$ was $68\,l \cdot min^{-1}$ (59% of measured MVV). He did not exhibit ventilatory limitation. $\delta\dot{V}_E/\delta\dot{V}O_2$ was normal. $V_{Tmax}$ and $f_{Rmax}$ were both within their expected ranges. $T_I/T_E$ was normal, indicating a normal ventilatory response pattern.

**Table 6.5.** Case 5: tabular data

| | | | |
|---|---|---|---|
| **Identification** | **ID no.** | **Age (years)** | **Gender (M/F)** |
| Illustrative case | 5 | 58 | M |
| **Anthropometric** | | **Technical** | |
| Height (in.) | 71 | Barometer (mmHg) | 749 |
| Height (m) | 1.80 | Ambient temperature (°C) | 23 |
| Weight (lb) | 257 | $F_IO_2$ (%) | 21% |
| Weight (kg) | 117 | Valve dead space (ml) | 80 |
| | | $\ddot{W}$ (W · min$^{-1}$) | 15 |
| Body mass index (kg · m$^{-2}$) | 36 | $\dot{W}_{max}$ (W) | 131 |
| **Pulmonary function** | **Predicted** | **Observed** | **%Predicted** |
| FVC (l) | 4.52 | 4.43 | 98% |
| $FEV_1$ (l) | 3.42 | 3.04 | 89% |
| $FEV_1$/FVC (%) | 76% | 69% | |
| MVV (l · min$^{-1}$) | 88 | 115 | 130% |
| **Aerobic capacity** | **Predicted** | **Observed** | **%pred$\dot{V}o_{2max}$** |
| $\dot{V}o_{2max}$ (l · min$^{-1}$) | 2.34 | 1.61 | 69% |
| $\dot{V}o_2\theta$ (l · min$^{-1}$) | 0.94 | 0.95 | 41% |
| $\delta\dot{V}o_2/\delta W$ (ml · min$^{-1}$ · W$^{-1}$) | 10.3 | 9.8 | |
| $\dot{V}o_{2unloaded}$ (l · min$^{-1}$) | | 0.62 | |
| **Cardiovascular response** | **Predicted** | **Observed** | **%Predicted** |
| $f_{Cmax}$ (min$^{-1}$) | 162 | 166 | 102% |
| Cardiac reserve (min$^{-1}$) | 0 | –4 | |
| $\dot{V}o_2/f_{Cmax}$ (ml) | 14.4 | 9.7 | 67% |
| $f_{Crest}$ (min$^{-1}$) | | 105 | |
| Resting ECG | SR 103/min, axis +60, P-QRS-T configuration normal | | |
| Exercise ECG | No dysrhythmia and no evidence of myocardial ischemia | | |
| | **Rest** | **Exercise (max.)** | **Recovery (2 min)** |
| Systolic BP (mmHg) | 128 | 192 | 160 |
| Diastolic BP (mmHg) | 100 | 99 | 86 |
| **Ventilatory response** | **Predicted** | **Observed** | **%MVV** |
| $\dot{V}_{Emax}$ (l · min$^{-1}$) | 115 | 68 | 59% |
| Ventilatory reserve (l · min$^{-1}$) | >15 | 47 | |
| $V_{Tmax}$ (l) | 2.22 | 1.95 | |
| $f_{Rmax}$ (min$^{-1}$) | <50 | 34 | |
| $T_I/T_E$ at end exercise | 0.8 | 0.9 | |

Table 6.5. (*cont.*)

| Gas exchange | Rest | Threshold | Maximum |
|---|---|---|---|
| $\dot{V}_E/\dot{V}O_2$ | 35 | 34 | 41 |
| $\dot{V}_E/\dot{V}CO_2$ | 36 | 32 | 31 |
| $P_{ET}O_2$ (mmHg) | 109 | 108 | 116 |
| $P_{ET}CO_2$ (mmHg) | 35 | 37 | 34 |
| $R$ | 0.98 | 1.06 | 1.33 |
| $SpO_2$ (%) | 97 | 98 | 98 |
| $PaO_2$ (mmHg) | 88 | | |
| $PaCO_2$ (mmHg) | 40 | | |
| $P_{(A-a)}O_2$ (mmHg) | 19 | | |
| $P_{(a-ET)}CO_2$ (mmHg) | 5 | | |
| $V_D/V_T$ (%) | 30% | | |
| **Muscle metabolism** | **Rest** | **Exercise (4 min)** | **Recovery (2 min)** |
| Lactate ($mg \cdot dl^{-1}$) | | | 42 |
| Ammonia ($\mu g \cdot dl^{-1}$) | | | |
| Creatine kinase ($U \cdot l^{-1}$) | | | |
| | **Predicted** | **Observed** | |
| $RQ_{mus}$ ($\delta\dot{V}CO_2/\delta\dot{V}O_2$) | 0.95 | 1.00 | |
| **Symptom perception** | **Rest** | **Exercise (max.)** | |
| Effort (observer impression) | | Excellent | |
| Symptoms (subjective) | | Dyspnea | |
| Perceived exertion (Borg scale/20) | | 13 | |
| Breathlessness (VAS scale/100) | | 71 | |

### Gas exchange

Ventilatory equivalents and end-tidal gas tensions showed normal response patterns. $V_D/V_T$ was 30% at rest, which was normal. $P_{(A-a)}O_2$ was 19 mmHg at rest, which was also normal. Oxygenation was normal throughout the study, as judged by pulse oximetry.

### Muscle metabolism

$RQ_{mus}$ was normal, as judged by the lower slope of the relationship between $\dot{V}CO_2$ and $\dot{V}O_2$. He exhibited a normal increase in blood lactate.

### Symptom perception

His RPE was 13/20, which was inappropriately low compared with the cardiovascular response. His $\beta$–score was 71/100, which was appropriate compared with the proportion of his ventilatory capacity utilized.

## Interpretation

Moderately reduced aerobic capacity and reduced metabolic threshold. He exhibited cardiovascular limitation at an abnormally low oxygen uptake. This could represent severe physical deconditioning or early cardiovascular disease. His mildly hypertensive response suggests a poorly compliant peripheral vascular system. However, he showed no evidence of dysrhythmia and no evidence of

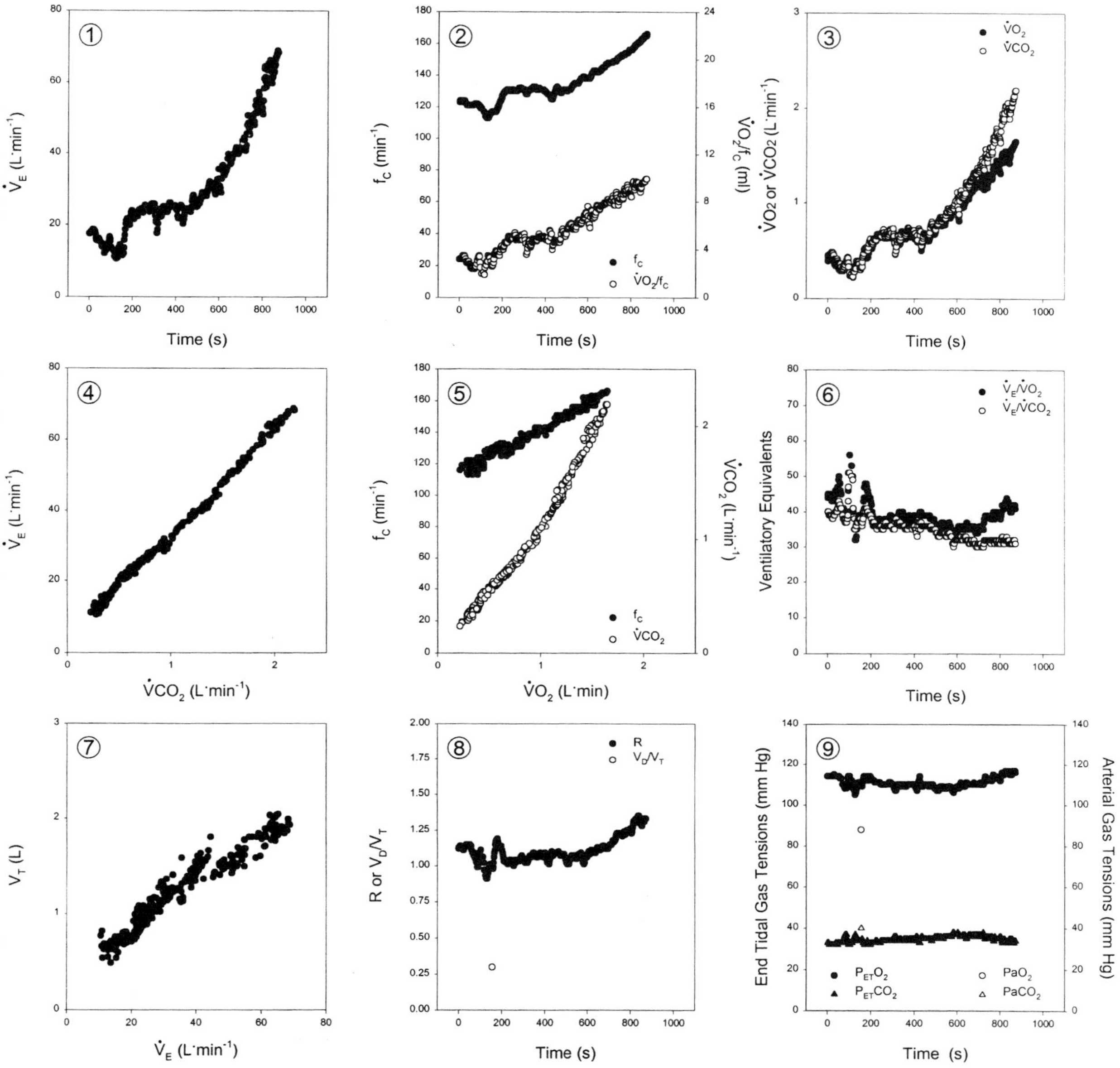


**Figure 6.5** Case 5. Nine-panel display. The data were obtained for a period of equilibration at rest then 3 min of unloaded pedaling followed by a ramp increase in work rate of 15 W · min$^{-1}$ to symptom-limited maximum.

myocardial ischemia during this study. He did display resting tachycardia and mild hyperventilation consistent with anxiety with the beginning of testing. The ventilatory response was otherwise normal. Gas exchange mechanisms and muscle metabolism appeared normal. Symptom perception was essentially normal, except for stoicism with respect to perceived exertion.

### Addendum

An echocardiogram was recommended to rule out cardiomyopathy or valvular heart disease. An exercise prescription was also given to the patient with the expectation of reversing any component of physical deconditioning.

## Case 6: Muscle fatigue and breathlessness (CXT: diagnostic)

### Purpose

This 65-year-old man was referred with severe muscle fatigue and unexplained breathlessness on exertion. He was overweight and had a restrictive abnormality on pulmonary function testing. He was taking no regular medications. He gave a 28 pack-year smoking history but quit 23 years prior to testing. He attempted walking about 30 min twice weekly.

### Method

A diagnostic exercise test was chosen utilizing a ramp work rate protocol on a cycle ergometer. Based on initial physical assessment and reported exercise habits, a ramp rate of $15\,W \cdot min^{-1}$ was chosen. Ventilation was measured using a bi-directional flow transducer. The metabolic measuring system was set in breath-by-breath mode. Peripheral measurements included ECG, systemic arterial pressure, and pulse oximetry. A cannula was inserted in the right radial artery and sequential samples of arterial blood were obtained for the measurement of lactate, ammonia, and creatine kinase.

After a period of equilibration at rest, he performed unloaded pedaling for 3 min followed by the ramp increase in work rate. He gave an excellent effort, achieving a maximum work rate of 112 W. He stopped exercise complaining of leg fatigue and breathlessness. There were no technical problems and no medical complications during the study.

### Results

#### Tabular data

See Table 6.6.

#### Graphical data

See Figure 6.6.

#### Aerobic capacity

$\dot{V}O_{2max}$ was $1.10\,l \cdot min^{-1}$ (52% of reference). This was moderately reduced. $\dot{V}O_2\theta$ was detected with fair confidence at an oxygen uptake of $0.50\,l \cdot min^{-1}$ (24% of reference $\dot{V}O_{2max}$). This was severely reduced. Work efficiency was abnormal, as judged by the relationship between $\dot{V}O_2$ and $\dot{W}$, which had a slope of $5.9\,ml \cdot min^{-1} \cdot W^{-1}$ compared with the normal value of $10.3\,ml \cdot min^{-1} \cdot W^{-1}$. $\dot{V}O_2$ for unloaded pedaling was lower than expected.

#### Cardiovascular response

$f_{Cmax}$ was $121\,min^{-1}$ (78% of reference). He did not exhibit cardiovascular limitation. $\dot{V}O_2/f_{Cmax}$ was 9.1 ml (67% of reference); however, $\delta f_C/\delta\dot{V}O_2$ was normal, consistent with a normal cardiovascular response pattern for the duration of the study. The ECG showed no dysrhythmia and no evidence of myocardial ischemia. Systemic arterial pressures were normal.

**Table 6.6.** Case 6: tabular data

| **Identification** | **ID no.** | **Age (years)** | **Gender (M/F)** |
|---|---|---|---|
| Illustrative case | 6 | 65 | M |
| **Anthropometric** | | **Technical** | |
| Height (in.) | 72 | Barometer (mmHg) | 762 |
| Height (m) | 1.83 | Ambient temperature (°C) | 23 |
| Weight (lb) | 251 | $F_IO_2$ (%) | 21% |
| Weight (kg) | 114 | Valve dead space (ml) | 80 |
| | | $\ddot{W}$ ($W \cdot min^{-1}$) | 15 |
| Body mass index ($kg \cdot m^{-2}$) | 34 | $\dot{W}_{max}$ (W) | 112 |
| **Pulmonary function** | **Predicted** | **Observed** | **%Predicted** |
| FVC (l) | 4.67 | 2.76 | 59% |
| $FEV_1$ (l) | 3.28 | 2.03 | 62% |
| $FEV_1$/FVC (%) | 70% | 74% | |
| MVV ($l \cdot min^{-1}$) | 86 | 74 | 86% |
| **Aerobic capacity** | **Predicted** | **Observed** | **%pred$\dot{V}O_{2max}$** |
| $\dot{V}O_{2max}$ ($l \cdot min^{-1}$) | 2.12 | 1.10 | 52% |
| $\dot{V}O_2\theta$ ($l \cdot min^{-1}$) | 0.85 | 0.50 | 24% |
| $\delta\dot{V}O_2/\delta W$ ($ml \cdot min^{-1} \cdot W^{-1}$) | 10.3 | 5.9 | |
| $\dot{V}O_{2unloaded}$ ($l \cdot min^{-1}$) | | 0.44 | |
| **Cardiovascular response** | **Predicted** | **Observed** | **%Predicted** |
| $f_{Cmax}$ ($min^{-1}$) | 155 | 121 | 78% |
| Cardiac reserve ($min^{-1}$) | 0 | 34 | |
| $\dot{V}O_2/f_{Cmax}$ (ml) | 13.7 | 9.1 | 67% |
| $f_{Crest}$ ($min^{-1}$) | | 80 | |
| Resting ECG | SR 80/min, axis +60, P-QRS-T configuration normal | | |
| Exercise ECG | No dysrhythmia and no evidence of myocardial ischemia | | |
| | **Rest** | **Exercise (max.)** | **Recovery (2 min)** |
| Systolic BP (mmHg) | 130 | 190 | |
| Diastolic BP (mmHg) | 80 | 90 | |
| **Ventilatory response** | **Predicted** | **Observed** | **%MVV** |
| $\dot{V}_{Emax}$ ($l \cdot min^{-1}$) | 74 | 61 | 82% |
| Ventilatory reserve ($l \cdot min^{-1}$) | $>15$ | 13 | |
| $V_{Tmax}$ (l) | 1.38 | 1.50 | |
| $f_{Rmax}$ ($min^{-1}$) | $<50$ | 47 | |
| $T_I/T_E$ at end exercise | 0.8 | 0.9 | |

**Table 6.6.** *(cont.)*

| Gas exchange | Rest | Threshold | Maximum |
|---|---|---|---|
| $\dot{V}_E/\dot{V}O_2$ | 55 | 36 | 57 |
| $\dot{V}_E/\dot{V}CO_2$ | 48 | 32 | 33 |
| $P_{ET}O_2$ (mmHg) | 106 | 110 | 122 |
| $P_{ET}CO_2$ (mmHg) | 36 | 37 | 33 |
| $R$ | 0.98 | 1.11 | 1.68 |
| $SpO_2$ (%) | 96 | 96 | 99 |
| $PaO_2$ (mmHg) | 64 | | 75 |
| $PaCO_2$ (mmHg) | 40 | | 38 |
| $P_{(A-a)}O_2$ (mmHg) | 45 | | 53 |
| $P_{(a-ET)}CO_2$ (mmHg) | 4 | | 5 |
| $V_D/V_T$ (%) | 37% | | 26% |
| **Muscle metabolism** | **Rest** | **Exercise (4 min)** | **Recovery (2 min)** |
| Lactate (mg · dl$^{-1}$) | 3 | 21 | 62 |
| Ammonia (µg · dl$^{-1}$) | 70 | 79 | 161 |
| Creatine kinase (U · l$^{-1}$) | 153 | 154 | 161 |
| | **Predicted** | **Observed** | |
| $RQ_{mus}$ ($\delta\dot{V}CO_2/\delta\dot{V}O_2$) | 0.95 | 1.00 | |
| **Symptom perception** | **Rest** | **Exercise (max.)** | |
| Effort (observer impression) | | Good | |
| Symptoms (subjective) | | Dyspnea, fatigue | |
| Perceived exertion (Borg scale/20) | | 20 | |
| Breathlessness (VAS scale/100) | | 90 | |

## Ventilatory response

$\dot{V}_{Emax}$ was 61 l · min$^{-1}$ (82% of measured MVV). He approached ventilatory limitation. $\delta\dot{V}_E/\delta\dot{V}O_2$ was increased, suggesting an exaggerated ventilatory response. He displayed a relatively high $f_{Rmax}$ compared with his aerobic capacity but $V_{Tmax}$ was within the expected range.

## Gas exchange

Ventilatory equivalents and end-tidal gas tensions suggested mildly abnormal gas exchange. $V_D/V_T$ was 37% at rest, which was normal and 26% at maximum exercise, which was also normal in relation to his $\dot{V}O_{2max}$ and his age. $P_{(A-a)}O_2$ was 40 mmHg at rest, which was abnormally high, and 53 mmHg at end exercise, which was also abnormally high. These findings suggest low $\dot{V}/\dot{Q}$ mismatch or increased physiological shunt. Despite these features, oxygenation was normal throughout the study, as judged by pulse oximetry.

## Muscle metabolism

$RQ_{mus}$ was normal, as judged by the lower slope of the $\dot{V}CO_2$–$\dot{V}O_2$ relationship. He displayed premature and exaggerated increases in lactate and ammonia levels during exercise of relatively low work rate. Creatine kinase levels were normal.

## Symptom perception

His RPE was 20/20, which was inappropriately high compared with the cardiovascular response. His

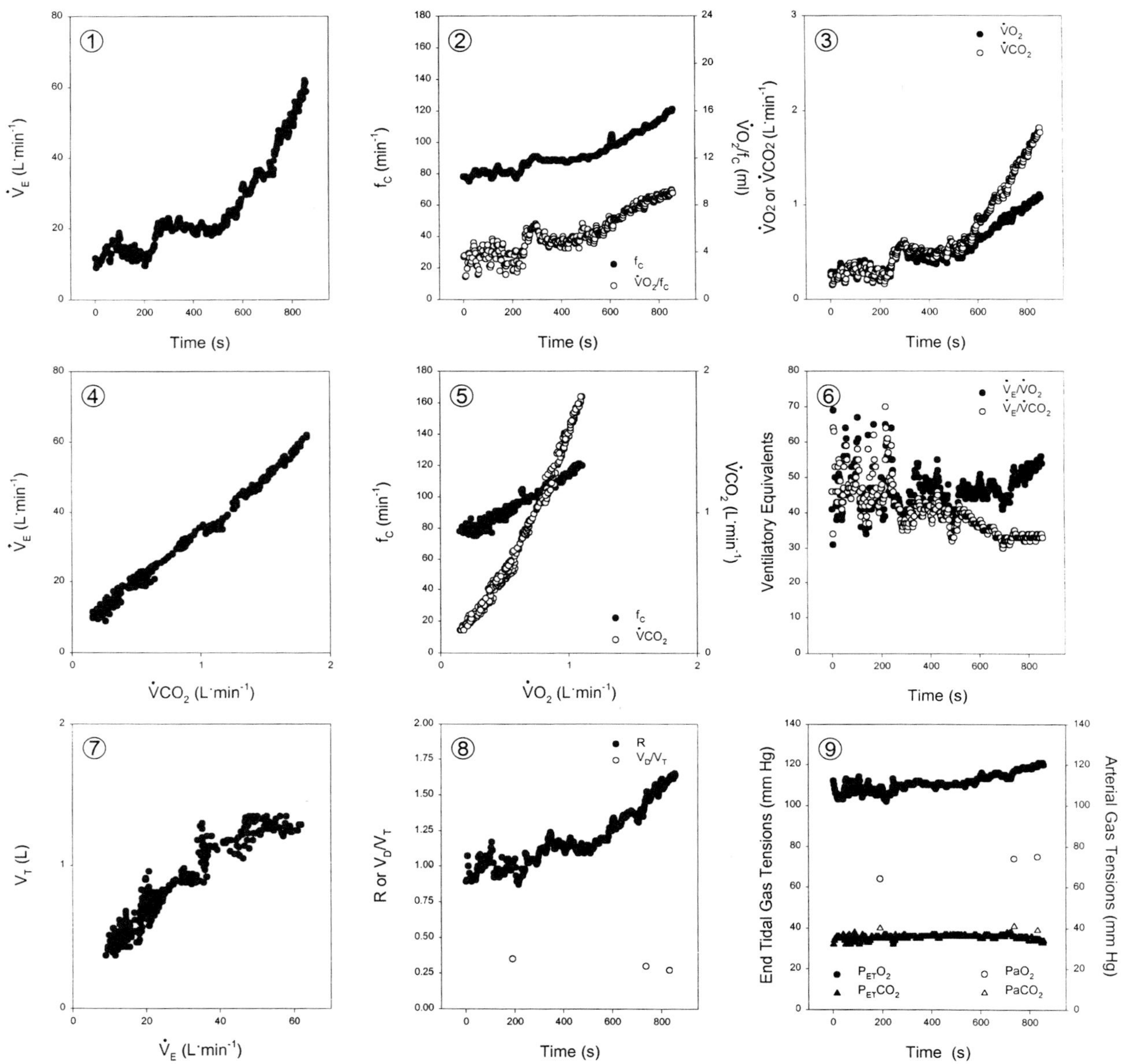


**Figure 6.6** Case 6. Nine-panel display. The data were obtained for a period of equilibration at rest then 3 min of unloaded pedaling followed by a ramp increase in work rate of 30 W · min$^{-1}$ to symptom-limited maximum.

$\beta$-score was 90/100, which was appropriate compared with the proportion of his ventilatory capacity utilized.

## Interpretation

Moderately reduced aerobic capacity with severely reduced metabolic threshold. There was evidence of premature increases in lactate and ammonia at low exercise work rate. In the absence of significant abnormalities in the cardiovascular response, these findings suggest a derangement of peripheral muscle metabolism such as one might see with mitochondrial or other myopathies. The increase in lactate is also reflected in the exaggerated ventilatory response and relative tachypnea at end exercise. The increased physiological shunt could be explained by basal atelectasis related to his obesity. His symptom perception reflects the physiological abnormalities described above.

## Addendum

He went on to have a quadriceps muscle biopsy which showed chronic inflammatory myopathy with some denervation changes.

# Appendix A Glossary (terms, symbols, definitions)

**Table A1.** Exercise test (XT) classification

| Term | Symbol or abbreviation | Definition |
|---|---|---|
| Performance exercise test | PXT | The PXT is typically performed on the apparently healthy population, often as part of preventive strategies, for health promotion, and to provide guidance for fitness improvement or as a basis for training athletes. Fitness assessment, progress monitoring, and exercise-training prescription are some of the uses of the PXT |
| Clinical exercise test | CXT | The CXT is usually reserved for individuals presenting with signs or symptoms of illness or disease. Exercise texts conducted in this discipline are generally for diagnostic purposes, for progress monitoring, or for rehabilitative exercise prescription |
| Field exercise test | FXT | The FXT is used when availability of more sophisticated instrumentation or practicality precludes the use of laboratory tests. Field tests are appropriate when testing individuals or groups of people and can provide quantitative and objective measures of exercise performance within the performance or clinical disciplines |
| Laboratory exercise test | LXT | The LXT is conducted in a controlled environment with sophisticated instruments enabling greater precision and accuracy in the measurement of a large number of physiological response variables. For these reasons, the LXT is preferred whenever feasible |

**Table A2.** Physiological response variables

| Symbol | Term | Units | Definition |
|---|---|---|---|
| $\alpha$ | Solubility coefficient | $ml \cdot mmHg^{-1}$<br>$ml \cdot kPa^{-1}$ | The amount of a specific gas that will dissolve in a specific liquid at a given partial pressure |
| $\beta$– | Breathlessness | | A measure of dyspnea usually administered with a visual analog scale (VAS) during and/or at the end of an incremental exercise test |
| $C_{(a-\bar{v})}O_2$ | Arterial–venous difference in oxygen content | $ml \cdot ml^{-1}$<br>$ml \cdot dl^{-1}$<br>$l \cdot l^{-1}$ | The difference in the oxygen content of the arterial and mixed venous blood, the latter typically sampled from the pulmonary artery |
| $\delta f_C / \delta \dot{V}O_2$ | Slope of the cardiovascular response | $l^{-1}$ | The linear increase of heart rate with increasing oxygen uptake. The slope is defined by the Fick equation and thus is related to the cardiac stroke volume and arterial–venous difference in oxygen content |
| $\delta \dot{V}_E / \delta \dot{V}O_2$ | Slope of the ventilatory response | | The nonlinear increase of minute ventilation with increasing oxygen uptake. The slope is determined by the Bohr equation and thus is related to the respiratory exchange ratio, the level at which the arterial partial pressure of $CO_2$ is controlled, and the ratio of dead space to tidal volume |
| $\delta \dot{V}O_2 / \delta \dot{W}$ ($\eta^{-1}$) | Slope of the metabolic response | $ml \cdot min^{-1} \cdot W^{-1}$ | The robustly linear increase in $\dot{V}O_2$ with increases in work rate observed in the normal response to incremental exercise. The slope has a normal value of about $10.3\,ml \cdot min^{-1} \cdot W^{-1}$ |
| $d_R$ | Running distance | m<br>yd<br>mile | Distance completed in running tests |
| $d_W$ | Walking distance | m<br>yd<br>mile | Distance completed in walking tests |
| $d_{W6}$ | Six-minute walking distance | m<br>yd | The distance covered in 6 min by an individual walking at his or her own chosen pace. The distance is recorded without regard to the number and duration of stops to rest |
| ECG | Electrocardiogram | mV and mm | The summation of uncancelled electrical vectors occurring during the cardiac cycle as measured at the body surface by certain configurations of skin electrodes |
| EELV | End-expiratory lung volume | ml<br>l | The volume of gas remaining in the lung at the end of expiration. At rest this volume equates to the functional residual capacity |
| EILV | End-inspiratory lung volume | ml<br>l | The volume of gas in the lung at the end of inspiration |
| $f_C$ | Heart rate | $min^{-1}$ | The frequency of cardiac cycles (beats) expressed per minute |
| $f_{Cmax}$ | Maximum heart rate | $min^{-1}$ | The highest heart rate achieved with an exhausting effort in an incremental exercise test |

**Table A2.** (*cont.*)

| Symbol | Term | Units | Definition |
|---|---|---|---|
| $f_{Cres}$ | Heart rate reserve | $min^{-1}$ | The difference between resting and maximum heart rate |
| $FEV_1$ | Forced expiratory volume in 1 s | l | The volume of air expelled from the lungs during the first second of a forced expiration from total lung capacity |
| $FEF_{25-75}$ | Forced expiratory flow | $l \cdot s^{-1}$ | The mean expiratory flow measured between 75% and 25% of the vital capacity during a forced expiration |
| $F_ACO_2$ | Fractional concentration of alveolar carbon dioxide | % | The fractional concentration of carbon dioxide in alveolar gas |
| $F_{\bar{E}}CO_2$ | Fractional concentration of mixed expired carbon dioxide | % | The fractional concentration of carbon dioxide in mixed expired gas |
| $F_{\bar{E}}N_2$ | Fractional concentration of mixed expired nitrogen | % | The fractional concentration of nitrogen in mixed expired gas |
| $F_{\bar{E}}O_2$ | Fractional concentration of mixed expired oxygen | % | The fractional concentration of oxygen in mixed expired gas |
| $F_ICO_2$ | Fractional concentration of inspired carbon dioxide | % | The fractional concentration of carbon dioxide in the inspired gas |
| $F_IN_2$ | Fractional concentration of inspired nitrogen | % | The fractional concentration of nitrogen in the inspired gas |
| $F_IO_2$ | Fractional concentration of inspired oxygen | % | The fractional concentration of oxygen in the inspired gas |
| $f_R$ | Respiratory rate | $min^{-1}$ | The frequency of ventilatory cycles (breaths) expressed per minute |
| $HCO_3^-$ | Bicarbonate | | The bicarbonate anion |
| La | Lactate | | The lactate anion |
| MVV | Maximum voluntary ventilation | $l \cdot min^{-1}$ | A highly effort-dependent maneuver requiring subjects to exert a maximal ventilatory effort by forcibly increasing tidal volume and respiratory rate for 12 or 15 s. The MVV is one method for estimating ventilatory capacity |
| $\eta$ | Work efficiency | $W \cdot ml^{-1} \cdot min$ | A measure of the external work obtained for a given metabolic cost |
| $\eta^{-1}$ | Work efficiency | $ml \cdot min^{-1} \cdot W^{-1}$ | A measure of the metabolic cost of performing external work |
| $NH_3$ | Ammonia | | The ammonia molecule |
| ~P | High-energy phosphate bond | | High-energy phosphate bonds such as are found in ATP and ADP |
| Pa | Systemic arterial pressure | mmHg (Torr) kPa | Systemic systolic blood pressure ($Pa_{sys}$) coincides with left ventricular contraction. Systemic diastolic blood pressure ($Pa_{dia}$) coincides with left ventricular relaxation immediately before systole |
| $P_{(A-a)}O_2$ | Alveolar–arterial oxygen partial pressure difference | mmHg (Torr) kPa | The difference in partial pressure (or tension) of oxygen between the arterial blood and the alveolar compartment of the lung, representing the completeness or effectiveness of oxygen exchange in the lung |

**Table A2.** (*cont.*)

| Symbol | Term | Units | Definition |
|---|---|---|---|
| $Pa\text{CO}_2$ | Arterial carbon dioxide partial pressure | mmHg (Torr) kPa | The partial pressure (or tension) of carbon dioxide in the systemic arterial blood |
| $P_A\text{CO}_2$ | Alveolar carbon dioxide partial pressure | mmHg (Torr) kPa | The partial pressure (or tension) of carbon dioxide in the alveolar gas |
| $P_{(a-ET)}\text{CO}_2$ | Arterial–end-tidal carbon dioxide partial pressure difference | mmHg (Torr) kPa | The difference in carbon dioxide partial pressure (or tension) between the arterial blood and the end-tidal gas, representing the extent to which ideal alveolar gas has been diluted with gas from the physiological dead space |
| $Pa\text{O}_2$ | Arterial oxygen partial pressure | mmHg (Torr) kPa | The partial pressure (or tension) of oxygen in the systemic arterial blood |
| $P_A\text{O}_2$ | Alveolar oxygen partial pressure | mmHg (Torr) kPa | The partial pressure (or tension) of oxygen in the alveolar gas |
| $P_B$ | Barometric pressure | mmHg (Torr) kPa | Pressure of the ambient air at a particular time and place |
| $P_{ET}\text{CO}_2$ | End-tidal carbon dioxide partial pressure | mmHg (Torr) kPa | The partial pressure (or tension) of carbon dioxide in gas exhaled at the end of a breath |
| $P_{ET}\text{O}_2$ | End-tidal oxygen partial pressure | mmHg (Torr) kPa | The partial pressure (or tension) of oxygen in gas exhaled at the end of a breath |
| $Ppa$ | Pulmonary arterial pressure | mmHg (Torr) kPa | The pressure in the pulmonary outflow tract and the main pulmonary arteries |
| $P_{\bar{v}}\text{O}_2$ | Mixed venous oxygen partial pressure | mmHg (Torr) kPa | The partial pressure of oxygen in mixed venous blood entering the right atrium and then flowing through the pulmonary arteries |
| $\dot{Q}_C$ | Cardiac output | $\text{ml} \cdot \text{min}^{-1}$ $\text{l} \cdot \text{min}^{-1}$ | The volume of blood ejected by either the left or right ventricle each minute. Cardiac output is the product of heart rate and cardiac stroke volume |
| $\dot{Q}\text{O}_{2\text{mus}}$ | Muscle oxygen consumption | $\text{l} \cdot \text{min}^{-1}$ $\text{ml} \cdot \text{min}^{-1}$ | Quantity of oxygen consumed by muscle per minute |
| $R$ | Respiratory exchange ratio | | The ratio of carbon dioxide output to oxygen uptake measured at the mouth in the non-steady state, representing whole-body carbon dioxide output and oxygen uptake |
| RPE | Rating of perceived exertion | | A subjective evaluation of an applied stimulus, e.g., exercise intensity |
| RQ | Respiratory quotient | | The ratio of carbon dioxide output to oxygen uptake measured at the mouth in the steady state or measured across an isolated organ or tissue |
| $\text{RQ}_{\text{mus}}$ | Muscle respiratory quotient | | The ratio of the increase in muscle $CO_2$ production to the concomitant increase in muscle oxygen consumption |
| $Sa\text{O}_2$ | Oxyhemoglobin saturation | % | Arterial oxyhemoglobin saturation measured by co-oximeter or calculated from $Pa\text{O}_2$ using a standard dissociation curve |
| $Sp\text{O}_2$ | Oxyhemoglobin saturation | % | Oxyhemoglobin saturation measured by pulse oximeter |

**Table A2.** *(cont.)*

| Symbol | Term | Units | Definition |
|---|---|---|---|
| SV | Cardiac stroke volume | ml | The volume of blood ejected by either the left or right ventricle with each systolic contraction |
| $t$ | Endurance time | min<br>s | The total time of exercise, excluding the warm-up period, for constant and incremental work rate protocols or for variable work rates such as walking and running tests |
| $T_E$ | Expiratory time | s | The time taken for expiration |
| $T_I$ | Inspiratory time | s | The time taken for inspiration |
| $T_I/T_E$ | Ratio of inspiratory to expiratory time | | Also called the *I/E* ratio, this variable indicates what proportion of the time taken for each breath is devoted to inspiration versus expiration. Hence, $T_I/T_E$ is a measure of breathing pattern |
| $t_{pc}$ | Pulmonary capillary transit time | s | Average time taken for blood to traverse the pulmonary capillary bed |
| $T_{TOT}$ | Total breath time | s | The time taken for a whole breath cycle, including inspiration and expiration |
| $\tau\dot{V}O_2$ | Time constant for oxygen uptake | s | Time constant for the kinetic response of oxygen uptake with a step change in external work rate |
| VAS | Visual analog scale | | A 100-mm line used to score breathlessness |
| $\dot{V}CO_2$ | Carbon dioxide output | $l \cdot min^{-1}$<br>$ml \cdot min^{-1}$ | The volume of carbon dioxide output per minute measured from the exhaled air |
| $\dot{V}CO_{2alv}$ | Alveolar carbon dioxide output | $l \cdot min^{-1}$<br>$ml \cdot min^{-1}$ | Volume of carbon dioxide released per minute into the alveolar compartment of the lung |
| $V_D$ | Dead space volume | ml<br>l | The volume of the physiological dead space ($V_{Dphysiol}$) comprises the anatomical dead space ($V_{Danat}$) plus the alveolar dead space ($V_{Dalv}$). $V_{Danat}$ represents the upper airway, trachea, and conducting bronchi and $V_{Dalv}$ represents nonperfused or underperfused areas of lung |
| *Vds* | Valve dead space | ml<br>l | Correction factor applied in the calculation of $V_D/V_T$ representing the additional dead-space volume due to the valve assembly and mouthpiece |
| $V_D/V_T$ | Dead space–tidal volume ratio | | The ratio between the dead-space volume and tidal volume where dead space is correctly represented by the physiological dead space ($V_{Dphysiol}$). This ratio indicates the efficiency of ventilation |
| $\dot{V}_E$ | Minute ventilation | $l \cdot min^{-1}$ | The total volume of air expired per minute from the lungs |
| $\dot{V}_{Ecap}$ | Ventilatory capacity | $l \cdot min^{-1}$ | The theoretical upper limit for minute ventilation. It may be estimated by the MVV maneuver or alternatively, with $FEV_1$ or the maximal inspiratory and expiratory flow–volume relationship |
| $\dot{V}_{Emax}$ | Maximum minute ventilation | $l \cdot min^{-1}$ | The highest value of minute ventilation attained and measured during incremental exercise |

**Table A2.** (*cont.*)

| Symbol | Term | Units | Definition |
|---|---|---|---|
| $\dot{V}_E\theta$ | Ventilatory threshold | $l \cdot min^{-1}$<br>$ml \cdot min^{-1}$<br>$ml \cdot kg^{-1} \cdot min^{-1}$ | Level of exercise above which there is acidemia and carotid body stimulation of ventilation with predictable consequences on gas exchange |
| $\dot{V}_E : V$ | Expiratory flow:volume relationship | $l \cdot s^{-1}$ | The maximal expiratory flow profile over the range of lung volumes from residual volume to total lung capacity. Also known as the flow–volume loop |
| $\dot{V}_E/\dot{V}CO_2$ | Ventilatory equivalent for carbon dioxide | | A measure of breathing efficiency derived by dividing the instantaneous minute ventilation by the carbon dioxide output |
| $\dot{V}_E/\dot{V}O_2$ | Ventilatory equivalent for oxygen | | A measure of breathing efficiency derived by dividing the instantaneous minute ventilation by the oxygen uptake |
| $\dot{V}_I : V$ | Inspiratory flow:volume relationship | $l \cdot s^{-1}$ | The maximal inspiratory flow profile over the range of lung volumes from total lung capacity to residual volume. Also known as the flow–volume loop |
| $\dot{V}O_2$ | Oxygen uptake | $l \cdot min^{-1}$<br>$ml \cdot min^{-1}$<br>$ml \cdot kg^{-1} \cdot min^{-1}$ | Volume of oxygen taken up per minute measured from the exhaled air |
| $\dot{V}O_{2alv}$ | Alveolar oxygen uptake | $l \cdot min^{-1}$<br>$ml \cdot min^{-1}$<br>$ml \cdot kg^{-1} \cdot min^{-1}$ | Volume of oxygen taken up per minute from the alveolar compartment of the lung |
| $\dot{V}O_{2deb}$ | Oxygen debt | ml<br>l | Excess volume of oxygen taken up after switching to a lower work rate |
| $\dot{V}O_{2def}$ | Oxygen deficit | ml<br>l | Shortfall of oxygen taken up after switching to a higher work rate |
| $\dot{V}O_2/f_C$ | Oxygen pulse | ml | A measure of cardiovascular efficiency indicating the metabolic value that derives from every heart beat. The oxygen pulse is derived by dividing the instantaneous oxygen uptake by heart rate |
| $\dot{V}O_2/f_R$ | Oxygen breath | ml | A measure of breathing efficiency indicating the metabolic value that derives from each breath. The oxygen breath is derived by dividing the instantaneous oxygen uptake by respiratory rate |
| $\dot{V}O_{2max}$ | Aerobic capacity | $l \cdot min^{-1}$<br>$ml \cdot min^{-1}$<br>$ml \cdot kg^{-1} \cdot min^{-1}$ | The highest oxygen uptake measured during an incremental exercise test for a specific mode of exercise. Aerobic capacity is another term for maximum oxygen uptake |
| $\dot{V}O_{2max}$ | Maximal oxygen uptake | $l \cdot min^{-1}$<br>$ml \cdot min^{-1}$<br>$ml \cdot kg^{-1} \cdot min^{-1}$ | The highest oxygen uptake achievable for a given individual based on age, gender, body size, and exercise mode |
| $\dot{V}O_{2max}$ | Maximum oxygen uptake | $l \cdot min^{-1}$<br>$ml \cdot min^{-1}$<br>$ml \cdot kg^{-1} \cdot min^{-1}$ | The highest oxygen uptake measured during an incremental exercise test for a specific mode of exercise. Maximum oxygen uptake is distinctly different from maximal oxygen uptake |

**Table A2.** *(cont.)*

| Symbol | Term | Units | Definition |
|---|---|---|---|
| $\dot{V}O_{2peak}$ | Peak oxygen uptake | $l \cdot min^{-1}$<br>$ml \cdot min^{-1}$<br>$ml \cdot kg^{-1} \cdot min^{-1}$ | A term sometimes used synonymously with $\dot{V}O_{2max}$, indicating the highest oxygen uptake achieved in a task-specific exercise test. The term is superfluous, in accordance with the definition of $\dot{V}O_{2max}$ noted above |
| $\dot{V}O_{2res}$ | Oxygen uptake reserve | $l \cdot min^{-1}$<br>$ml \cdot min^{-1}$<br>$ml \cdot kg^{-1} \cdot min^{-1}$ | The difference between resting and maximum oxygen uptake |
| $\dot{V}/\dot{Q}$ | Ventilation–perfusion ratio | | The ratio of ventilation to perfusion usually described for a particular region of the lung. When considering the respiratory system as a whole this ratio is the minute ventilation ($\dot{V}_E$) divided by cardiac output ($\dot{Q}_C$) |
| $\dot{V}O_2\theta$ | Metabolic threshold | $l \cdot min^{-1}$<br>$ml \cdot min^{-1}$<br>$ml \cdot kg^{-1} \cdot min^{-1}$ | Level of exercise above which a sustained increase in blood lactate occurs with predictable consequences on gas exchange |
| $V_T$ | Tidal volume | ml<br>l | The volume of a single breath. By convention, $V_T$ is expressed as the expired volume. The expired volume is typically larger than the inspired volume due to the effects of temperature, humidity, and the altered composition of expired gas that result from exchange of oxygen and carbon dioxide in the lungs |
| $\dot{W}$ | Work rate | W<br>$J \cdot s^{-1}$<br>$kg \cdot m \cdot min^{-1}$ | Power: the rate of performing work |
| $\ddot{W}$ | Work rate increment | $W \cdot min^{-1}$ | The rate at which a work rate is increased, e.g., $25\,W \cdot min^{-1}$ is a work rate increment |
| $\dot{W}_{ext}$ | External work rate | W<br>$J \cdot s^{-1}$<br>$kg \cdot m \cdot min^{-1}$ | Rate of performing external physical work such as can be measured using an ergometer |
| $\dot{W}_{mus}$ | Muscle work rate | W<br>$J \cdot s^{-1}$<br>$kg \cdot m \cdot min^{-1}$ | Rate of performing muscular work |

# Appendix B Calculations and conversions

## Oxygen cost of exercise

### Leg cycling

Two equations are often used to determine the $O_2$ cost of exercise. Whilst they differ conceptually, the prediction of $O_2$ cost is similar. In Equation B1, the coefficient 10.3 represents the empirically derived $\dot{V}O_2$ to work rate slope ($ml \cdot min^{-1} \cdot W^{-1}$). The 5.8 coefficient with body weight (BW) accounts for the oxygen cost of cycling at 0 W ($ml \cdot min^{-1}$). This oxygen cost of lifting the legs, along with the constant 151 ($ml \cdot min^{-1}$), includes the resting $\dot{V}O_2$.

$$\dot{V}O_2 = (10.3 \cdot \dot{W}) + (5.8 \cdot BW) + 151 \quad (B1)$$

where $\dot{V}O_2$ is in $ml \cdot min^{-1}$, $\dot{W}$ is work rate in watts, and BW is body weight in kg.

Alternatively, Equation B2 uses the empirically derived oxygen cost of performing 1 kg · m of work (1.8 $ml \cdot min^{-1}$) plus 0.2 $ml \cdot min^{-1}$ for the added cost of moving the legs to obtain the coefficient 2 used with the work rate value in $kg \cdot m \cdot min^{-1}$. An estimate of the resting $\dot{V}O_2$ is the *y*-intercept value calculated by multiplying the $\dot{V}O_2$ estimate of the resting metabolic rate (3.5 $ml \cdot kg^{-1} \cdot min^{-1}$) multiplied by the body weight.

$$\dot{V}O_2 = (2 \cdot \dot{W}) + (3.5 \cdot BW) \quad (B2)$$

where $\dot{V}O_2$ is in $ml \cdot min^{-1}$, $\dot{W}$ is work rate in $kg \cdot m \cdot min^{-1}$, and BW is body weight in kg.

**Example:** What is the expected $O_2$ cost of cycling at 100 W (612 $kg \cdot m \cdot min^{-1}$) for a 70-kg subject?

Using Equation B1: $\dot{V}O_2 = (10.3 \cdot 100) + (5.8 \cdot 70) + 151$

$\dot{V}O_2 = 1587\ ml \cdot min^{-1}$

Using Equation B2: $\dot{V}O_2 = (2 \cdot 612) + (3.5 \cdot 70)$

$\dot{V}O_2 = 1469\ ml \cdot min^{-1}$

***Note:** Some practitioners may be inclined to use one of the above equations to estimate $\dot{V}O_{2max}$. This is an inappropriate use of these equations, since they were designed to estimate the $\dot{V}O_2$ of steady-state exercise. Consequently, $\dot{V}O_{2max}$ would be overestimated by these equations.*

### Treadmill walking

The oxygen cost for treadmill walking (speeds ranging between 50 and 100 $m \cdot min^{-1}$ (1.9–3.7 m.p.h.) can be conveniently broken down into three additive components – the horizontal (H) component, the vertical (V) component, and the resting (R) component – as follows.

$$\dot{V}O_2 = \dot{V}O_2H + \dot{V}O_2V + \dot{V}O_2R \quad (B3)$$

where all $\dot{V}O_2$ units are $ml \cdot kg^{-1} \cdot min^{-1}$.

$$\dot{V}O_2H = speed \cdot 0.1 \quad (B4)$$

where speed is expressed in $m \cdot min^{-1}$.

***Note:** To convert m.p.h. to $m \cdot min^{-1}$, multiply m.p.h. by 26.8.*

$$\dot{V}O_2V = speed \cdot 1.8 \cdot grade \quad (B5)$$

where speed is expressed in $m \cdot min^{-1}$ and grade is percentage grade divided by 100.

$$\dot{V}O_2R = 3.5 \quad (B6)$$

**Example:** What is the oxygen cost of walking 3.1 m.p.h. at 6% grade?

Using Equations B3–B6:
$\dot{V}O_2 = \dot{V}O_2H + \dot{V}O_2V + \dot{V}O_2R$

$\dot{V}O_2H = (3.1 \cdot 26.8 \cdot 0.1) = 8.3$
$\dot{V}O_2V = (3.1 \cdot 26.8 \cdot 1.8 \cdot 0.06) = 9.0$
$\dot{V}O_2R = 3.5$

$\dot{V}O_2 = 8.3 + 9.0 + 3.5$
$\dot{V}O_2 = 20.8\ ml \cdot kg^{-1} \cdot min^{-1}$

*Note: As noted above for leg cycling, some practitioners may be inclined to estimate* $\dot{V}O_{2max}$ *from Equation B3. This will overestimate* $\dot{V}O_{2max}$, *since Equation B3 was designed to estimate the* $\dot{V}O_2$ *of steady-state exercise.*

## Treadmill running

The oxygen cost for treadmill running, defined as speeds greater than $134\ m \cdot min^{-1}$ (5 m.p.h.) or when subjects are jogging at speeds between 80 and $134\ m \cdot min^{-1}$, may be broken down into three additive components as with treadmill walking: the horizontal (H) component, the vertical (V) component, and the resting (R) component. However, two differences exist between the walking and the running equations. The first is the coefficient for speed in the horizontal component which increases from 0.1 to $0.2\ ml \cdot kg^{-1} \cdot min^{-1}$ per $m \cdot min^{-1}$. The second is for the vertical component in which the oxygen cost is reduced by half, i.e., multiplied by 0.5.

$$\dot{V}O_2 = \dot{V}O_2H + \dot{V}O_2V + \dot{V}O_2R \qquad (B7)$$

where all $\dot{V}O_2$ units are $ml \cdot kg^{-1} \cdot min^{-1}$.

$$\dot{V}O_2H = speed \cdot 0.2 \qquad (B8)$$

where speed is expressed in $m \cdot min^{-1}$.

***Note:*** *to convert m.p.h. to* $m \cdot min^{-1}$, *multiply m.p.h. by 26.8.*

$$\dot{V}O_2V = speed \cdot 1.8 \cdot grade \cdot 0.5 \qquad (B9)$$

where speed is expressed by $m \cdot min^{-1}$ and grade is percentage grade divided by 100.

$\dot{V}O_2R = 3.5$

**Example:** What is the oxygen cost of running 7.5 m.p.h. at 8% grade?

Using Equations B7–B9
$\dot{V}O_2H = (7.5 \cdot 26.8 \cdot 0.2) = 40.2$
$\dot{V}O_2V = (7.5 \cdot 26.8 \cdot 1.8 \cdot 0.08 \cdot 0.5) = 14.5$
$\dot{V}O_2R = 3.5$

$\dot{V}O_2 = 40.2 + 14.5 + 3.5$
$\dot{V}O_2 = 58.2\ ml \cdot kg^{-1} \cdot min^{-1}$

***Note:*** *The same caution regarding estimation of* $\dot{V}O_{2max}$ *indicted above applies to equations used to estimate the oxygen cost of treadmill running.*

## Arm cycling

The equation for estimating the oxygen cost of arm cycling is similar to that for leg cycling. However, since the oxygen cost for arm cycling is higher than for leg cycling at comparable work rates, the coefficient for work rate is correspondingly higher, as shown in Equation B10 (compared with Equation B2).

$$\dot{V}O_2 = (3 \cdot \dot{W}) + (3.5 \cdot BW) \qquad B10$$

where $\dot{V}O_2$ is in $ml \cdot min^{-1}$, $\dot{W}$ is work rate in $kg \cdot m \cdot min^{-1}$, and BW is body weight in kg.

**Example:** What is the expected $O_2$ cost of arm cranking at 100 W ($612\ kg \cdot m \cdot min^{-1}$) for a 70-kg subject?

Using Equation B10:
$\dot{V}O_2 = (3 \cdot 612) + (3.5 \cdot 70)$
$\dot{V}O_2 = 2081\ ml \cdot min^{-1}$

## Stepping

The oxygen cost of stepping may be calculated in a manner similar to that shown for treadmill walking.

$$\dot{V}O_2 = \dot{V}O_2H + \dot{V}O_2V + \dot{V}O_2R \qquad (B11)$$

where all $\dot{V}O_2$ units are $ml \cdot kg^{-1} \cdot min^{-1}$.

In this case, however, the resting component is zero as it is included in the $\dot{V}O_2H$ and $\dot{V}O_2V$ components.

$$\dot{V}O_2H = (0.35 \cdot \text{stepping frequency}) \quad (B12)$$

where $\dot{V}O_2$ is in $ml \cdot kg^{-1} \cdot min^{-1}$ and stepping frequency is steps $\cdot$ $min^{-1}$. The 0.35 coefficient converts stepping frequency into $ml \cdot kg^{-1} \cdot min^{-1}$.

$$\dot{V}O_2V = \text{step height} \cdot \text{stepping frequency} \cdot 1.33 \cdot 1.8 \quad (B13)$$

where $\dot{V}O_2$ is in $ml \cdot kg^{-1} \cdot min^{-1}$, step height is in m, 1.33 represents the $O_2$ cost of stepping up and down (1.0 for stepping up and 0.33 for stepping down), while 1.8 represents the $O_2$ cost of performing 1 kg $\cdot$ m of work.

**Example 1:** What is the oxygen cost of stepping at 24 steps $min^{-1}$ on a bench 41.3 cm high?

Using Equations B11–B13:
$\dot{V}O_2 = \dot{V}O_2H + \dot{V}O_2V + \dot{V}O_2R$

$\dot{V}O_2H = (0.35 \cdot 24) = 8.4$
$\dot{V}O_2V = (0.413 \cdot 24 \cdot 1.33 \cdot 1.8) = 23.7$
$\dot{V}O_2R = 0$

$\dot{V}O_2 = 8.4 + 23.7 + 0$
$\dot{V}O_2 = 32.1\ ml \cdot kg^{-1} \cdot min^{-1}$

**Example 2:** What is the oxygen cost of climbing a flight of 15 stairs in 40 s for a 75-kg subject? The rise of each stair is 7 in. (17.8 cm).

Using Equations B11–B13:
$\dot{V}O_2 = \dot{V}O_2H + \dot{V}O_2V + \dot{V}O_2R$

$\dot{V}O_2H = (0.35 \cdot 15 \cdot (40/60)) = 7.8$
Modifying Equation B13 for stepping up only:
$\dot{V}O_2V = (0.178 \cdot 22.5 \cdot 1.0 \cdot 1.8) = 7.2$
$\dot{V}O_2R = 0$

$\dot{V}O_2 = 7.8 + 7.2 + 0$
$\dot{V}O_2 = 15.0\ ml \cdot kg^{-1} \cdot min^{-1}$

## Estimation of $\dot{V}O_{2max}$ from predictive tests

This section of Appendix B contains equations for predicting $\dot{V}O_{2max}$ from various field and laboratory tests designed for that purpose.

### Cooper 12-minute run test

$$\dot{V}O_{2max} = (0.02233 \cdot d_R) - 11.3 \quad (B14a)$$

where $\dot{V}O_{2max}$ is in $ml \cdot kg^{-1} \cdot min^{-1}$ and $d_R$ is the distance run in 12 min expressed in m.

**Example:** a subject runs 2400 m in the 12-min time period. What is the predicted $\dot{V}O_{2max}$?

Using Equation B14a:
$\dot{V}O_{2max} = (0.02233 \cdot 2400) - 11.3$
$\dot{V}O_{2max} = 42.3\ ml \cdot kg^{-1} \cdot min^{-1}$

(Cooper, K. (1968). A means of assessing maximal oxygen intake correlation between field and treadmill testing. *J. Am. Med. A.*, **203**, 201–4.)

### Cooper 1.5-minute run test

$$\dot{V}O_{2max} = 483/t + 3.5 \quad (B14b)$$

where $\dot{V}O_{2max}$ is in $ml \cdot kg^{-1} \cdot min^{-1}$ and $t$ is time to run 1.5 miles.

**Example:** a person runs 1.5 miles in 12 min. What is the predicted $\dot{V}O_{2max}$?

Using Equation B14b:
$\dot{V}O_{2max} = 483/12 + 3.5$
$\dot{V}O_{2max} = 43.8\ ml \cdot kg^{-1} \cdot min^{-1}$

### Rockport walking test

$$\dot{V}O_{2max} = 132.853 - (0.1696 \cdot BW) - (0.3877 \cdot age) + (6.315 \cdot gender) - (3.2649 \cdot time) - (0.1565 \cdot f_C) \quad (B15)$$

where $\dot{V}O_2$ is in $ml \cdot kg^{-1} \cdot min^{-1}$; BW is body weight in kg; age is in years; gender has a coefficient of 0 for females and 1 for males; time is in min for the time to complete the 1-mile walk; $f_C$ is heart rate in $min^{-1}$.

**Example:** A 45-year-old, 90-kg female walks 1 mile in 19 min 40 s with an ending heart rate of 156 $min^{-1}$. What is the predicted $\dot{V}O_{2max}$?

Using Equation B15:
$\dot{V}O_{2max} = 132.853 - (0.0769 \cdot 90) - (0.3877 \cdot 45) + (6.315 \cdot 0) - (3.2649 \cdot 19.67) - (0.1565 \cdot 156)$

$\dot{V}O_{2max} = 19.9\ ml \cdot kg^{-1} \cdot min^{-1}$

(Kline, G. M., Porcari, J. P., Hintermeister, R. et al. (1987). Estimation of $\dot{V}O_{2max}$ from a one-mile track walk, gender, age, and body weight. *Med. Sci. Sports Exerc.*, **19**, 253–9.)

### Storer maximal cycle test

Females:

$$\dot{V}O_{2max} = (9.39 \cdot \dot{W}) + (7.7 \cdot BW) - (5.88 \cdot age) + 136.7 \quad (B16)$$

Males:

$$\dot{V}O_{2max} = (10.51 \cdot \dot{W}) + (6.35 \cdot BW) - (10.49 \cdot age) + 519.3 \quad (B17)$$

In both equations, $\dot{V}O_{2max}$ is in $ml \cdot min^{-1}$, $\dot{W}$ is maximal work rate in watts, BW is body weight in kg, and age is in years.

**Example:** For an 80-kg male subject aged 35 years who has a maximal work rate of 220 W:

Using Equation B17:
$\dot{V}O_{2max} = (10.51 \cdot 220) + (6.35 \cdot 80) - (10.49 \cdot 35) + 519.3$
$\dot{V}O_{2max} = 2972\ ml \cdot min^{-1}$

(Storer, T. W., Davis, J. A. & Caiozzo, V. J. (1990). Accurate prediction of $\dot{V}O_{2max}$ in cycle ergometry. *Med. Sci. Sports Exerc.*, **22**, 704–12.)

### Queen's College step test

Males:

$$\dot{V}O_{2max} = 111.33 - (0.42 \cdot f_{Crec}) \quad (B18)$$

Females:

$$\dot{V}O_{2max} = 65.81 - (0.1847 \cdot f_{Crec}) \quad (B19)$$

where $\dot{V}O_{2max}$ is expressed in $ml \cdot kg \cdot min^{-1}$ and $f_{Crec}$ is heart rate recorded between 5 and 20 s of recovery.

(McArdle, W. D., Katch, F. I., Pechar, G. S., Jacobson, L., & Ruck, S. (1972). Reliability and interrelationships between maximal oxygen uptake, physical work capacity, and step test scores in college women. *Med. Sci. Sports Exerc.*, **4**, 182–6.)

### Siconolfi step test

$$\dot{V}O_{2max} = (0.302 \cdot nomogram\dot{V}O_{2max}) - (0.019 \cdot age) + 1.593 \quad (B20)$$

where $\dot{V}O_{2max}$ is expressed in $l \cdot min^{-1}$, nomogram $\dot{V}O_{2max}$ refers to the Åstrand–Ryhming nomogram (see Figure C5, Appendix C), and age is in years.

(Siconolfi, S. F., Garber, C. E., Laster, T. M. & Carleton, R. A. (1985). A simple, valid step test for estimating maximal oxygen uptake in epidemiological studies. *Am. J. Epidemiol.*, **121**, 382–90.)

### Balke treadmill test

$$\dot{V}O_2 = speed \cdot (0.073 + grade/100) \cdot 1.8 \quad (B21)$$

where $\dot{V}O_2$ is expressed in $ml \cdot kg^{-1} \cdot min^{-1}$; speed is fixed at 90 $m \cdot min^{-1}$; grade is grade divided by 100 percent at the end of the test; and 1.8 is the oxygen requirement in $ml \cdot min^{-1}$ of 1 kg · m of work.

It must be noted that this equation is exclusively for use with the original protocol published by Balke & Ware using a fixed 3.3 m.p.h. treadmill speed with a grade increment of 1% · $min^{-1}$ up to a heart rate of 180 $min^{-1}$. Readers are cautioned to apply the above equation only with the original protocol. It is not appropriate with any of the many modifications in common practice today.

(Balke, B. & Ware, R. (1959). An experimental study of Air Force personnel. *US Armed Forces Med. J.*, **10**, 675–88.)

### Bruce treadmill test

The Bruce treadmill protocol is one of the most often used treadmill protocols used today. Equations for predicting $\dot{V}O_{2max}$ are available for sedentary and active men; there is also a generalized equation for healthy men and women with a gender coefficient, and an equation for cardiac patients, as given in Equations B22a–d below.

Sedentary men:

$$\dot{V}o_{2max} = (3.298 \cdot t) + 4.07 \tag{B22a}$$

Active men:

$$\dot{V}o_{2max} = (3.778 \cdot t) + 0.19 \tag{B22b}$$

Generalized:

$$\dot{V}o_{2max} = (3 \cdot 36 \cdot t) - (2.82 \cdot \text{gender}) + 6.70 \tag{B22c}$$

Cardiac patients:

$$\dot{V}o_{2max} = (2.327 \cdot \text{time}) + 9.48 \tag{B22d}$$

where $\dot{V}o_{2max}$ is in $ml \cdot kg^{-1} \cdot min^{-1}$; $t$ is time in min and for Equation B22c, gender is 1 for males and 2 for females.

## Calculation of standardized gas volumes

### General gas law

$$V2 = V1 \cdot \frac{P1}{P2} \cdot \frac{T2}{T1} \tag{B23}$$

### Conversion from ATPS to BTPS

$$V_{BTPS} = V_{ATPS} \cdot \left(\frac{P_B - P_{H2O}}{P_B - 47}\right) \cdot \left(\frac{310}{273 + T_E}\right) \tag{B24}$$

where $V_{BTPS}$ is a volume (l) corrected to body temperature and pressure, saturated with water vapor; $V_{ATPS}$ is a volume (l) collected under conditions of ambient temperature and pressure, saturated with water vapor; $P_B$ is the barometric pressure (mmHg); $P_{H2O}$ is the water vapor pressure (mmHg) at the specified temperature; $T_E$ is the temperature of the exhaled air in °C; 47 is the water vapor pressure (mmHg) at body temperature (37 °C), and 310 is body temperature in degrees Kelvin (°K)=°C + 273.

### Conversion from ATPS to STPD

$$V_{STPD} = V_{ATPS} \cdot \left(\frac{P_B - P_{H2O}}{P_B}\right) \cdot \left(\frac{273}{273 + T_E}\right) \tag{B25}$$

where $V_{STPD}$ is a volume (l) corrected to standard temperature and pressure, dry; $V_{ATPS}$ is a volume (l) collected under conditions of ambient temperature and pressure saturated with water vapor; $P_B$ is the barometric pressure (mmHg); $P_{H2O}$ is the water vapor pressure (mmHg) at the specified temperature; 273 is zero °C expressed in degrees Kelvin (°K), and $T_E$ is the temperature of the exhaled air in °C.

### Conversion from BTPS to STPD

$$V_{STPD} = V_{BTPS} \cdot \left(\frac{P_B - 47}{P_B}\right) \cdot \left(\frac{273}{310}\right) \tag{B26}$$

where symbols and values are the same as described above.

## Calculation of oxygen uptake ($\dot{V}o_2$)

Oxygen uptake is equal to the oxygen breathed in minus the oxygen breathed out. Therefore:

$$\dot{V}o_2 = (\dot{V}_I \cdot F_I o_2) - (\dot{V}_E \cdot F_{\bar{E}} o_2) \tag{B27}$$

where $\dot{V}o_2$ is oxygen uptake in $l \cdot min^{-1}$; $\dot{V}_I$ is the inspired minute volume ($l \cdot min^{-1}$), $\dot{V}_E$ is the expired minute volume ($l \cdot min^{-1}$), $F_{\bar{E}}o_2$ is the mixed expired oxygen fraction, and $F_I o_2$ is the inspired oxygen fraction.

Expired air contains more $CO_2$, less $O_2$, and a slightly different concentration of nitrogen ($N_2$) than the inspired air due to gas exchange in the lung. Since nitrogen is neither produced nor taken up metabolically, the change in its concentration is due to changing proportions of $CO_2$ and $O_2$. The differences in $CO_2$ and $O_2$ concentrations in the expired versus inspired air result in the volumes of the expired and inspired air being unequal. This difference is in direct proportion to the difference in the fractional concentration of nitrogen in the inspired versus the expired air. Since $N_2$ is inert,

$$\dot{V}_I \cdot F_I N_2 = \dot{V}_E \cdot F_{\bar{E}} N_2 \tag{B28}$$

where $F_I N_2$ is the inspired nitrogen fraction and $F_{\bar{E}} N_2$ is the expired nitrogen fraction. Thus:

$$\dot{V}_I = \dot{V}_E \cdot \left(\frac{F_{\bar{E}} N_2}{F_I N_2}\right) \tag{B29}$$

This calculation, used to calculate inspired volume, $\dot{V}_I$, when only $\dot{V}_E$ is measured, has been attributed to Haldane and referred to as the Haldane transformation.

Substituting for $\dot{V}_I$ in Equation B27,

$$\dot{V}O_2 = \left[\left(\dot{V}_E \cdot \left(\frac{F_{\bar{E}}N_2}{F_I N_2}\right) \cdot F_I O_2\right)\right] - (\dot{V}_E \cdot F_{\bar{E}}O_2) \quad \text{(B30)}$$

Since the composition of inspired air remains relatively constant, with $F_I O_2 = 0.2093$ and $F_I N_2 = 0.7904$, and since $F_{\bar{E}}N_2 = (1 - F_{\bar{E}}O_2 - F_{\bar{E}}CO_2)$, substituting in Equation B30:

$$\dot{V}O_2 = \left(\dot{V}_E \cdot \frac{(1 - F_{\bar{E}}O_2 - F_{\bar{E}}CO_2)}{0.7904} \cdot 0.2093\right) - (\dot{V}_E \cdot F_{\bar{E}}O_2) \quad \text{(B31)}$$

Reducing:

$$\dot{V}O_2 = \dot{V}_E \cdot [(1 - F_{\bar{E}}O_2 - F_{\bar{E}}CO_2) \cdot 0.265) - F_{\bar{E}}O_2] \quad \text{(B32)}$$

By convention $\dot{V}O_2$ is expressed under standard conditions (STPD).

## Calculation of carbon dioxide output ($\dot{V}CO_2$)

$$\dot{V}CO_2 = \dot{V}_E \cdot F_{\bar{E}}CO_2 \quad \text{(B33)}$$

By convention $\dot{V}CO_2$ is expressed under standard conditions (STPD).

## Calculation of the respiratory exchange ratio (*R*)

$$R = \frac{\dot{V}CO_2}{\dot{V}O_2} \quad \text{(B34)}$$

**Table B1.** Conversion constants for selected measurement units useful in an exercise-testing laboratory. The SI[a] base units (le Système International d'Unités) are in italics

| Measurement | To convert | Into | Multiply by |
|---|---|---|---|
| Energy | kilocalories | foot-pound | 3087 |
| | kilocalories | kilogram-meters per second | 426.85 |
| Force | *newtons* | kilogram-meter per second per second | 1.0 |
| Length | kilometers | feet | 3281 |
| | kilometers | inches | $3.937 \cdot 10^4$ |
| | kilometers | miles | 0.6214 |
| | kilometers | yards | 1094 |
| | *meters* | feet | 3.281 |
| | *meters* | inches | 39.37 |
| | *meters* | miles (stat) | $6.214 \cdot 10^{-4}$ |
| | *meters* | yards | 1.094 |
| | miles (statute) | feet | 5280 |
| | miles (statute) | inches | $6.336 \cdot 10^4$ |
| | miles (statute) | kilometers | 1.609 |
| | miles (statute) | *meters* | 1609 |
| | miles (statute) | yards | 1760 |
| | millimeters | feet | $3.281 \cdot 10^{-3}$ |
| | millimeters | inches | 0.03937 |
| | millimeters | miles | $6.214 \cdot 10^{-7}$ |
| | millimeters | yards | $1.094 \cdot 10^{-3}$ |
| | yards | centimeters | 91.44 |
| | yards | kilometers | $9.144 \cdot 10^{-4}$ |
| | yards | *meters* | 0.9144 |
| | yards | miles (stat) | $5.682 \cdot 10^{-4}$ |
| | yards | millimeters | 914.4 |
| Power | *watts* | foot-pound per minute | 44.27 |
| | *watts* | foot-pound per second | 0.7378 |
| | *watts* | horsepower | $1.341 \cdot 10^{-3}$ |
| | *watts* | joules per second | 1 |
| | *watts* | kilocalories per minute | 0.01433 |
| | *watts* | kilogram-meter per minute | 6.12 |
| Pressure | millimeters of mercury | *pascals* | 133.32 |
| | millimeters of mercury | kilopascals | 0.13332 |
| | millimeters of mercury | torr | 1.0 |
| Revolutions | number of revolutions | degrees | 360 |
| | revolutions per minute | degrees per second | 6 |
| | revolutions per minute | revolutions per second | 0.01667 |

**Table B1.** *(cont.)*

| Measurement | To convert | Into | Multiply by |
|---|---|---|---|
| Speed | kilometers per hour | centimeters per second | 27.78 |
| | kilometers per hour | feet per minute | 54.68 |
| | kilometers per hour | feet per second | 0.9113 |
| | kilometers per hour | meters per minute | 16.67 |
| | kilometers per hour | meters per second | 0.2778 |
| | kilometers per hour | miles per hour | 0.6214 |
| | meters per second | feet per minute | 196.8 |
| | meters per second | feet per second | 3.281 |
| | meters per second | kilometers per hour | 3.6 |
| | meters per second | kilometers per minute | 0.06 |
| | meters per second | miles per hour | 2.237 |
| | meters per second | miles per minute | 0.03728 |
| | meters per minute | centimeters per second | 1.667 |
| | meters per minute | feet per minute | 3.281 |
| | meters per minute | feet per second | 0.05468 |
| | meters per minute | kilometers per hour | 0.06 |
| | meters per minute | miles per hour | 0.03728 |
| | miles per hour | centimeters per second | 44.70 |
| | miles per hour | feet per minute | 88 |
| | miles per hour | feet per second | 1.467 |
| | miles per hour | kilometers per hour | 1.609 |
| | miles per hour | kilometers per minute | 0.02682 |
| | miles per hour | meters per minute | 26.82 |
| | miles per hour | miles per minute | 0.1667 |
| | miles per minute | kilometers per minute | 1.609 |
| | miles per minute | miles per hour | 60 |
| Temperature | temperature (°C) | temperature (°F) | $(°C \times 1.8) + 32$ |
| | temperature (°F) | temperature (°C) | $(°F - 32) \cdot 0.5556$ |
| Volume | liters | cubic centimeters | 1000 |
| | liters | cubic feet | 0.03531 |
| | liters | cubic inches | 61.02 |
| | liters | cubic meters | 0.001 |
| | liters | American gallons | 0.2642 |
| | liters | American pints | 2.113 |
| | liters | American quarts | 1.057 |
| Weight[b] | grams | milligrams | 1000 |
| | grams | ounces (avdp) | 0.03527 |
| | grams | pounds | $2.205 \cdot 10^{-3}$ |
| | *kilograms* | grams | 1000 |
| | *kilograms* | joules per meter (*newtons*) | 9.807 |

**Table B1.** *(cont.)*

| Measurement | To convert | Into | Multiply by |
|---|---|---|---|
| | *kilograms* | pounds | 2.205 |
| | pounds | joules per meter (*newtons*) | 4.448 |
| | pounds | *kilograms* | 0.4536 |
| | pounds | ounces | 16 |
| Work | *joules* | foot-pounds | 0.7376 |
| | *joules* | kilocalories | $2.389 \cdot 10^{-4}$ |
| | *joules* | kilogram-meters | 0.1020 |
| | *joules* | newton-meters | 1.0 |
| | kilogram-meters | *joules* | 9.804 |
| | kilogram-meters | kilocalories | $2.342 \cdot 10^{-3}$ |

[a]SI Units: a system of reporting units of measurement that is uniform in concept and style and accepted internationally. The base units italicized above are preferred units of measurement.
[b]Weight is more strictly defined as mass accelerated by gravity. Grams and kilograms are units of mass whereas pounds and ounces are usually considered as weights.

# Appendix C Reference values

## Maximum oxygen uptake ($\dot{V}O_{2max}$)

There have been many reports of reference values for $\dot{V}O_{2max}$. Most have been conducted using males and females from the USA, Canada, and European countries. The ethnicity and activity levels of the subjects are often not well defined. All prediction equations include an age factor. Some include height, others body weight or lean body mass. Some derive $\dot{V}O_{2max}$ in $l \cdot min^{-1}$ while others derive $\dot{V}O_{2max}$ in $ml \cdot kg^{-1} \cdot min^{-1}$.

Interestingly, if certain studies are compared, there is remarkable agreement in the prediction of $\dot{V}O_{2max}$ in $ml \cdot kg^{-1} \cdot min^{-1}$ based on age and gender. Figure C1 illustrates reference values for $\dot{V}O_{2max}$ in $ml \cdot kg^{-1} \cdot min^{-1}$ in relation to age and gender based on five such studies. Table C1 shows experimental details from these five studies, including numbers of subjects and the mode of exercise testing. The data from these studies have been combined by averaging the intercepts and slopes to derive equations for men and women, as shown in Table C1 and Figure C1. Once a reference value for $\dot{V}O_{2max}$ has been obtained in $ml \cdot kg^{-1} \cdot min^{-1}$, then an absolute value in $l \cdot min^{-1}$ can be derived assuming ideal body weight based on height (see below). Thereafter the height-adjusted $\dot{V}O_{2max}$ can be adjusted for actual body weight. Obesity increases $\dot{V}O_{2max}$ in $l \cdot min^{-1}$ while negatively impacting physical fitness. This can be illustrated by again expressing the weight-adjusted reference value for $\dot{V}O_{2max}$ in $ml \cdot kg^{-1} \cdot min^{-1}$ (see below).

The exercise practitioner can use any of these individual prediction equations or consider using the composite equations that represent all of the summated data. Whichever approach is adopted, the reader is reminded that the reference value of $\dot{V}O_{2max}$ used should be derived from a study population which matches as closely as possible the subject or subjects currently being assessed.

### Calculation

If the composite equations illustrated in Table C1 and Figure C1 are used, the following approach is recommended:

1. Use the age and gender of the subject to derive $\dot{V}O_{2max}$ in $ml \cdot kg^{-1} \cdot min^{-1}$ using Equations C1 or C2, and Figure C1.
   Males:
   $$\dot{V}O_{2max} = 50.02 - (0.394 \cdot age) \quad (C1)$$
   Females:
   $$\dot{V}O_{2max} = 42.83 - (0.371 \cdot age) \quad (C2)$$
   where $\dot{V}O_{2max}$ is maximal oxygen uptake expressed in $ml \cdot kg^{-1} \cdot min^{-1}$ and age is expressed in years.
2. Use the reference equations C3 and C4 derived from Metropolitan Life Tables to calculate ideal body weight (IBW) from height in meters.
   Males:
   $$IBW = (71.6 \cdot Ht) - 51.8 \quad (C3)$$
   Females:
   $$IBW = (62.6 \cdot Ht) - 45.5 \quad (C4)$$
   where IBW is ideal body weight in kg and Ht is height in meters.

3. Multiply the reference value for $\dot{V}O_{2max}$ derived in step 1 by the IBW derived in step 2 to derive a reference value for $\dot{V}O_{2max}$ in $l \cdot min^{-1}$ that assumes an ideal body weight. Figure C2 shows these height-adjusted reference values for males and females respectively.
4. Adjust the height-adjusted reference value for $\dot{V}O_{2max}$ derived in step 3 for actual body weight (ABW) using Equation C5. Figure C3 shows weight-adjusted reference values for males and females respectively.

$$(wt\text{-}adj)\dot{V}O_{2max} = (ht\text{-}adj)\dot{V}O_{2max} + ((ABW - IBW) \cdot 0.0058) \quad (C5)$$

where $(wt\text{-}adj)\dot{V}O_{2max}$ is weight-adjusted $\dot{V}O_{2max}$, $(ht\text{-}adj)\dot{V}O_{2max}$ is height-adjusted $\dot{V}O_{2max}$, ABW is actual body weight, and IBW is ideal body weight in kg.

Alternatively, the weight-adjusted $\dot{V}O_{2max}$ for any individual can be derived directly by combining steps 1, 2, 3, and 4, as shown in Equations C6 and C7.

Males:

$$(wt\text{-}adj)\dot{V}O_{2max} = ((0.0716 \cdot Ht) - 0.0518) \cdot (44.22 - (0.394 \cdot age)) + (0.0058 \cdot ABW) \quad (C6)$$

Females:

$$(wt\text{-}adj)\dot{V}O_{2max} = ((0.0626 \cdot Ht) - 0.0455) \cdot (37.03 - (0.371 \cdot age)) + (0.0058 \cdot ABW) \quad (C7)$$

where $(wt\text{-}adj)\dot{V}O_{2max}$ is weight-adjusted $\dot{V}O_{2max}$, *Ht* is height in meters, age is expressed in years, and ABW is actual body weight in kg.

5. If desired, the reference value for $\dot{V}O_{2max}$ derived in step 4 can be converted from $l \cdot min^{-1}$ to $ml \cdot kg \cdot min^{-1}$ by dividing by actual body weight (ABW). Figure C4 shows these reference values for males and females respectively.

## References

1. Pollock, M. L., Schmidt, D. H. & Jackson, A. S. (1980). Measurement of cardiorespiratory fitness and body composition in the clinical setting. *Comp. Ther.*, **6**, 9.
2. Jones, N. L., Makrides, L., Hitchcock, C., Chypchar, T. & McCartney, N. (1985). Normal standards for an incremental progressive cycle ergometer test. *Am. Rev. Respir. Dis.*, **131**, 700–8.
3. Hansen, J. E., Sue, D. Y. & Wasserman, K. (1984). Predicted values for clinical exercise testing. *Am. Rev. Respir. Dis.*, **129** suppl., S49–55.
4. Shvartz, E. & Reibold, R. C. (1990). Aerobic fitness norms for males and females aged 6 to 75 years. *Aviat. Space Environ. Med.*, **61**, 3–11.
5. Davis, J. A., Storer, T. W., Caiozzo, V. J. & Pham, P. H. Unpublished data.
6. Metropolitan Life Insurance Company (1959). New weight standards for men and women. *Stat. Bull. Metropol. Life Insur. Co.*, **40**, 1.

## Lower 95% confidence interval for $\dot{V}O_{2max}$

Four gender-specific equations for predicting reference values for $\dot{V}O_{2max}$ using nonexercise variables are given below. These are based on healthy, nonsmoking, sedentary males ($n = 103$) and females ($n = 101$), aged 20–70 years, who performed a maximal cycle exercise test (Davis et al., unpublished data). Since the sample population was homogeneous with respect to health and activity level, the standard error of estimate (SEE) derived from each equation allows calculation of the lower 95% confidence interval (95% CI). Thus, subtracting the 95% CI from the predicted $\dot{V}O_{2max}$ identifies the lower limit for $\dot{V}O_{2max}$ expected for any given subject. A measured $\dot{V}O_{2max}$ falling below this lower limit is potentially due to disease, not a sedentary lifestyle.

The equations given here are unique in that they are the only ones currently available that can correctly estimate the lower limit of normal for a given subject. While these prediction equations are specific to cycle ergometer exercise, a practitioner may consider increasing the calculated $\dot{V}O_{2max}$ values from these equations by 10–15% in order to compare $\dot{V}O_{2max}$ values obtained from treadmill exercise testing.

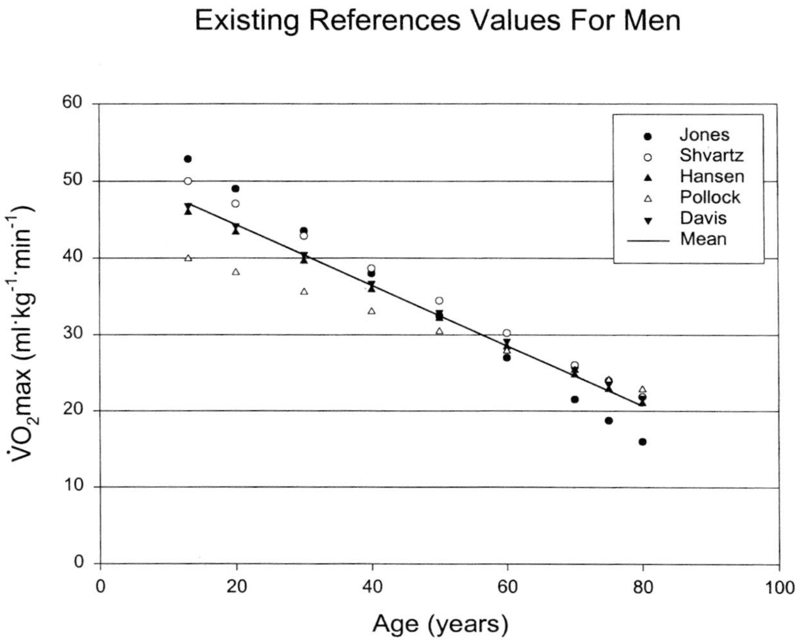


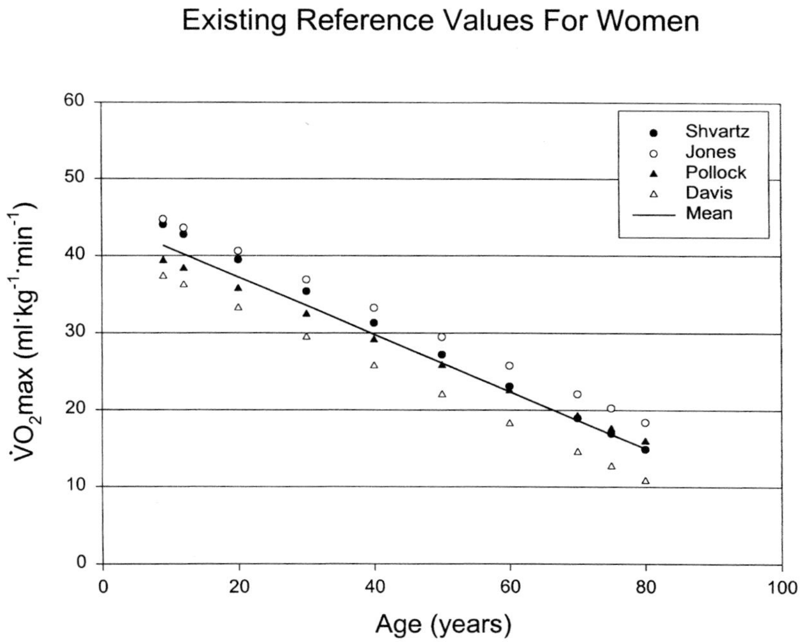


**Figure C1** Reference values for maximum oxygen uptake based on gender and age. Maximum oxygen uptake is expressed in ml · kg$^{-1}$ · min$^{-1}$. The sources of these data are described in Table C1. The data have been combined by averaging the intercepts and slopes to give the composite Equations C1 and C2.

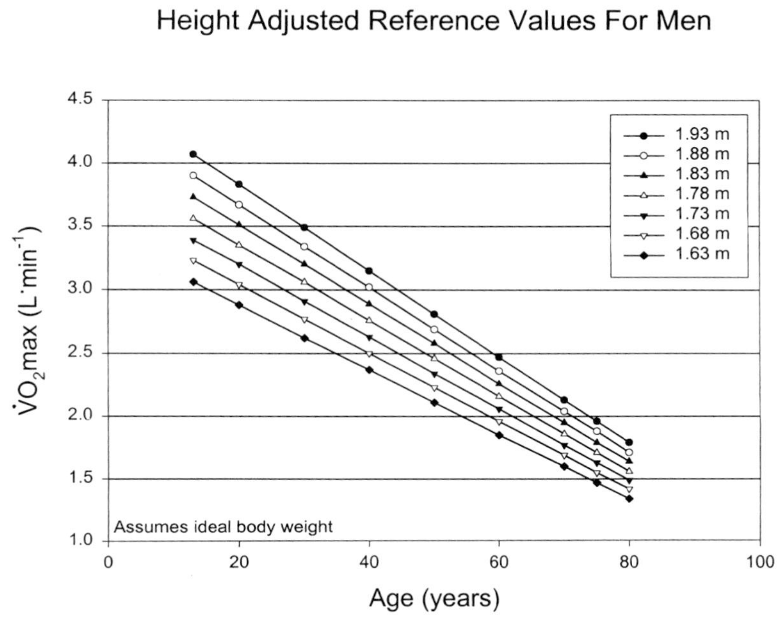


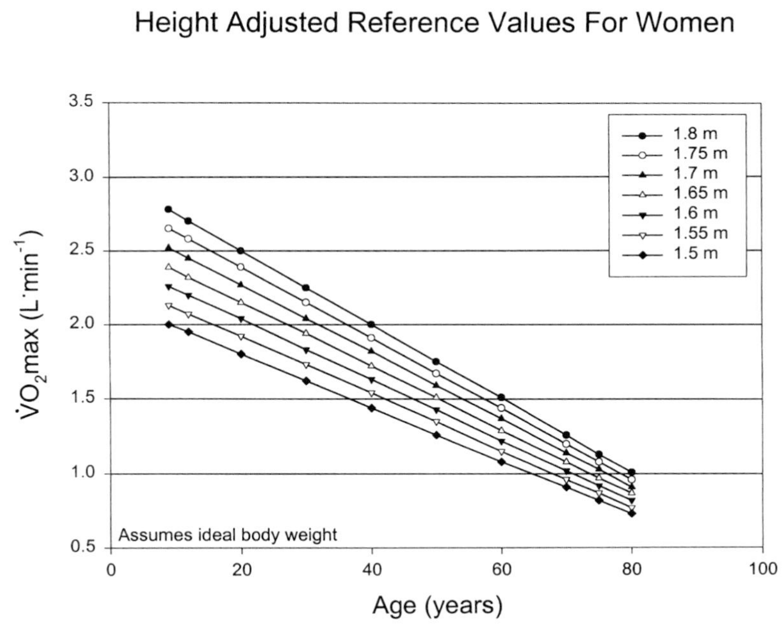


**Figure C2** Reference values for maximum oxygen uptake based on gender, age, and height. Maximum oxygen uptake is expressed in $l \cdot min^{-1}$. These data assume that a subject is of ideal body weight, as calculated using Equations C3 and C4.

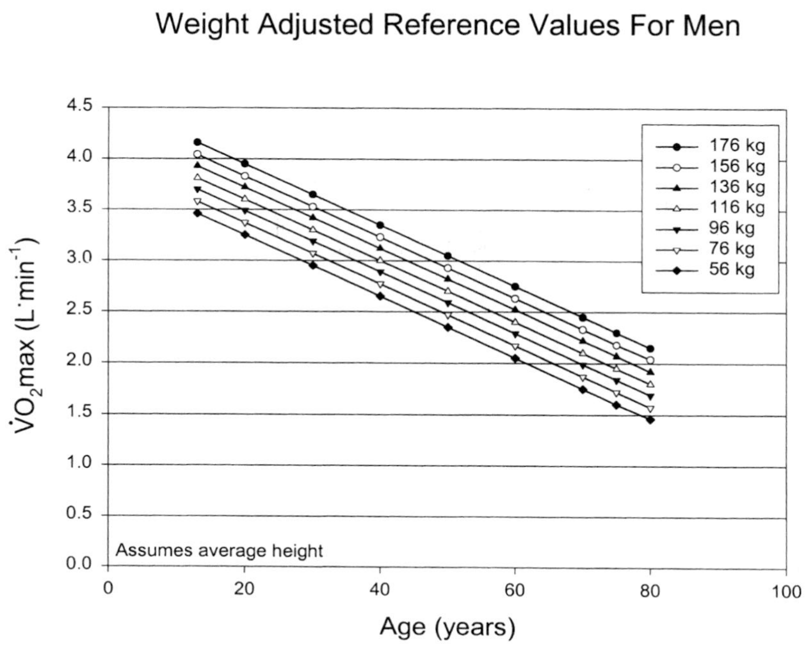


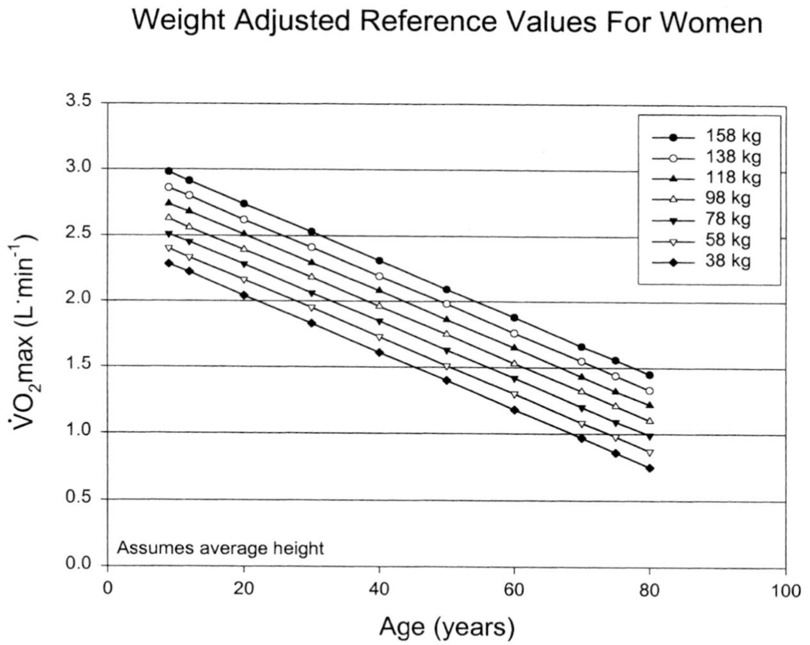


**Figure C3** Reference values for maximum oxygen uptake based on gender, age, and body weight. Maximum oxygen uptake is expressed in $l \cdot min^{-1}$. These data assume average heights of 1.78 m (70 in.) for men and 1.65 m (65 in.) for women.

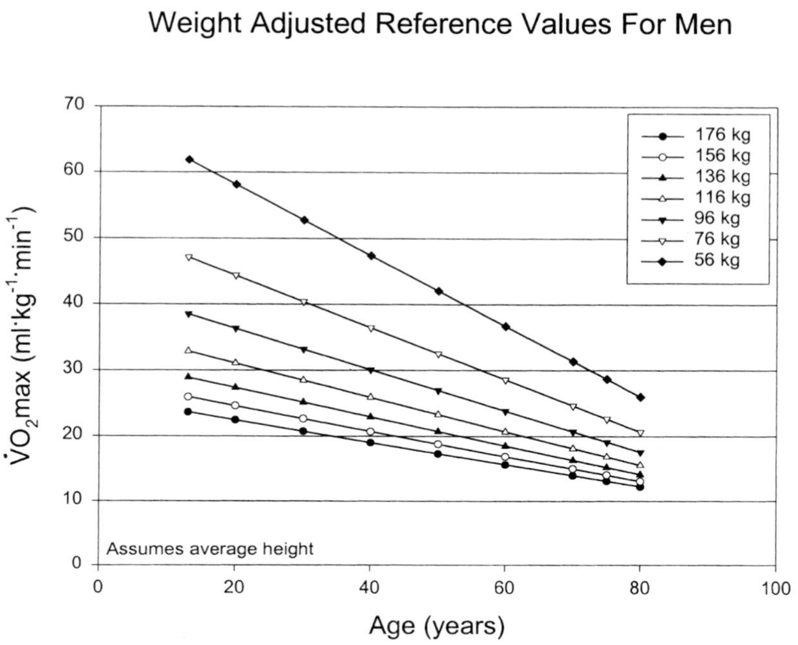


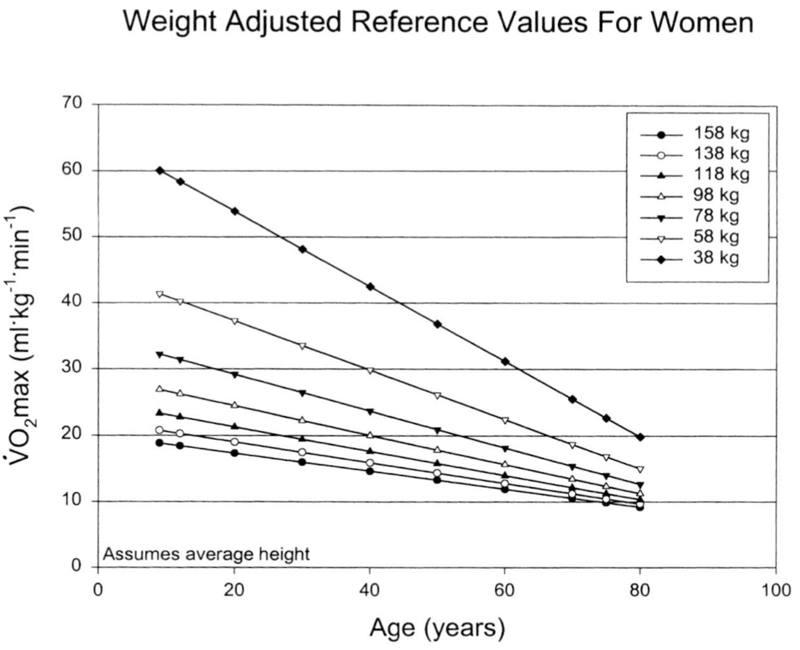


**Figure C4** Reference values for maximum oxygen uptake based on gender, age, and body weight. Maximum oxygen uptake is expressed in ml · kg$^{-1}$ · min$^{-1}$. These data assume average heights of 1.78 m (70 in.) for men and 1.65 m (65 in.) for women. Note that when $Vo_{2max}$ is expressed in ml · kg$^{-1}$ · min$^{-1}$, excess body weight results in spuriously low reference values whereas underweight subjects may have spuriously high reference values.

**Table C1.** Sources of reference values for $\dot{V}o_{2max}$ (ml · kg$^{-1}$ · min$^{-1}$)

| Study | Year | Equation | Number of subjects | Country of origin | Age range | Activity level | Exercise mode | Subject characteristics |
|---|---|---|---|---|---|---|---|---|
| **Males** | | | | | | | | |
| Pollock et al. | 1980 | 43.20 – (0.255 · age) | | | | | | |
| Hansen et al. | 1984 | 50.75 – (0.372 · age) | 77 | USA | 34–74 | | Cycle | Included smokers, obese, hypertensives |
| Jones et al. | 1985 | 60.00 – (0.550 · age) | 50 | | 15–71 | 54% active | Cycle | 13% smokers |
| Shvartz & Reibold | 1990 | 44.54 – (0.420 · age) | 98 samples | USA, Canada, Europe | 6–75 | Sedentary or mildly active | Cycle (32 samples) Treadmill (25 samples) Stepping (5 samples) | Analyzed 62 studies conducted in USA, Canada and seven European countries |
| Davis et al. | 2000 | 51.63 – (0.375 · age) | 103 | USA | 20–70 | Sedentary | Cycle | Sedentary, nonsmokers |
| Composite equation | | 50.02 – (0.394 · age) | | | | | | |

| Study | Year | Equation | Number of subjects | Country of origin | Age range | Activity level | Exercise mode | Comments |
|---|---|---|---|---|---|---|---|---|
| **Females** | | | | | | | | |
| Pollock et al. | 1980 | 42.30 – (0.330 · age) | | | | | | |
| Jones et al. | 1985 | 48.00 – (0.370 · age) | 50 | | 15–71 | 54% active | | 13% smokers |
| Shvartz & Reibold | 1990 | 40.31 – (0.410 · age) | 43 samples | USA, Canada, Europe | 6–75 | Sedentary or mildly active | Cycle (32 samples) Treadmill (25 samples) Stepping (5 samples) | Analyzed 62 studies conducted in USA, Canada and seven European countries |
| Davis et al. | 2000 | 40.69 – (0.373 · age) | 101 | USA | 20–70 | Sedentary | Cycle | Sedentary, nonsmokers |
| Composite equation | | 42.83 – (0.371 · age) | | | | | | |

Refer to text for references.

## Åstrand–Ryhming nomogram

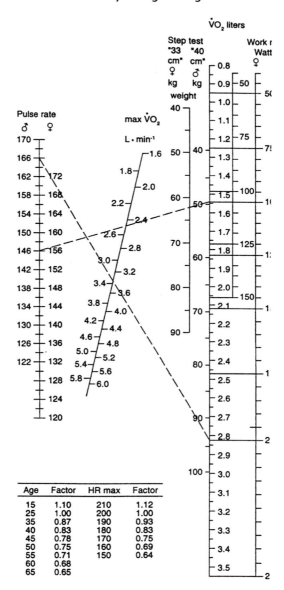

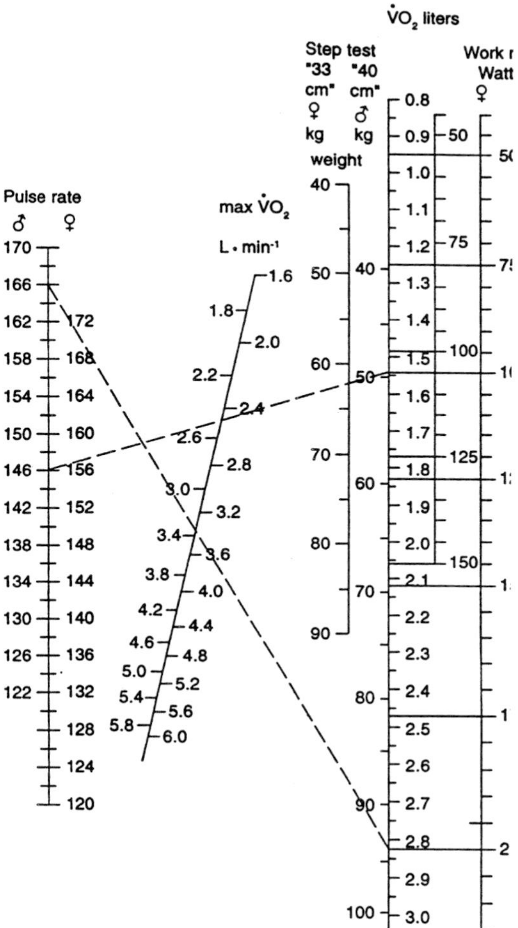


| Age | Factor | HR max | Factor |
|---|---|---|---|
| 15 | 1.10 | 210 | 1.12 |
| 25 | 1.00 | 200 | 1.00 |
| 35 | 0.87 | 190 | 0.93 |
| 40 | 0.83 | 180 | 0.83 |
| 45 | 0.78 | 170 | 0.75 |
| 50 | 0.75 | 160 | 0.69 |
| 55 | 0.71 | 150 | 0.64 |
| 60 | 0.68 | | |
| 65 | 0.65 | | |

**Figure C5** Åstrand–Ryhming nomogram for the calculation of aerobic capacity ($\dot{V}o_{2max}$) from values of heart rate ($f_C$) and oxygen uptake ($Vo_2$) at a submaximal work rate during a cycle, treadmill, or step test. In exercise tests where oxygen uptake is not determined, it can be estimated by reading horizontally from the 'body weight' scale (step test) or work rate ($\dot{W}$) scale (cycle test) to the oxygen uptake ($\dot{V}o_2$) scale.

Subsequent to the development of the original Åstrand–Rhyming nomogram, factors for correcting the nomogram-determined $Vo_{2max}$ were computed for age and maximal heart rate (when known). These correction factors appear in the box in the lower left corner of the nomogram. The value for $Vo_{2max}$ obtained from the nomogram is multiplied by *either* the factor for age *or* the factor for maximal heart rate, if known. This takes into account the reduction of maximal heart rate with age. Modified with permission from: Åstrand, P.-O. & Rhyming, I. (1954). A nomogram for calculation of aerobic capacity (physical fitness) from pulse rate during submaximal work. *J. Appl. Physiol.*, 7, 218–21.

## Nomogram for Spirometric Indices of Lung Function (Males of European descent)

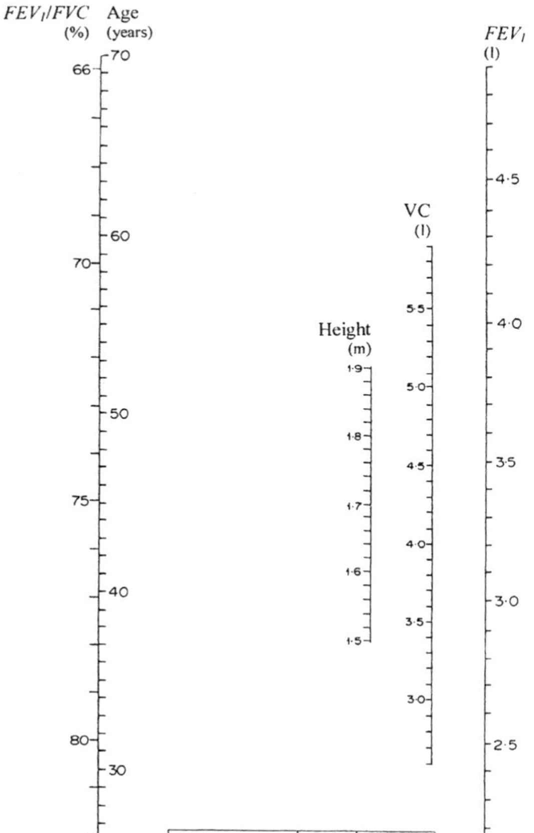


| Index | SD | Units |
|---|---|---|
| $FEV_1$ | 0.50 | liters |
| $VC$ | 0.58 | liters |
| $FEV_1/FVC$ | 7.2 | % |

**Figure C6** Nomogram relating vital capacity (VC), forced expired volume in one second ($FEV_1$) and $FEV_1$/FVC (%) to age (years) and height (m) for healthy adult males of European descent. $FEV_1$/FVC% is related only to age. Modified with permission from Cotes, J. E. (1979). *Lung function. Assessment and application in medicine.* Oxford: Blackwell Scientific Publications.

## Nomogram for Spirometric Indices of Lung Function (Females of European descent)

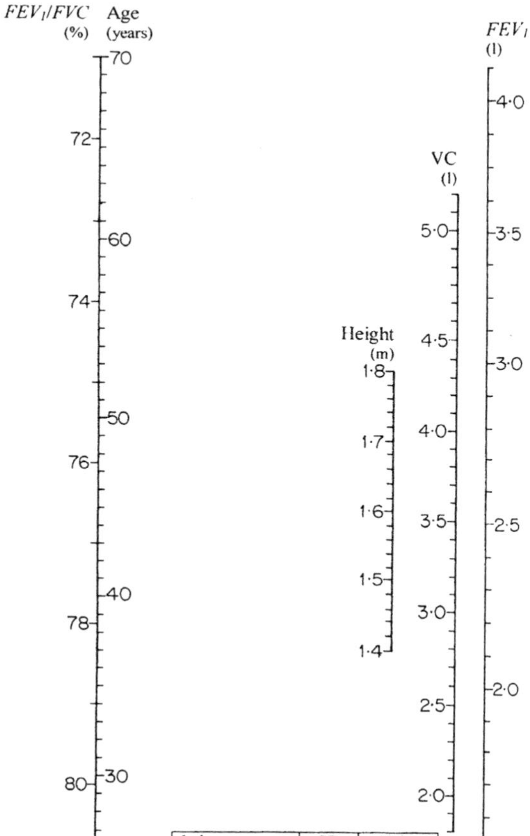


| Index | SD | Units |
|---|---|---|
| $FEV_1$ | 0.36 | liters |
| $VC$ | 0.47 | liters |
| $FEV_1/FVC$ | 6.2 | % |

**Figure C7** Nomogram relating vital capacity (VC), forced expired volume in one second ($FEV_1$) and $FEV_1$/FVC (%) to age (years) and height (m) for healthy adult females of European descent. $FEV_1$/FVC% is related only to age. Modified with permission from Cotes, J. E. (1979). *Lung function. Assessment and application in medicine.* Oxford: Blackwell Scientific Publications.

## Nomogram for Spirometric Indices of Lung Function (Males of African descent)

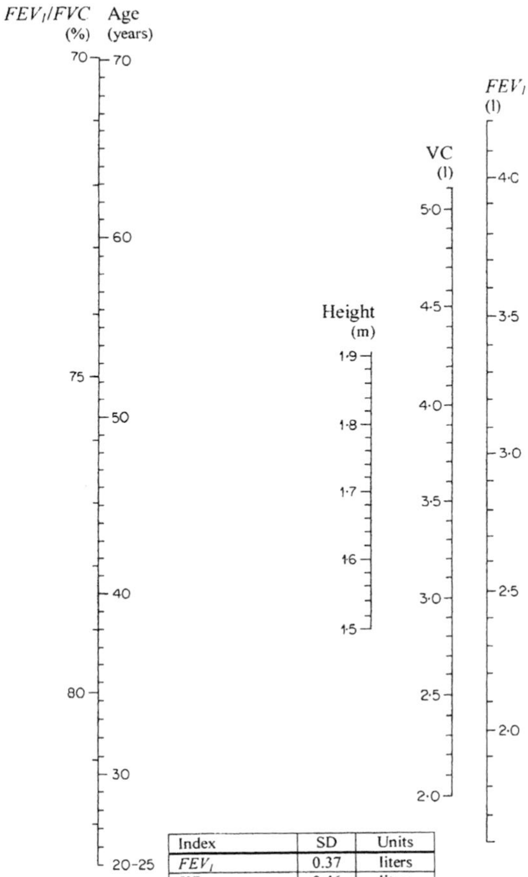


| Index | SD | Units |
|---|---|---|
| *FEV₁* | 0.37 | liters |
| *VC* | 0.46 | liters |
| *FEV₁/FVC* | 8.7 | % |

**Figure C8** Nomogram relating vital capacity (VC), forced expired volume in one second ($FEV_1$) and $FEV_1$/FVC (%) to age (years) and height (m) for healthy adult males of African descent. $FEV_1$/FVC% is related only to age. Modified with permission from Cotes, J. E. (1979). *Lung function. Assessment and application in medicine.* Oxford: Blackwell Scientific Publications. The data are from Miller, G. J., Cotes, J. E., Hall, A. M., Salvosa, C. B. & Ashworth, M. T. (1972). Lung function and exercise performance in healthy men and women of African ethnic origin. *Quart. J. Exp. Physiol.*, **57**, 325–41.

## Nomogram for Spirometric Indices of Lung Function (Females of African descent)

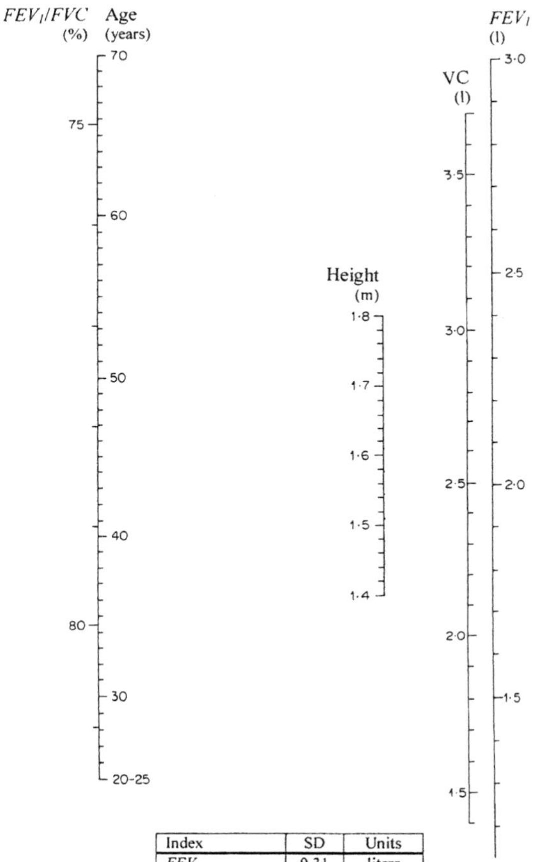


| Index | SD | Units |
|---|---|---|
| *FEV₁* | 0.31 | liters |
| *VC* | 0.38 | liters |
| *FEV₁/FVC* | 7.6 | % |

**Figure C9** Nomogram relating vital capacity (VC), forced expired volume in one second ($FEV_1$) and $FEV_1$/FVC (%) to age (years) and height (m) for healthy adult females of African descent. $FEV_1$/FVC% is related only to age. Modified with permission from Cotes, J. E. (1979). *Lung function. Assessment and application in medicine.* Oxford: Blackwell Scientific Publications. The data are from Miller, G. J., Cotes, J. E., Hall, A. M., Salvosa, C. B. & Ashworth, M. T. (1972). Lung function and exercise performance in healthy men and women of African ethnic origin. *Quart. J. Exp. Physiol.*, **57**, 325–41.

### Males

$\dot{V}O_{2max} = (0.0186 \cdot ht) - (0.0283 \cdot age) + 0.5947$

$R = 0.79$; SEE = 0.363; 95% CI = 0.601

where $\dot{V}O_{2max}$ is in $l \cdot min^{-1}$, ht is standing height in cm, age is in years, $R$ is the multiple correlation coefficient, SEE is the standard error of the estimate and CI is the confidence interval.

Alternatively, better prediction of $\dot{V}O_{2max}$ is obtained when values for fat-free mass are available and used in the following equation:

$\dot{V}O_{2max} = (0.0234 \cdot FFM) - (0.0272 \cdot age) + 2.3245$

R = 0.82; SEE = 0.335; 95% CI = 0.556

where $\dot{V}O_{2max}$ is in $l \cdot min^{-1}$, FFM is the fat-free mass in kg and age is in years.

### Females

$\dot{V}O_{2max} = (0.0085 \cdot ht) - (0.02166 \cdot age) + 0.9536$

$R = 0.76$; SEE = 0.227; 95% CI = 0.377

where $\dot{V}O_{2max}$ is in $l \cdot min^{-1}$, ht is standing height in cm and age is in years.

Alternatively, better prediction of $\dot{V}O_{2max}$ is obtained when values for fat-free mass are available and used in the following equation:

$\dot{V}O_{2max} = (0.0157 \cdot FFM) - (0.0172 \cdot age) + 1.6394$

$R = 0.79$; SEE = 0.215; 95% CI = 0.357

where $\dot{V}O_{2max}$ is in $l \cdot min^{-1}$, FFM is the fat-free mass in kg and age is in years.

## Classification of cardiorespiratory fitness based on maximum oxygen uptake

Tables C2 for males and C3 for females indicate fitness categories in quintiles based on $\dot{V}O_{2max}$ expressed in $ml \cdot kg^{-1} \cdot min^{-1}$. The American Heart Association and Cooper data are based on treadmill exercise. The Åstrand data are based on cycle ergometer exercise and fit subjects in the younger age groups. It is important to use mode-specific reference values when attempting to classify performance based on $\dot{V}O_{2max}$ obtained from an exercise test. This suggests use of American Heart Association or Cooper data for classifying $\dot{V}O_{2max}$ obtained from treadmill tests and the Åstrand data when classifying $\dot{V}O_{2max}$ obtained from cycle ergometer tests.

## Metabolic threshold ($\dot{V}O_2\theta$)

The following equations predict reference values and the lower 95% confidence limit for $\dot{V}O_2\theta$. These equations were developed from maximal cycle ergometer exercise tests on 103 male and 101 female subjects aged 20–70 years who were healthy, nonsmoking, and sedentary (Davis et al., 1997). The equations were cross-validated on an independent sample, demonstrating high multiple correlation coefficients and low standard errors of estimate suggesting generalizability. These equations are the only ones currently available that allow correct calculation of the lower limit of normal since they were developed on sedentary, healthy, nonsmoking subjects. It must be noted that the $\dot{V}CO_2$–$\dot{V}O_2$ relationship was used to identify $\dot{V}O_2\theta$ (see Chapter 4). The lower limit of normal is determined by first calculating $\dot{V}O_2\theta$ using the appropriate equation below, and then subtracting the corresponding 95% CI.

### Males

$\dot{V}O_2\theta = (0.0093 \cdot height) - (0.0136 \cdot age) + 0.4121$

$R = 0.70$; SEE = 0.228; 95% CI = 0.378

where $\dot{V}O_{2max}$ is in $l \cdot min^{-1}$, height is standing height in cm, age is in years, $R$ is the multiple correlation coefficient, SEE is the standard error of the estimate and CI is the confidence interval.

### Females

$\dot{V}O_2\theta = (0.0064 \cdot height) - (0.0053 \cdot age) + 0.1092$

$R = 0.59$; SEE = 0.131; 95% CI = 0.217

where $\dot{V}O_{2max}$ is in $l \cdot min^{-1}$, height is standing height in cm and age is in years.
(Davis, J. A., Storer, T. W. & Caiozzo, V. J. (1997). Prediction of normal values for lactate threshold estimated by gas exchange in men and women. *Eur. J. Appl. Physiol.*, **76**, 157–64.)

## 6-Min walking test

The following equations may be used to compare patient performance on the 6-min walk test with reference values and the lower 95% confidence limit for healthy adults aged 40–80 years.
(Enright, P. L. & Sherrill, D. L. (1998). Reference equations for the six-minute walk in healthy adults. *Am. J. Respir. Crit. Care Med.*, **158**, 1384–7.)

### Males

$$d_{W6} = (7.57 \cdot \text{height}) - (5.02 \cdot \text{age}) - (1.76 \cdot \text{weight}) - 309$$

where $d_{W6}$ is the 6-min walking distance in m; height is standing height in cm measured in stocking feet; age is in years; and weight is body weight in kg.

Alternatively, body mass index (BMI) may be used in place of height and weight, yielding the following equation:

$$d_{W6} = 1140 - (5.61 \cdot \text{BMI}) - (6.94 \cdot \text{age})$$

where $d_{W6}$ is the 6-min walking distance in m; BMI is the body mass index ($kg \cdot m^{-2}$) and age is in years.

The lower 95% confidence limit may be calculated by subtracting 153 m from the result of either equation.

### Females

$$d_{W6} = (2.11 \cdot \text{height}) - (2.29 \cdot \text{age}) - (5.78 \cdot \text{weight}) + 667$$

where $d_{W6}$ is the 6-min walking distance in m; height is standing height in cm measured in stocking feet; age is in years; and weight is body weight in kg.

Alternatively, BMI may be used in place of height and weight, yielding the following equation:

$$d_{W6} = 1017 - (6.24 \cdot \text{BMI}) - (5.83 \cdot \text{age})$$

where $d_{W6}$ is the 6-min walking distance in m; BMI is the body mass index ($kg \cdot m^{-2}$) and age is in years.

The lower 95% confidence limit may be calculated by subtracting 139 m from the result of either equation.

**Table C2.** Fitness categories for males, based on $\dot{V}o_{2max}$ expressed in $ml \cdot kg^{-1} \cdot min^{-1}$

| Age | Low | Fair | Average | Good | High |
|---|---|---|---|---|---|
| **20–29 years** | | | | | |
| AHA[a] | ⩽24 | 25–33 | 34–42 | 43–52 | ⩾53 |
| Cooper et al.[b] | ⩽32 | 33–35 | 36–43 | 44–47 | ⩾48 |
| Åstrand[c] | ⩽38 | 39–43 | 44–51 | 52–56 | ⩾57 |
| **30–39 years** | | | | | |
| AHA | ⩽22 | 23–30 | 31–38 | 39–48 | ⩾49 |
| Cooper et al. | ⩽30 | 31–35 | 36–40 | 41–45 | ⩾46 |
| Åstrand | ⩽34 | 35–39 | 40–47 | 48–51 | ⩾52 |
| **40–49 years** | | | | | |
| AHA | ⩽19 | 20–26 | 27–35 | 36–44 | ⩾45 |
| Cooper et al. | ⩽29 | 30–33 | 34–39 | 40–44 | ⩾45 |
| Åstrand | ⩽30 | 31–35 | 36–43 | 44–47 | ⩾48 |
| **50–59 years** | | | | | |
| AHA | ⩽17 | 18–24 | 25–33 | 34–42 | ⩾43 |
| Cooper et al. | ⩽25 | 26–30 | 31–35 | 36–43 | ⩾44 |
| Åstrand | ⩽25 | 26–31 | 32–39 | 40–43 | ⩾44 |
| **60–69 years** | | | | | |
| AHA | ⩽15 | 16–22 | 23–30 | 31–40 | ⩾41 |
| Cooper et al. | ⩽19 | 20–25 | 26–32 | 33–40 | ⩾41 |
| Åstrand | ⩽21 | 22–26 | 27–35 | 36–39 | ⩾40 |

[a] American Heart Association (1972). *Exercise Testing and Training of Apparently Healthy Individuals: A Handbook for Physicians.* Dallas, TX: American Heart Association.

[b] Cooper, K. H., Pollock, M. L., Wilmore, J. H. & Fox, S. M. (1978). *Health and Fitness through Physical Activity*, New York, NY: John Wiley, pp. 266–85. Original data have been rounded for consistency with the other fitness classification sources.

[c] Åstrand, I. (1960). Aerobic work capacity in men and women with special reference to age. *Acta Physiol. Scand.*, **49** (Suppl. 169). For purposes of comparison, the Åstrand data, originally published in units of $l \cdot min^{-1}$, have been converted to $ml \cdot kg^{-1} \cdot min^{-1}$ by assuming body weights of 72 kg for males and 58 kg for females.

**Table C3.** Fitness categories for females, based on $\dot{V}O_{2max}$ expressed in $ml \cdot kg^{-1} \cdot min^{-1}$

| Age | Low | Fair | Average | Good | High |
|---|---|---|---|---|---|
| **20–29 years** | | | | | |
| AHA[a] | ≤13 | 24–30 | 31–37 | 38–48 | ≥49 |
| Cooper et al.[b] | ≤23 | 24–28 | 29–33 | 34–37 | ≥38 |
| Åstrand[c] | ≤28 | 29–34 | 35–43 | 44–48 | ≥49 |
| **30–39 years** | | | | | |
| AHA | ≤19 | 20–27 | 28–33 | 34–44 | ≥45 |
| Cooper et al. | ≤22 | 23–26 | 27–32 | 33–36 | ≥37 |
| Åstrand | ≤27 | 28–33 | 34–41 | 42–47 | ≥48 |
| **40–49 years** | | | | | |
| AHA | ≤16 | 17–23 | 24–30 | 31–41 | ≥42 |
| Cooper et al. | ≤20 | 21–24 | 25–30 | 31–34 | ≥35 |
| Åstrand | ≤25 | 26–31 | 32–40 | 41–45 | ≥46 |
| **50–59 years** | | | | | |
| AHA | ≤14 | 15–20 | 21–27 | 28–37 | ≥38 |
| Cooper et al. | ≤19 | 20–22 | 23–28 | 29–32 | ≥33 |
| Åstrand | ≤21 | 22–28 | 29–36 | 37–41 | ≥42 |
| **60–69 years** | | | | | |
| AHA | ≤12 | 13–17 | 18–23 | 24–34 | ≥35 |
| Cooper et al. | ≤17 | 18–20 | 21–24 | 25–29 | ≥30 |

[a] American Heart Association (1972). *Exercise Testing and Training of Apparently Healthy Individuals: A Handbook for Physicians.* Dallas, TX: American Heart Association.

[b] Cooper, K. H., Pollock, M. L., Wilmore, J. H. & Fox, S. M. (1978). *Health and Fitness through Physical Activity*, New York, NY: John Wiley, pp. 266–85. Original data have been rounded for consistency with the other fitness classification sources.

[c] Åstrand, I. (1960). Aerobic work capacity in men and women with special reference to age. *Acta Physiol. Scand.*, **49** (Suppl. 169). For purposes of comparison, the Åstrand data, originally published in units of $l \cdot min^{-1}$, have been converted to $ml \cdot kg^{-1} \cdot min^{-1}$ by assuming body weights of 72 kg for males and 58 kg for females.

**Table C4.** Classification of cardiorespiratory fitness based on Cooper 12-minute run test. Values represent distance (miles) run in 12 min

| Age/gender | Very poor | Poor | Fair | Good | Excellent | Superior |
|---|---|---|---|---|---|---|
| **13–19 years** | | | | | | |
| Males | ≤1.29 | 1.30–1.37 | 1.38–1.56 | 1.57–1.72 | 1.73–1.86 | ≥1.87 |
| Females | ≤0.99 | 1.00–1.18 | 1.19–1.29 | 1.30–1.43 | 1.44–1.51 | ≥1.52 |
| **20–29 years** | | | | | | |
| Males | ≤1.21 | 1.22–1.31 | 1.32–1.49 | 1.50–1.64 | 1.65–1.76 | ≥1.77 |
| Females | ≤0.95 | 0.96–1.11 | 1.12–1.22 | 1.23–1.34 | 1.35–1.45 | ≥1.46 |
| **30–39 years** | | | | | | |
| Males | ≤1.17 | 1.18–1.30 | 1.31–1.45 | 1.46–1.56 | 1.57–1.69 | ≥1.70 |
| Females | ≤0.93 | 0.95–1.05 | 1.06–1.18 | 1.19–1.29 | 1.30–1.39 | ≥1.40 |
| **40–49 years** | | | | | | |
| Males | ≤1.13 | 1.14–1.24 | 1.25–1.39 | 1.40–1.53 | 1.54–1.65 | ≥1.66 |
| Females | ≤0.87 | 0.88–0.98 | 0.99–1.11 | 1.12–1.24 | 1.25–1.34 | ≥1.35 |
| **50–59 years** | | | | | | |
| Males | ≤1.02 | 1.03–1.16 | 1.17–1.30 | 1.31–1.44 | 1.45–1.58 | ≥1.59 |
| Females | ≤0.83 | 0.84–0.93 | 0.94–1.05 | 1.06–1.18 | 1.19–1.30 | ≥1.31 |
| **60 years/over** | | | | | | |
| Males | ≤0.86 | 0.87–1.02 | 1.03–1.20 | 1.21–1.32 | 1.33–1.55 | ≥1.56 |
| Females | ≤0.77 | 0.78–0.86 | 0.87–0.98 | 0.99–1.09 | 1.10–1.18 | ≥1.19 |

*Source:* Cooper, K. H. (1982). *The Aerobics Program for Total Well-Being.* New York: Bantam Books/M. Evans.

**Table C5.** Classification of cardiorespiratory fitness based on Cooper 12-minute cycle test (three-speed or less). Values represent distance (miles) cycled in 12 min

| Age/gender | Very poor | Poor | Fair | Good | Excellent |
|---|---|---|---|---|---|
| **13–19 years** | | | | | |
| Males | ⩽2.74 | 2.75–3.74 | 3.75–4.74 | 4.75–5.74 | ⩾5.75 |
| Females | ⩽1.74 | 1.75–2.74 | 2.75–3.74 | 3.75–4.74 | ⩾4.75 |
| **20–29 years** | | | | | |
| Males | ⩽2.49 | 2.50–3.49 | 3.50–4.49 | 4.50–5.49 | ⩾5.50 |
| Females | ⩽1.49 | 1.50–2.49 | 2.50–3.49 | 3.50–4.49 | ⩾4.50 |
| **30–39 years** | | | | | |
| Males | ⩽2.24 | 2.25–3.24 | 3.25–4.24 | 4.25–5.24 | ⩾5.25 |
| Females | ⩽1.24 | 1.25–2.24 | 2.25–3.24 | 3.25–4.24 | ⩾4.25 |
| **40–49 years** | | | | | |
| Males | ⩽1.99 | 2.00–2.99 | 3.00–3.99 | 4.00–4.99 | ⩾5.00 |
| Females | ⩽0.99 | 1.00–1.99 | 2.00–2.99 | 3.00–3.99 | ⩾4.00 |
| **50–59 years** | | | | | |
| Males | ⩽1.74 | 1.75–1.49 | 2.50–3.49 | 3.50–4.49 | ⩾4.50 |
| Females | ⩽0.74 | 0.75–1.49 | 1.50–2.49 | 2.50–3.49 | ⩾3.50 |
| **60 years/over** | | | | | |
| Males | ⩽1.74 | 1.75–2.24 | 2.25–2.99 | 3.00–3.99 | ⩾4.00 |
| Females | ⩽0.74 | 0.75–1.24 | 1.25–1.99 | 2.00–2.99 | ⩾3.00 |

Cycle as far as you can in 12 min in an area where traffic is not a problem. Try to cycle on a hard, flat surface, with the wind (less than 10 m.p.h.), and use a bike with no more than three gears. If the wind is blowing harder than 10 m.p.h., take the test another day. Measure the distance you cycle in 12 min by either the speedometer/odometer on the bike (which may not be accurate) or by another means, such as a car odometer or an engineering wheel.

*Source:* Cooper, K. H. (1982). *The Aerobics Program for Total Well-Being.* New York: Bantam Books/M. Evans.

**Table C6.** Classification of cardiorespiratory fitness based on Cooper 12-minute swimming test. Values represent distance (yards) swum in 12 min

| Age/gender | Very poor | Poor | Fair | Good | Excellent |
|---|---|---|---|---|---|
| **13–19 years** | | | | | |
| Males | ⩽499 | 500–599 | 600–699 | 700–799 | ⩾800 |
| Females | ⩽399 | 400–499 | 500–599 | 600–699 | ⩾700 |
| **20–29 years** | | | | | |
| Males | ⩽399 | 400–499 | 500–599 | 600–699 | ⩾700 |
| Females | ⩽299 | 300–399 | 400–499 | 500–599 | ⩾600 |
| **30–39 years** | | | | | |
| Males | ⩽349 | 350–449 | 450–549 | 550–649 | ⩾650 |
| Females | ⩽249 | 250–349 | 350–449 | 450–549 | ⩾550 |
| **40–49 years** | | | | | |
| Males | ⩽299 | 300–399 | 400–499 | 500–599 | ⩾600 |
| Females | ⩽199 | 200–299 | 300–399 | 400–499 | ⩾500 |
| **50–59 years** | | | | | |
| Males | ⩽249 | 250–349 | 350–449 | 450–549 | ⩾550 |
| Females | ⩽149 | 150–249 | 250–349 | 350–449 | ⩾450 |
| **60 years/over** | | | | | |
| Males | ⩽249 | 250–299 | 300–399 | 400–499 | ⩾500 |
| Females | ⩽149 | 150–199 | 200–299 | 300–399 | ⩾400 |

The swimming test requires you to swim as far as you can in 12 min using whatever stroke you prefer and resting as necessary but trying for a maximum effort. The easiest way to take the test is in a pool with known dimensions and it helps to have another person record the laps and time. Be sure to use a watch with a sweep second hand.
*Source:* Cooper, K. H. (1982). *The Aerobics Program for Total Well-Being.* New York: Bantam Books/M. Evans.

**Table C7.** Classification of cardiorespiratory fitness based on Cooper 1.5-mile run test. Values represent time (min:s) elapsed in completing 1.5 miles

| Age/gender | Very poor | Poor | Fair | Good | Excellent | Superior |
|---|---|---|---|---|---|---|
| **13–19 years** | | | | | | |
| Males | ⩾15:31 | 15:30–12:11 | 12:10–10:49 | 10:48–9:41 | 9:40–8:37 | ⩽8:36 |
| Females | ⩾18:31 | 18:30–16:55 | 16:54–14:31 | 14:30–12:30 | 12:29–11:50 | ⩽11:49 |
| **20–29 years** | | | | | | |
| Males | ⩾16:01 | 16:00–14:01 | 14:00–12:01 | 12:00–10:46 | 10:45–9:45 | ⩽9:44 |
| Females | ⩾19:01 | 18:31–19:00 | 15:55–18:30 | 13:31–15:54 | 12:30–13:30 | ⩽12:29 |
| **30–39 years** | | | | | | |
| Males | ⩾16:31 | 16:30–14:44 | 14:45–12:31 | 12:30–11:01 | 11:00–10:00 | ⩽9:59 |
| Females | ⩾19:31 | 19:01–10:30 | 16:31–19:00 | 14:31–16:30 | 13:00–14:30 | ⩽12:59 |
| **40–49 years** | | | | | | |
| Males | ⩾17:31 | 17:30–15:36 | 15:35–13:01 | 13:00–11:31 | 11:30–10:30 | ⩽10:29 |
| Females | ⩾20:01 | 20:00–19:31 | 19:30–17:31 | 17:30–15:56 | 15:55–13:45 | ⩽13:44 |
| **50–59 years** | | | | | | |
| Males | ⩾19:01 | 19:00–17:01 | 17:00–14:31 | 14:30–12:31 | 12:30–11:00 | ⩽10:59 |
| Females | ⩾20:31 | 20:30–20:01 | 20:00–19:01 | 19:00–16:31 | 16:30–14:30 | ⩽14:29 |
| **60 years/over** | | | | | | |
| Males | ⩾20:01 | 20:00–19:01 | 19:00–16:16 | 16:15–14:00 | 13:59–11:15 | ⩽11:14 |
| Females | ⩾21:01 | 21:31–21:00 | 20:30–19:31 | 19:30–17:30 | 17:30–16:30 | ⩽16:29 |

*Source:* Cooper, K. H. (1982). *The Aerobics Program for Total Well-Being.* New York: Bantam Books/M. Evans.

**Table C8.** Classification of cardiorespiratory fitness based on Cooper 3-mile walk test. Values represent time (min:s) to complete 3-mile walk

| Age/gender | Very poor | Poor | Fair | Good | Excellent |
|---|---|---|---|---|---|
| **13–19 years** | | | | | |
| Males | ⩾45:01 | 45:00–41:01 | 41:00–37:31 | 37:30–33:00 | ⩽32:59 |
| Females | ⩾47:01 | 47:00–43:01 | 43:00–39:31 | 39:30–35:00 | ⩽34:59 |
| **20–29 years** | | | | | |
| Males | ⩾46:01 | 46:00–42:01 | 42:00–38:31 | 38:30–34:00 | ⩽33:59 |
| Females | ⩾48:01 | 48:00–44:01 | 44:00–40:31 | 40:30–36:00 | ⩽35:59 |
| **30–39 years** | | | | | |
| Males | ⩾49:01 | 49:00–44:31 | 44:30–40:01 | 40:00–35:00 | ⩽34:59 |
| Females | ⩾51:01 | 51:00–46:31 | 46:30–42:01 | 42:00–37:30 | ⩽37:29 |
| **40–49 years** | | | | | |
| Males | ⩾52:01 | 52:00–47:01 | 47:00–42:01 | 42:00–36:30 | ⩽36:29 |
| Females | ⩾54:01 | 54:00–49:01 | 49:00–44:01 | 44:00–39:00 | ⩽38:59 |
| **50–59 years** | | | | | |
| Males | ⩾55:01 | 55:00–50:01 | 50:00–45:01 | 45:00–39:00 | ⩽38:59 |
| Females | ⩾57:01 | 57:00–52:01 | 52:00–47:01 | 47:00–42:00 | ⩽41:59 |
| **60 years/over** | | | | | |
| Males | ⩾60:01 | 60:00–54:01 | 54:00–48:01 | 48:00–41:00 | ⩽40:59 |
| Females | ⩾63:01 | 63:00–57:01 | 57:00–51:01 | 51:00–45:00 | ⩽44:59 |

The walking test requires participants to cover 3 miles in the fastest time possible without running.
*Source:* Cooper, K. H. (1982). *The Aerobics Program for Total Well-Being.* New York: Bantam Books/M. Evans.

**Table C9.** Predicted $\dot{V}o_{2max}$ ($ml \cdot kg^{-1} \cdot min^{-1}$) based on the Cooper's qualitative categories

| Age/gender | Very poor | Poor | Fair | Good | Excellent | Superior |
|---|---|---|---|---|---|---|
| **13–19 years** | | | | | | |
| Males | ⩽34.9 | 35.0–38.3 | 38.4–45.1 | 45.2–50.9 | 51.0–55.9 | ⩾56.0 |
| Females | ⩽24.9 | 25.0–30.9 | 31.0–34.9 | 35.0–38.9 | 39.0–41.9 | ⩾42.0 |
| **20–29 years** | | | | | | |
| Males | ⩽32.9 | 33.0–36.4 | 36.5–42.4 | 42.5–46.4 | 46.5–52.4 | ⩾52.5 |
| Females | ⩽23.5 | 23.6–28.9 | 29.0–32.9 | 33.0–36.9 | 37.0–40.9 | ⩾41.0 |
| **30–39 years** | | | | | | |
| Males | ⩽31.4 | 31.5–35.4 | 35.5–40.9 | 41.0–44.9 | 45.0–49.4 | ⩾49.5 |
| Females | ⩽22.7 | 22.8–26.9 | 27.0–31.4 | 31.5–35.6 | 35.7–40.0 | ⩾40.1 |
| **40–49 years** | | | | | | |
| Males | ⩽30.1 | 30.2–33.5 | 33.6–38.9 | 39.0–43.7 | 43.8–48.0 | ⩾48.1 |
| Females | ⩽20.9 | 21.0–24.4 | 24.5–28.9 | 29.0–32.8 | 32.9–36.9 | ⩾37.0 |
| **50–59 years** | | | | | | |
| Males | ⩽26.0 | 26.1–30.9 | 31.0–35.7 | 35.8–40.9 | 41.0–45.3 | ⩾45.4 |
| Females | ⩽20.1 | 20.2–22.7 | 22.8–26.9 | 27.0–31.4 | 31.5–35.7 | ⩾35.8 |
| **60 years/over** | | | | | | |
| Males | ⩽20.4 | 20.5–26.0 | 26.1–32.2 | 32.2–36.4 | 36.5–44.2 | ⩾44.3 |
| Females | ⩽17.4 | 17.5–20.1 | 20.2–24.4 | 24.5–30.2 | 30.3–31.4 | ⩾31.5 |

*Source:* Cooper, K. H. (1982). *The Aerobics Program for Total Well-Being.* New York: Bantam Books/M. Evans.

**Table C10.** Assessment of operative risk for thoracic surgery by exercise testing

| | Low | Intermediate | High | Very high |
|---|---|---|---|---|
| $\dot{V}O_{2max}$ ($l \cdot min^{-1}$) | ⩾1.50 | 1.49–1.00 | ⩽0.99 | |
| | | C 0%[a] | C 70%[a] | |
| $\dot{V}O_{2max}$ ($ml \cdot kg^{-1} \cdot min^{-1}$) | ⩾20 | 19–15 | 14–10[d] | ⩽9 |
| | C 10%[b] | Mt 0%; Mb 0%[c] | Mt 0%; Mb 11%[c]; C 100%[b] | Mt 29%; Mb 43%[c] |
| $\dot{V}O_2\theta$ ($ml \cdot kg^{-1} \cdot min^{-1}$) | ⩾15 | 14–10 | ⩽9 | |
| | | Mt 1%[e] | Mt 18%[e] | |
| $\dot{V}O_2/f_{Cmax}$ (ml) | ⩾10.0 | | ⩽9.9 | |
| | C 0%[d] | | C 100%[d] | |

where Mt is mortality, Mb is morbidity, C is a complication.

[a] Eugene, J., Brown, S. E., Light, R. W., Milne, N. E. & Stemmer, E. A. (1982). Maximum oxygen consumption: a physiologic guide to pulmonary resection. *Surg. Forum*, **33**, 260–2.

[b] Smith, T. P., Kinasewitz, G. T., Tucker, W. Y., Spillers, W. P. & George, R. B. (1984). Exercise capacity as a predictor of post-thoracotomy morbidity. *Am. Rev. Respir. Dis.*, **129**, 730–4.

[c] Bechard, D. & Westein, L. (1987). Assessment of exercise oxygen consumption as preoperative criterion for lung resection. *Ann. Thorac. Surg.*, **44**, 344–9.

[d] Epstein, S. K., Faling, L. J., Daly, B. D. T. & Celli, B. R. (1993). Predicting complications after pulmonary surgery. *Chest*, **104**, 694–700.

[e] Older, P., Smith, R., Courtney, P. & Hone, R. (1993). Preoperative evaluation of cardiac failure and ischemia in elderly patients by cardiopulmonary exercise texting.

**Table C11.** Effect of cadence (r.p.m.) errors on work rate ($\dot{W}$) and the oxygen uptake ($\dot{V}O_2$) that may be predicted from those work rates

| | r.p.m. | | | Work rate ($\dot{W}$) | | |
|---|---|---|---|---|---|---|
| Load (kp) | Assumed value ($min^{-1}$) | Actual value ($min^{-1}$) | Flywheel circumference (m) | Assumed value (W) | Actual value (W) | Error (%) |
| 2 | 60 | 59 | 6 | 117.6 | 115.7 | −2 |
| 2 | 60 | 58 | 6 | 117.6 | 113.7 | −3 |
| 2 | 60 | 57 | 6 | 117.6 | 111.8 | −5 |
| 2 | 60 | 56 | 6 | 117.6 | 109.8 | −7 |
| 2 | 60 | 55 | 6 | 117.6 | 107.8 | −8 |
| 2 | 60 | 54 | 6 | 117.6 | 105.9 | −10 |

Thus, a counting error of 6 r.p.m. will result in over- or underestimating the actual work rate by 10%. This error may obscure any real gain in $\dot{V}O_{2max}$ as determined from tests predicting that value from work rate and heart rate.

# Appendix D Protocols and supplemental materials

**Table D1.** Balke treadmill protocol

| Stage | Time (min) | Speed (m.p.h.) | Grade (%) | $\dot{V}O_2$ (ml · kg$^{-1}$ · min$^{-1}$) | METs | Change in $\dot{V}O_2$ (ml · kg$^{-1}$ · min$^{-1}$) |
|---|---|---|---|---|---|---|
| 1 | 1 | 3.3 | 1 | 13.9 | 4 | 0 |
| 2 | 1 | 3.3 | 2 | 15.5 | 4.4 | 1.6 |
| 3 | 1 | 3.3 | 3 | 17.1 | 4.9 | 1.6 |
| 4 | 1 | 3.3 | 4 | 18.7 | 5.3 | 1.6 |
| 5 | 1 | 3.3 | 5 | 20.3 | 5.8 | 1.6 |
| 6 | 1 | 3.3 | 6 | 21.9 | 6.3 | 1.6 |
| 7 | 1 | 3.3 | 7 | 23.5 | 6.7 | 1.6 |
| 8 | 1 | 3.3 | 8 | 25.1 | 7.2 | 1.6 |
| 9 | 1 | 3.3 | 9 | 26.7 | 7.6 | 1.6 |
| 10 | 1 | 3.3 | 10 | 28.3 | 8.1 | 1.6 |
| 11 | 1 | 3.3 | 11 | 29.9 | 8.5 | 1.6 |
| 12 | 1 | 3.3 | 12 | 31.4 | 9.0 | 1.6 |
| 13 | 1 | 3.3 | 13 | 33.0 | 9.4 | 1.6 |
| 14 | 1 | 3.3 | 14 | 34.6 | 9.9 | 1.6 |
| 15 | 1 | 3.3 | 15 | 36.2 | 10.3 | 1.6 |
| 16 | 1 | 3.3 | 16 | 37.8 | 10.8 | 1.6 |
| 17 | 1 | 3.3 | 17 | 39.4 | 11.3 | 1.6 |
| 18 | 1 | 3.3 | 18 | 41.0 | 11.7 | 1.6 |
| 19 | 1 | 3.3 | 19 | 42.6 | 12.2 | 1.6 |
| 20 | 1 | 3.3 | 20 | 44.2 | 12.6 | 1.6 |

This table indicates 20 possible stages for the original Balke protocol. The treadmill speed is kept constant, at 3.3 m.p.h. (88.4 m · min$^{-1}$). Note that the increments in expected $VO_2$ are equal and relatively small (1.6 ml · kg$^{-1}$ · min$^{-1}$), entirely due to the change in grade. While this protocol may be appropriate for older, deconditioned, or patient groups, it is too long for more fit populations. As suggested in Chapter 3, an exercise test protocol should be chosen so that it terminates in 8–12 min for each subject. Many modifications of this 1-min incremental protocol have been developed in which the speed and/or grade is changed to achieve the 8–12-min termination time. Figure D4 illustrates how to develop a spreadsheet that will calculate an appropriate grade increment based on treadmill speed, desired protocol duration, and a reference value for $VO_{2max}$.

**Table D2.** Bruce treadmill protocol

| Stage | Time (min) | Speed (m.p.h.) | Speed (m · min⁻¹) | Grade (%) | $\dot{V}o_2$ (ml · kg$^{-1}$ · min$^{-1}$) | METs | Change in $\dot{V}o_2$ (ml · kg$^{-1}$ · min$^{-1}$) |
|---|---|---|---|---|---|---|---|
| Ia | 3 | 1.7 | 45.6 | 0 | 8.1 | 2.3 | 0 |
| Ib | 3 | 1.7 | 45.6 | 5 | 12.2 | 3.5 | 4.1 |
| Ic | 3 | 1.7 | 45.6 | 10 | 16.3 | 4.6 | 4.1 |
| II | 3 | 2.5 | 67.0 | 12 | 24.7 | 7.0 | 8.4 |
| III | 3 | 3.4 | 91.1 | 14 | 35.6 | 10.2 | 10.9 |
| IV | 3 | 4.2 | 112.6 | 16 | 47.2 | 13.5 | 11.6 |
| V | 3 | 5.0 | 134.0 | 18 | 52.0 | 14.9 | 4.8 |
| VI | 3 | 5.5 | 147.4 | 20 | 59.5 | 17.0 | 7.5 |

The Bruce treadmill protocol is the most frequently used treadmill protocol in clinical exercise testing. This table contains both the standard Bruce protocol (stages I–VI) and a modified version designed for patient groups (stages Ia–Ic and beyond). The protocol may be continued with additional 3-min stages in which speed is increased 0.5 m.p.h. (13.4 m · min$^{-1}$) and 2% grade for each stage. The protocol has unequal increments in $\dot{V}o_2$ and may produce uncomfortable walking/running conditions due to awkward speeds (4.2 m.p.h.) and steep grades, the latter possibly causing calf or low back pain. The 3-min stages may obscure detection of the metabolic threshold as compared to protocols with 1-min stages.

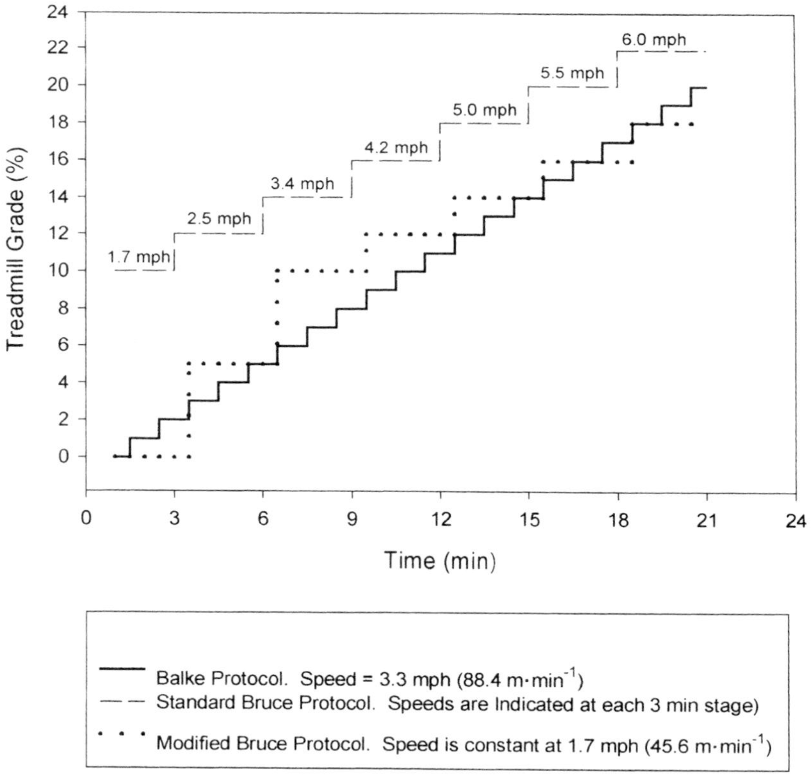


**Figure D1** The Balke, standard Bruce, and modified Bruce treadmill protocols.

## Standard instructions for the 6-minute walk test

The following or similar narrative should be used prior to the administration of each 6-minute walk test so that every patient receives the same instructions each time the test is administered. The narrative is best recorded on audiotape and played to the subject immediately before every test.

*This is a 6-minute walking test. Before you start, please listen carefully to the following instructions. During this test you should try to walk as far as you possibly can in 6 minutes. You can choose your walking pace according to how you feel but try to achieve a steady pace throughout the test. Do not be concerned if you have to slow down or stop to rest. If you do stop to rest, try to start walking again as soon as possible. Remember that the goal of this test is to cover as much distance as possible in 6 minutes. I will start timing your walk as soon as you begin. Please start walking now.*

## Blood pressure measurement procedures

Subjects should have been allowed to rest (seated, with feet flat on the floor) for at least 5 min before blood pressure measurements are obtained.

1. Obtain measurements with the subject in a relaxed, comfortable position with the arm bare (*do not apply the cuff or stethoscope head over clothing*).
2. Choose the correct cuff size for the size of the subject's arm.
3. The bladder width should encircle 40% of the circumference of the arm. Table D3 will assist the user in choosing the correct cuff size based on measurement of the subject's arm circumference.
4. Palpate and, if necessary, mark the brachial artery in the antecubital fossa.
5. Apply the correct-size cuff to the arm with the bladder centered over the brachial artery. Leave about 2 cm (1 in.) between the bottom of the cuff and the brachial artery. *Do not apply over clothing.* If sleeves are rolled up, be sure that they are not too tight as this will yield inaccurate readings.
6. Estimate the systolic pressure by palpating the radial or brachial pulse as you inflate the cuff. Note the pressure on the manometer when the palpated pulse disappears. Record and wait 30 s.
7. Insert stethoscope earpieces. Remember to turn earpieces slightly forward to facilitate fit in the outer ear canals.
8. Place the bell head of the stethoscope over the brachial artery with light pressure.
9. Elevate the arm to heart level.
10. After the 30-s pause, inflate the cuff again to a level 30 mmHg above the pressure at which the palpated pulse disappeared.
11. Deflate the cuff slowly at a rate of $2\ \mathrm{mmHg \cdot s^{-1}}$, allowing the mercury column to fall completely to zero. *Do not reinflate during the course of a measurement.*
12. Record the pressure at which you hear the first blood pressure sounds for two consecutive beats. This "onset of sounds" (K1) represents the systolic blood pressure.
13. Record the pressure at which the sounds disappear (K5) as the diastolic blood pressure.
14. Wait 1–2 min, then repeat steps 8–13 in the same arm.
15. Repeat steps 4–13 in the opposite arm.
16. If you have difficulty hearing a blood pressure, deflate the cuff to zero and wait 30 s. Reinflate the cuff with the participant's arm raised above her/his head. Lower the arm to heart level, apply stethoscope and proceed from step 10.
17. Record both blood pressure measurements for each arm on the data sheet.
18. Inform the subject of the results. Use Table D4 to indicate whether the blood pressure is within desirable limits *on this particular day.*

**Table D3.** Guide to assist in choosing correct sphygmomanometer cuff size

| | | | |
|---|---|---|---|
| Cuff width (cm) | 12 | 15 | 18 |
| Ideal arm circumference (cm) | 30.0 | 37.5 | 45.0 |
| Arm circumference range (cm) | 26–33 | 33–41 | >41 |

**Table D4.** Desirable upper limits for systemic arterial systolic and blood pressures

| Age range (years) | Desirable limits for blood pressure (mmHg) |
|---|---|
| Adults | ≤140/90 |
| Ages 14–18 | ≤135/90 |
| Ages 10–14 | ≤125/85 |
| Ages 6–10 | ≤120/80 |
| Less than age 6 | ≤110/75 |

## Calibration of Monark cycle ergometer

**Table D5.** Cycle ergometer calibration data sheet

| Calibration weight (kg) | Sector reading Date | Date | Date |
|---|---|---|---|
| 0.5 | | | |
| 1.0 | | | |
| 1.5 | | | |
| 2.0 | | | |
| 2.5 | | | |
| 3.0 | | | |
| 3.5 | | | |
| 4.0 | | | |
| 4.5 | | | |
| 6.0 | | | |
| 6.5 | | | |
| 7.0 | | | |

Among the most common mechanically braked ergometers used in laboratory settings today is the Monark ergometer. Developed by von Döbeln nearly 50 years ago, this ergometer uses gravity and a known mass to indicate the workload. Calibration procedures for this common ergometer are presented here and require only about 5 min to complete. The following will be needed:

1. Set of calibration weights of at least the following configuration:
   (a) one 500-g weight (0.5 kg).
   (b) several (four would be ideal) 1-kg weights.
   (c) one 5-kg weight.
2. A thin cord, wire, or a piece of a clothes hanger from which to hang the calibration weights.
3. A data sheet to record your measurements.

### Procedures

Refer to Figure D2.

1. Remove the lower end of the friction belt from the spring by loosening the tension knob.
2. Ensure that the pendulum hangs freely.
3. Adjust the marked sector so that the red index line on the pendulum lines up exactly with the "0" mark on the sector.

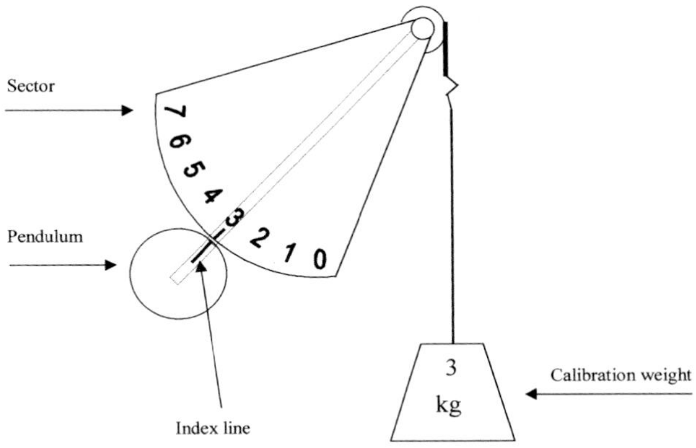


**Figure D2** Calibration of a mechanically braked cycle ergometer.

4. Hang one of the calibration weights from the belt hanging over the pulley wheel.
5. The pendulum will now move away from gravity and should line up with the mark on the sector corresponding to the weight. For example, a 3-kg weight should line up with the "3" mark on the sector.
6. Repeat these procedures for weights ranging between 0.5 kg and 7 kg, recording results on the data sheet (Table D5).
7. Before making any adjustment, make sure that the weight is hanging freely, the pendulum is hanging freely, and the initial position of the index line on the pendulum is actually at "0" on the sector.
8. If necessary, the center of gravity of the pendulum weight may be moved up or down (move down if the index line on the pendulum is *above* the sector mark corresponding to the calibration weight).

   ***Note:*** *The above procedures are known as static calibration and do not take into account friction resistance offered by the cycle's drive train, i.e., the chain, sprocket, bearings, and bottom bracket. Performing regular maintenance and lubrication of these moving parts can minimize these sources of error. Dynamic calibration may also be performed using a dynamic torque meter (see Chapter 2).*

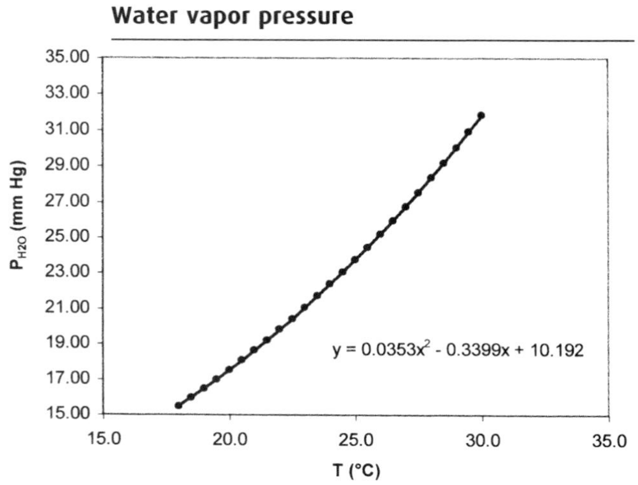


**Figure D3** Regression of water vapor pressures at different temperatures between 18°C and 30°C. Data points were fitted with a second-order polynomial to yield the equation shown.

The plot of $P_{H_2O}$ versus gas temperature, shown in Figure D3, is well fit with a second-order polynomial with the equation

$$y = 0.0353x^2 - 0.3399x + 10.192 \quad \text{(D1)}$$

This equation may be conveniently used in calculators or spreadsheets for calculating BTPS and STPD gas correction factors with no loss in precision (Table D6).

**Table D6.** Water vapor pressure ($P_{H_2O}$) of saturated gas at various temperatures (°C)

| Gas temperature (°C) | $P_{H_2O}$ (mmHg) | Gas temperature (°C) | $P_{H_2O}$ (mmHg) |
|---|---|---|---|
| 18.0 | 15.48 | 24.5 | 23.06 |
| 18.5 | 15.97 | 25.0 | 23.76 |
| 19.0 | 16.48 | 25.5 | 24.47 |
| 19.5 | 17.00 | 26.0 | 25.21 |
| 20.0 | 17.54 | 26.5 | 25.96 |
| 20.5 | 18.08 | 27.0 | 26.74 |
| 21.0 | 18.65 | 27.5 | 27.54 |
| 21.5 | 19.23 | 28.0 | 28.35 |
| 22.0 | 19.83 | 28.5 | 29.18 |
| 22.5 | 20.44 | 29.0 | 30.04 |
| 23.0 | 21.07 | 29.5 | 30.92 |
| 23.5 | 21.71 | 30.0 | 31.82 |
| 24.0 | 22.38 | 37.0 | 47.00 |

## Detailed crash cart contents

Although the arrangement of supplies can be varied to suit the practitioners' particular needs and preferences, the following contains a workable and complete list of crash cart contents suitable for most exercise-testing applications.

### Top of cart

Contaminated needle box
Defibrillator with two rolls of extra paper
Electrolyte gel for defibrillator
1 package defibrillation/pacing pads
1 small package ECG electrodes
Gloves, mask, eye shield
Intubation tray
Electrical suction pump (or connection to wall suction)
Suction canister
Suction connecting tubing

### Left side of cart

Ambu bag with trach adapter
IV pole (attached to cart)
$O_2$ mask with tubing
E-size oxygen cylinder (or connection to wall-piped oxygen)
Two-stage regulator for oxygen tank
$O_2$ flow meter
Tank wrench

### Back of cart

CPR board
Clipboard with 1 arrest form
Crash cart supply list

### First Drawer

This drawer contains crash cart medications. One way to arrange these contents is by purpose, i.e., drugs to correct dysrhythmias, drugs to increase blood pressure and cardiac output, drugs to increase heart rate, etc. (Table D7).

### Second drawer

Alcohol and iodine (Betadine) swabs
3 blood gas kits
5 green IV labels
10 gummed labels, plain
Needles:
  10 18-gauge by 1.5 in.
  4 22-gauge by 4 in. spinal needles
  15 20-gauge by 1 in.
  10 22-gauge by 1 in.
5 iodine (povidone) ointment packs
5 sterile $H_2O$, 30 ml
5 sterile saline, 30 ml
Syringes, 3 ml (2); 10 ml (10); 20 ml (2); TB (5)
5 heplock
5 multidose adapters
5 interlink syringe cannula
5 Leuer-lock cannula

### Third drawer

5 each 2 × 2 and 4 × 4 gauze sponges
Blood sample tubes, 3 each
  red top: 10 and 15 ml
  green top: 7 ml
  blue top: 4.5 ml
  lavender top: 7 ml
  corvac: 7 ml
Butterfly/scalp vein needles 2 each – 19 and 21 gauge
4 ECG monitoring electrodes
2 irrigating syringes (60 ml)
IV catheters, 3 each; 16 gauge, 18 gauge and 20 gauge
3 IV start kits
1 tube lidocaine jelly
1 bottle Betadine
4 suction kits 14–16 Fr.
1 Yankauer suction tip
3 tourniquets
Tape: 2 rolls each 1 and 2 in. size
  Paper, plastic, and adhesive
3 liquid adhesive, single dose

### Fourth drawer

Sterile gloves sizes 6.5 through 8.5
2 Kelly clamps (disposable)

**Table D7.** Drugs recommended for a crash cart listed alphabetically by proprietary name

| Drug | Quantity | Amount | Strength |
|---|---|---|---|
| Aminophylline 250 mg | 1 | 10 ml vial | $25\,mg \cdot ml^{-1}$ |
| Atropine 1 mg | 4 | 10 ml syringe | $0.1\,mg \cdot ml^{-1}$ |
| Calcium chloride 1 g | 2 | 10 ml syringe | $100\,mg \cdot ml^{-1}$ |
| Dextrose 50% | 2 | 50 ml | $25\,g \cdot 50\,ml^{-1}$ |
| Diazepam 10 mg/2 ml | 1 | 2 ml vial | $5\,mg \cdot ml^{-1}$ |
| Diphenhydramine 50 mg $ml^{-1}$ | 1 | 1 ml vial | $50\,mg \cdot ml^{-1}$ |
| Dopamine (premixed bag) | 1 | 400 mg/250 ml D5W | $16\,mg \cdot ml^{-1}$ |
| Epinephrine 1:1000 | 1 | 1 ml amp | $1\,mg \cdot ml^{-1}$ |
| Epinephrine 1:1000 | 1 | 30 ml vial | $1\,mg \cdot ml^{-1}$ |
| Epinephrine 1:10 000 (1 mg) | 5 | 10 ml $1\frac{1}{2}$ in. short needle | 1 mg/10 ml |
| Flumazenil 0.5 mg | 1 | 5 ml vial | $0.1\,mg \cdot ml^{-1}$ |
| Furosemide 100 mg | 1 | 10 ml vial | $10\,mg \cdot ml^{-1}$ |
| Isoproterenol 1 mg | 1 | 5 ml amp | 1 mg/5 ml |
| Lidocaine (premixed bag) | 1 | 2 g/250 ml D5W | $8\,mg \cdot ml^{-1}$ |
| Lidocaine 100 mg | 3 | 5 ml syringe | $20\,mg \cdot ml^{-1}$ |
| Magnesium sulfate 50% (5 g) (must be diluted) | 1 | 10 ml vial | 5 g/10 ml |
| Methylprednisolone 1 g | 1 | 8 ml vial | 1 g/8 ml |
| Midazolam 2 mg/2 ml | 2 | 2 ml vial | $1\,mg \cdot ml^{-1}$ |
| Naloxone 0.4 mg | 2 | 1 ml vial | $0.4\,mg \cdot ml^{-1}$ |
| Norepinephrine 4 mg | 2 | 4 ml amp | $1\,mg \cdot ml^{-1}$ |
| Procainamide 1 g | 2 | 10 ml vial | $100\,mg \cdot ml^{-1}$ |
| Sodium bicarbonate 8.4% | 2 | 50 ml syringe | $1\,mmol \cdot l^{-1} \cdot ml^{-1}$ |
| Sodium chloride | 4 | 10 ml vial | 0.9% (normal) |
| Verapamil 5 mg/2 ml | 2 | 2 ml vial | 5 mg/2 ml |

1 suture scissors (disposable)
2 5-in-1 connectors
1 razor
Silk suture, 2 each; 2-0, 3-0, 4-0
1 Salem sump tube, no. 16
5 surgical lubricant
Scalpels no. 11 and no. 15 (disposable)
1 chest tube clamp
Oral airways (small, medium, large)
1 nasal airway (no. 7)
2 sterile towels

### Fifth drawer

IV solutions
- 2 50 cc 5% dextrose in water (D5W)
- 2 500 cc 5% dextrose in water (D5W)
- 1 1000 cc % dextrose in water (D5W)
- 3 500 cc 0.9% (normal) saline
- 2 250 cc % dextrose in water (D5W)

2 3-way stopcocks
2 dual injection sets
4 macro tubing sets
3 mini drip sets
2 "Y" blood recipient sets and 80 μm blood sets
4 long extension sets
1 blood set with pump
1 pressure bag
1 flashlight with 2 extra batteries (date all batteries)
1 Long armboard

### Bottom shelf

1 thorocotomy tray
1 trach tray
1 cut-down tray
1 Foley tray with cath no. 14
Manual blood pressure cuff
Extension cord
Pacemaker box

**Table D8.** Potential errors in the principal derived variables with given errors in the primary or measured variables

| | | Error in derived variables | | | |
|---|---|---|---|---|---|
| Primary variable | Measurement error | $\dot{V}_{E,BTPS}$ | $\dot{V}O_{2,STPD}$ | $\dot{V}CO_{2,STPD}$ | $R$ |
| $\dot{V}_{E,ATPS}$ | +5% | +5.0% | +5.0% | +5.0% | 0.0% |
| $F_{\bar{E}}O_2$ | +0.01 | 0.0% | −1.3%[a] | 0.0%[a] | +1.3% |
| $F_{\bar{E}}CO_2$ | +0.01 | 0.0% | −0.3%[a] | +1.0%[a] | +1.3% |
| $T$ | +1°C | −0.5% | −0.5% | −0.5% | 0.0% |
| $P_B$ | +5 mmHg | 0.0% | +0.67% | +0.67% | 0.0% |

[a] These percentage errors must be multiplied by $V_{E,ATPS}$ to obtain absolute errors in $\dot{V}O_2$ and $\dot{V}CO_2$.

This table illustrates an error analysis for the calculation of $\dot{V}_E$, $\dot{V}O_2$, $\dot{V}CO_2$, and $R$ from the primary or measured variables required for these calculations. Note that for the purposes of this analysis $\dot{V}_{E,ATPS}$ is considered as a primary variable although actually it is derived from measurements of $V_T$ and $f_R$. The combined effects of simultaneous errors in more than one measurement are not shown.

**Important points**

1. Errors in the measurement of $\dot{V}_{E,ATPS}$ produce proportional errors in $\dot{V}_{E,BTPS}$, $\dot{V}O_2$ and $\dot{V}CO_2$.
2. The greatest potential for errors lies in the effect of measurement of $F_{\bar{E}}O_2$ and $F_{\bar{E}}CO_2$ on $\dot{V}O_2$ and $\dot{V}CO_2$ respectively. Furthermore, these errors increase in proportion to minute ventilation.
3. Modest errors in the measurement of $T$ and $P_B$ produce only small errors in the derived variables.

**Example:** At a minute ventilation ($\dot{V}_{E,ATPS}$) of 60 l · min$^{-1}$ an error of +0.01 (absolute error of +1%) in the measurement of $F_{\bar{E}}O_2$ will result in a 0.78 l · min$^{-1}$ *under*estimate of $VO_2$ (error=1.3% multiplied by 60). If the true value of $\dot{V}O_2$ in this example is 2.23 l · min$^{-1}$ then the measured value will be 1.45 l · min$^{-1}$ which represents an absolute error of 35%. Similarly, an error of +0.01 (absolute error of +1%) in the measurement of $F_{\bar{E}}CO_2$ will result in a 0.60 l · min$^{-1}$ *over*estimate of $\dot{V}CO_2$ (error=1% multiplied by 60). If the true value of $\dot{V}CO_2$ in this example is 2.50 l · min$^{-1}$, then the measured value will be 3.10 l · min$^{-1}$, which represents an absolute error of 24%.

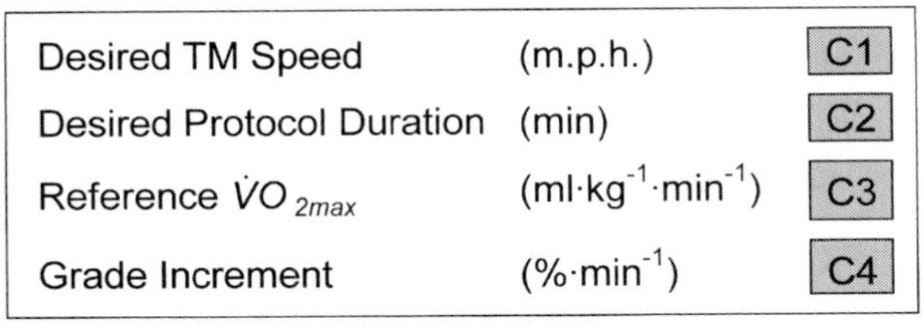
Desired TM Speed (m.p.h.) C1
Desired Protocol Duration (min) C2
Reference $\dot{V}O_{2max}$ (ml·kg$^{-1}$·min$^{-1}$) C3
Grade Increment (%·min$^{-1}$) C4

**Figure D4** Simple computer spreadsheet for the calculation of grade increments for a treadmill protocol using fixed walking speeds of 50–100 m · min$^{-1}$ (1.9–3.7 m.p.h.). Create the spreadsheet as shown in this figure then calculate the optimal grade increment by the following steps: (a) Enter the desired treadmill speed (m.p.h.) in cell C1. (b) Enter the desired protocol duration (usually 10 min) in cell C2. (c) Enter a reference value for $\dot{V}O_{2max}$ (ml · kg$^{-1}$ · min$^{-1}$) in cell C3. (d) Enter the following equation in cell C4 to show the optimal grade increment:=(C3–(C1*26.8*0.1)–3.5)/(C1*26.8*1.8)*100)/C2.

## Informed consent

The informed consent is an important part of the preliminary testing procedures. This document is designed to provide subjects or patients with adequate information about the testing procedures so that their consent to participate is *informed.* It is recommended that all subjects or patients read, understand, agree to, and sign the informed consent before testing. The informed consent should be documented and preserved. Since laws vary from state to state, individualized legal advice should be sought before adopting any form.

The basic elements of the informed consent include:

1. The content of the explanation of the test adequately and fairly describes its nature, including an identification of those procedures which are experimental.
2. A description of the procedures with an explanation of the potential risks and discomforts.
3. A description of the benefits to be expected either to the individual or to society.
4. When applicable, appropriate alternatives to having an exercise test that would be advantageous to the individual should be disclosed.
5. The explanation should be terms that a lay person can fully understand.
6. An offer should be provided to answer any inquiries concerning the procedures.
7. It must be made clear that participation is voluntary and that an individual may withdraw consent and discontinue participation any time without prejudice.
8. Compensation for participation should not constitute an undue inducement to participate in a procedure.
9. Consent should not include any exculpatory language through which the subject is made to waive, or appear to waive, any legal rights or to release the institution or its agents from liability or negligence.
10. Statements on privacy and confidentiality indicating that no information provided by the subject will be disclosed to others without the subject's written permission. Exceptions to privacy and confidentiality may be required if necessary to protect subjects' rights and/or safety (e.g., if injured) or if required by law.
11. A statement of emergency care and compensation that will be provided if the procedure results in an injury.
12. A statement indicating that the practitioner may abort the test if best judgment so indicates.

## Exercise Test Preparation

| |
|---|
| ***APPOINTMENT TIME:*** ______________________ ***DATE:*** ____________________ |

Dear ______________________________

Your exercise test is scheduled at the above time. Please be prompt and prepare for this test as indicated below. Please plan on this appointment lasting between 30 and 60 minutes.

*In order to ensure the utmost in accuracy we ask that you comply with the following:*

### Pre-Test Instructions

Be sure that you are rested. If you exercise the day before the test, be sure it is of light to moderate intensity and relatively short duration. You should not exercise within 12 hours of your test.

You should not have eaten within 3-4 hours of the test. However, it is important that a light meal such as fruit, juice, and/or unsweetened cereal be consumed to maintain adequate blood sugar levels.

Avoid alcohol, caffeine, and tobacco within 8 hours of the test.

Be sure you are adequately hydrated. Drink plenty of water during the hours before the test.

Wear loose fitting, comfortable clothing and appropriate footwear for exercise.

Do ___ Do NOT ___ discontinue the following medications: ________________________________________

for __________ hours/days before your scheduled appointment.

### Additional Preparation and Instructions:

Upon your arrival, you will be given a medical history questionnaire and a consent form. Please be sure to have all necessary information available such as social security number, drivers license number, and insurance information.

If you must cancel or reschedule your test, please do so at least 48 hours in advance.

I have read, understand, and agree to the above guidelines and policies.

______________________ __________

Signature Date

## Physical Activity Readiness Questionnaire (PAR-Q)

**Regular physical activity is fun and healthy, and increasingly more people are starting to become more active every day. Being more active is very safe for most people. However, some people should check with their doctor before they start becoming much more physically active.**

If you are planning to become much more physically active than you are now, start by answering the seven questions in the box below. If you are between the ages of 15 and 69, the PAR-Q will tell you if you should check with your doctor before you start. If you are over 69 years of age, and you are not used to being very active, Check with your doctor.

Common sense is your best guide when you answer these questions. Please read the questions carefully and answer each one honestly:
Check YES or NO

| YES | NO | |
|---|---|---|
| ☐ | ☐ | 1. Has a doctor ever said that you have a heart condition and recommended only medically supervised activity? |
| ☐ | ☐ | 2. Do you have chest pain brought on by physical activity? |
| ☐ | ☐ | 3. Have you developed chest pain in the past month? |
| ☐ | ☐ | 4. Have you on 1 or more occasions lost consciousness or fallen over as a result of dizziness? |
| ☐ | ☐ | 5. Do you have a bone or joint problem that could be aggravated by the proposed physical activity? |
| ☐ | ☐ | 6. Has a doctor ever recommended medication for your blood pressure or a heart condition? |
| ☐ | ☐ | 7. Are you aware, through your own experience or a doctor's advice, of any other physical reason that would prohibit you from exercising without medical supervision |

**If you answered YES to one or more questions:**

Talk with your doctor by phone or in person BEFORE you start becoming much more physically active or BEFORE you have a fitness appraisal. Tell your doctor about this PAR-Q and which questions you answered YES.

- You may be able to do any activity you want—as long as you start slowly and build up gradually. Or, you may need to restrict your activities to those which are safe for you. Talk with your doctor about the kinds of activities you wish to participate in and follow his/her advice.

**If you answered NO to all questions:**

If you answered NO honestly to <u>all</u> PAR-Q questions, you can be reasonably sure that you can:

- start becoming much more physically active – begin slowly and build-up gradually. This is the safest and easiest way to go.
- Take part in a fitness appraisal – this is an excellent way to determine your basic fitness so that you can plan the best way for you to live actively.

**DELAY becoming much more active:**

- If you are not feeling well because of a temporary illness such as a cold or fever – wait until you feel better; or
- If you may be pregnant – talk to your doctor before you start becoming more active.

**PLEASE NOTE:**

If your health changes so that you then answer YES to any of the above questions, tell your fitness or health professional. Ask whether you should change your physical activity plan.

I have read, understood, and completed this questionnaire. Any questions I had were answered to my full satisfaction.

Name: ______________________ Date: ______________________

Signature: ______________________ Signature of Parent: ______________________
Or Guardian (for participants under the age of majority)

Witness: ______________________

*NOTE: The law varies from state to state. No form should be adopted or used by any program without individualized legal advice.*

## AHA/ACSM Health/Fitness Facility Pre-Participation Screening Questionnaire

Assess your health needs by marking all true statements.

NAME: ______________________

DATE: ______________________

**History you have had:**

- ❑ a heart attack
- ❑ heart surgery
- ❑ cardiac catheterization
- ❑ coronary angioplasty (PTCA)
- ❑ pacemaker/implantable cardiac defibrillator/rhythm disturbance
- ❑ heart valve disease
- ❑ heart failure
- ❑ heart transplantation
- ❑ congenital heart disease

*If you marked any of the statements in this section, consult your healthcare provider before engaging in exercise. You may need to use a facility with a medically qualified staff.*

---

**Symptoms**

- ❑ You experience chest discomfort with exertion.
- ❑ You experience unreasonable breathlessness.
- ❑ You experience dizziness, fainting, blackouts.
- ❑ You take heart medications.

**Other health issues:**

- ❑ You have musculoskeletal problems.
- ❑ You have concerns about the safetv of exercise.
- ❑ You take prescription medication(s).
- ❑ You are pregnant.

---

**Cardiovascular risk factors**

- ❑ You are a man older than 45 years.
- ❑ You are a woman older than 55 years or you have had a hysterectomy or you are postmenopausal.
- ❑ You smoke.
- ❑ Your blood pressure is >140/90.
- ❑ You don't know your blood pressure.
- ❑ You take blood pressure medication.
- ❑ Your blood cholesterol level is >240 mg/dL.
- ❑ You don't know your cholesterol level.
- ❑ You have a close blood relative who had a heart attack before age 55 (father or brother) or age 65 (mother or sister).
- ❑ You are diabetic or take medicine to control your blood sugar.
- ❑ You are physically inactive (ie, you get <30 minutes of physical activity on at least 3 days per week).
- ❑ You are >20 pounds overweight.

*If you marked 2 or more of the statements in this section, consult your healthcare provider before engaging in exercise. You might benefit by using a facility with a professionally qualified exercise staff to guide your exercise program.*

---

None of the above is true.

*You should be able to exercise safely without consulting your healthcare provider in almost any facility that meets your exercise program needs.*

***AHA/ACSM indicates American Heart*** Association/American College of Sports Medicine.

## Cycle Ergometer Exercise Test Data Sheet

Date ___ / ___ / ___

Name ____________________ Subject ID# __________ Test # __________

Age __________ Gender __________ Height (in/cm) ________ Weight (lb/kg) ______

Medication ____________________ $FEV_1$ ($L$) __________ $MVV$ ($L{\cdot}min^{-1}$) ____

Ergometer __________ Seat Height (cm) ______ Protocol ____________________

| Standing/Seated Rest → | | | $f_C$ | $Pa_{sys}$ | $Pa_{dia}$ | | Comments |
|---|---|---|---|---|---|---|---|
| | | | | | | | |
| Time | Watts | RPM | | | | RPE | |
| 0-1 | | | | | | | |
| 1-2 | | | | | | | |
| 2-3 | | | | | | | |
| 3-4 | | | | | | | |
| 4-5 | | | | | | | |
| 5-6 | | | | | | | |
| 6-7 | | | | | | | |
| 7-8 | | | | | | | |
| 8-9 | | | | | | | |
| 9-10 | | | | | | | |
| 10-11 | | | | | | | |
| 11-12 | | | | | | | |
| 12-13 | | | | | | | |
| 13-14 | | | | | | | |
| 14-15 | | | | | | | |
| 15-16 | | | | | | | |
| 16-17 | | | | | | | |
| 17-18 | | | | | | | |
| 18-19 | | | | | | | End Time: |
| 19-20 | | | | | | | $f_C$ max: |
| 20-21 | | | | | | | $\dot{V}O_2$ max ($L{\cdot}min^{-1}$): |
| Recovery | | | | | | | |
| Time | | | $f_C$ | $Pa_{sys}$ | $Pa_{dia}$ | | Comments |
| 1 | | | | | | | |
| 3 | | | | | | | |
| 5 | | | | | | | |
| 7 | | | | | | | |

Reason for termination: ____________________

Physician comments: ____________________ Signed: __________

Test Results: Normal □ Borderline □ Abnormal □ Indeterminate □

Test Personnel: ____________________

# Treadmill Ergometer Exercise Test Data Sheet

Date ___ / ___ / ___

Name ____________________ Subject ID# __________ Test # __________

Age __________ Gender __________ Height (in/cm) ________ Weight (lb/kg) ______

Medication ____________________ $FEV_1$ $(L)$ __________ $MVV$ $(L{\cdot}min^{-1})$ ____

Protocol ____________________

| Standing/Seated Rest → | | | $f_C$ | $Pa_{sys}$ | $Pa_{dia}$ | | Comments |
|---|---|---|---|---|---|---|---|
| | | | | | | | |
| Time | Speed | Grade | | | | RPE | |
| 0-1 | | | | | | | |
| 1-2 | | | | | | | |
| 2-3 | | | | | | | |
| 3-4 | | | | | | | |
| 4-5 | | | | | | | |
| 5-6 | | | | | | | |
| 6-7 | | | | | | | |
| 7-8 | | | | | | | |
| 8-9 | | | | | | | |
| 9-10 | | | | | | | |
| 10-11 | | | | | | | |
| 11-12 | | | | | | | |
| 12-13 | | | | | | | |
| 13-14 | | | | | | | |
| 14-15 | | | | | | | |
| 15-16 | | | | | | | |
| 16-17 | | | | | | | |
| 17-18 | | | | | | | |
| 18-19 | | | | | | | End Time: |
| 19-20 | | | | | | | $f_C$ max: |
| 20-21 | | | | | | | $\dot{V}O_2$ max $(L{\cdot}min^{-1})$: |
| Recovery | | | | | | | |
| Time | | | $f_C$ | $Pa_{sys}$ | $Pa_{dia}$ | | Comments |
| 1 | | | | | | | |
| 3 | | | | | | | |
| 5 | | | | | | | |
| 7 | | | | | | | |

Reason for termination: ____________________

Physician comments: ____________________ Signed: __________

Test Results: Normal ☐ Borderline ☐ Abnormal ☐ Indeterminate ☐

Test Personnel: ____________________

**Borg Scale for Rating Perceived Exertion**

Please use this scale to indicate your perception of effort during the test. For example, use the descriptions to help you choose a number that describes how strenuous or heavy you feel the exercise is when shown this chart.

| | |
|---|---|
| 6 | No exertion at all |
| 7 | Extremely light |
| 8 | |
| 9 | Very light |
| 10 | |
| 11 | Light |
| 12 | |
| 13 | Somewhat hard |
| 14 | |
| 15 | Hard |
| 16 | |
| 17 | Very hard |
| 18 | |
| 19 | Extremely hard |
| 20 | Maximal exertion |

It is your own feeling of effort and exertion that is important, not what other people think. Look at the scale and the expressions and point to one of the numbers when requested.

## Borg CR10 Scale for Rating Perceived Exertion

Please use this scale to indicate your perception of effort during the test. For example, use the descriptions to help you choose a number that describes how weak or strong your discomfort is when you are shown this chart. It is your own feeling of effort and exertion that is important, not what other people think. Look at the scale and the expressions and point to one of the numbers when requested.

| | |
|---|---|
| 0 | Nothing at all |
| 0.3 | |
| 0.5 | Extremely weak |
| 1 | Very weak |
| 1.5 | |
| 2 | Weak |
| 2.5 | |
| 3 | Moderate |
| 4 | |
| 5 | Strong |
| 6 | |
| 7 | Very Strong |
| 8 | |
| 9 | |
| 10 | Extremely strong |

Proper instruction in use of this scale is important. Subjects should led to understand the interpretation of the descriptive terms that coincide with the numbers. Note that some subjects may be confused with the terms "weak" and "strong". They may report how they feel at a certain level of effort ("I feel weak here" or "I feel strong here") instead of correctly reporting sensations of discomfort (weak discomfort or strong discomfort) resulting from the level of exertion.

### Visual analog scale (VAS) for breathlessness

This scale represents varying degrees of breathlessness. Make a short pencil mark on the line at the point that indicates how breathless you feel at the time the scale is presented to you.

| | |
|---|---|
| NOT AT ALL<br>BREATHLESS | EXTREMELY<br>BREATHLESS |

EXERCISE PHYSIOLOGY LABORATORY - WORKSHEET

PATIENT LABEL

| DATE OF STUDY |
|---|
| |

| TYPE OF STUDY | |
|---|---|
| DIAGNOSTIC WITH ABG | |
| DIAGNOSTIC WITH OXIMETRY | |
| DIAGNOSTIC - MYOPATHY | |
| AMBULATORY O2 WITH ABG | |
| AMBULATORY O2 WITH OXIMETRY | |
| EIB TEST | |
| SIX MINUTE WALKING TEST | |
| RESEARCH PROTOCOL | |
| | |

| PULMONARY DIAGNOSIS | |
|---|---|
| COPD | |
| EMPHYSEMA | |
| ASTHMA | |
| PULMONARY FIBROSIS | |
| INTERSTITIAL LUNG DISEASE | |
| DYSPNEA | |
| INDUSTRIAL EXPOSURE | |
| HYPERVENTILATION | |
| | |

| CARDIOVASCULAR DIAGNOSIS | |
|---|---|
| CAD | |
| HYPERTENSION | |
| CARDIOMYOPATHY | |
| VALVULAR DISEASE | |
| CHF | |
| PVD | |
| | |

| MUSCULOSKELETAL DIAGNOSIS | |
|---|---|
| MYALGIA | |
| MYOPATHY | |
| CHRONIC FATIGUE | |
| JOINT INJURY | |
| MUSCLE INJURY | |
| BONE INJURY | |
| | |

| OTHER DIAGNOSIS | |
|---|---|
| ANXIETY | |
| OBESITY | |
| | |
| | |

| REFERRING PHYSICIAN | |
|---|---|
| | |
| | |
| | |
| | |
| | |
| | |
| | |
| | |
| | |
| | |
| | |

| REASON FOR REFERRAL | |
|---|---|
| EXERCISE LIMITATION | |
| DYSPNEA | |
| FATIGUE | |
| MYALGIA | |
| EXERCISE INDUCED WHEEZING | |
| CHEST PAIN | |
| EIB | |
| FITNESS ASSESSMENT | |
| REHABILITATION EVALUATION | |
| PRE-OPERATIVE EVALUATION | |
| FOLLOW-UP | |
| STUDY PROTOCOL | |
| | |

| HISTORY OF PRESENT ILLNESS |
|---|
| AGE: RACE: GENDER: M / F |

| ANTHROPOMETRIC | |
|---|---|
| HEIGHT (inches) | |
| WEIGHT (lb) | |

| MEDICATIONS | |
|---|---|
| DIGOXIN | |
| *BETA-ADRENOCEPTOR BLOCKER* | |
| LABETOLOL (TRANDATE) | |
| *CALCIUM CHANNEL BLOCKER* | |
| *METHYLXANTHINE* | |
| THEOPHYLLINE (THEODUR) | |
| *TRICYCLIC ANTIDEPRESSANT* | |
| DOXEPIN (SENEQUAN) | |
| *BENZODIAZEPINE* | |
| ALPRAZOLAM (XANAX) | |
| FLUOXETINE (PROZAC) | |
| | |
| | |
| | |

| SMOKING HISTORY | |
|---|---|
| NEVER | |
| CURRENT (/day) | |
| QUIT (year) | |
| PACK YEARS | |
| | |
| | |

| EXERCISE HISTORY | |
|---|---|
| NONE | |
| WALKING | |
| CYCLING | |
| SWIMMING | |
| | |
| FREQUENCY (times/week) | |
| DURATION (hours/week) | |
| | |

| COMMENTS |
|---|
| |

| TECHNICAL | |
|---|---|
| BAROMETRIC PRESSURE | |
| AMBIENT TEMPERATURE | |
| SADDLE HEIGHT | |

| PROTOCOL | |
|---|---|
| REST (MIN) | |
| WARMUP (min) | |
| RAMP RATE (watt/min) | |
| INCREMENT (watt/min) | |
| Wmax (watt) | |
| | |

| ARTERIAL BLOOD | |
|---|---|
| LEFT | |
| RIGHT | |
| RADIAL | |
| BRACHIAL | |
| SINGLE | |
| MULTIPLE (cannula) | |
| | |

| VENOUS BLOOD | |
|---|---|
| LEFT | |
| RIGHT | |
| ANTECUBITAL | |
| SINGLE | |
| MULTIPLE (cannula) | |
| | |

| CHECK LIST | |
|---|---|
| CONSENT | |
| RPE | |
| VAS | |

| EFFORT | |
|---|---|
| EXCELLENT | |
| GOOD | |
| FAIR | |
| POOR | |
| | |

| SYMPTOMS AT END EXERCISE | |
|---|---|
| DYSPNEA | |
| LEG FATIGUE | |
| LEG ACHE | |
| GENERAL FATIGUE | |
| CHEST PAIN | |
| LIGHT HEADED | |
| | |

| COMPLICATIONS | |
|---|---|
| NONE | |
| TECHNICAL | |
| DYSRHYTHMIA | |
| MYOCARDIAL ISCHEMIA | |
| HYPOTENSION | |
| BRONCHOSPASM | |
| | |

EXERCISE PHYSIOLOGY LABORATORY - DATA REDUCTION SHEET

| NAME (LAST, FIRST) | ID# | AGE (Y) | GENDER (M/F) | DATE OF STUDY (M / D / Y) |
|---|---|---|---|---|
| | | | | |
| **ANTHROPOMETRIC** | | **TECHNICAL** | | **DIAGNOSIS** |
| Height (in) | | Barometer (mm Hg) | | |
| Height (m) | | Ambient T (°C) | | |
| Weight (lb) | | $F_{IO_2}$ (%) | 21% | |
| Weight (kg) | | Valve dead space (ml) | 50 | |
| | | $\dot{W}$incr (watt·min$^{-1}$) | | |
| Body mass index (kg·m$^{-2}$) | | $\dot{W}$max (watt) | | |
| **PULMONARY FUNCTION** | **REFERENCE** | **OBSERVED** | **%REFERENCE** | **COMMENT** |
| FVC (l) | | | | |
| $FEV_1$ (l) | | | | |
| $FEV_1$/FVC (%) | | | | |
| MVV (l·min$^{-1}$) | | | | |
| **AEROBIC CAPACITY** | **REFERENCE** | **OBSERVED** | **%ref$\dot{V}O_2$max** | **$\dot{V}O_2$ (ml kg$^{-1}$ min$^{-1}$)** |
| $\dot{V}O_2$max (l·min$^{-1}$) | | | | |
| $\dot{V}O_2\theta$ (l·min$^{-1}$) | | | | |
| $\delta\dot{V}O_2/\delta\dot{W}$ (ml·min$^{-1}$·watt$^{-1}$) | 10.3 | | | |
| $\dot{V}O_2$unloaded (l·min$^{-1}$) | | | | |
| **CARDIOVASCULAR RESPONSE** | **REFERENCE** | **OBSERVED** | **%REFERENCE** | **COMMENT** |
| fcmax (min$^{-1}$) | | | | |
| Cardiac reserve (min$^{-1}$) | 0 | | | |
| $\dot{V}O_2$/fcmax (ml) | | | | |
| fcrest (min$^{-1}$) | | | | |
| Resting ECG | | | | |
| Exercise ECG | | | | |
| | **REST** | **EXERCISE (max)** | **RECOVERY (2 min)** | |
| Systolic BP (mm Hg) | | | | |
| Diastolic BP (mm Hg) | | | | |
| **VENTILATORY RESPONSE** | **REFERENCE** | **OBSERVED** | **%MVV** | **COMMENT** |
| $\dot{V}_E$max (l·min$^{-1}$) | | | | |
| Ventilatory reserve (l·min$^{-1}$) | >15 | | | |
| $V_T$max (l) | | | | |
| $f_R$max (min$^{-1}$) | <50 | | | |
| $T_I/T_E$ at end exercise | 0.8 | | | |
| **GAS EXCHANGE** | **REST** | **THRESHOLD** | **MAXIMUM** | **COMMENT** |
| $\dot{V}_E/\dot{V}O_2$ | | | | |
| $\dot{V}_E/\dot{V}CO_2$ | | | | |
| $P_{ET}O_2$ (mm Hg) | | | | |
| $P_{ET}CO_2$ (mm Hg) | | | | |
| R | | | | |
| $SpO_2$ (%) | | | | |
| $PaO_2$ (mm Hg) | | | | |
| $PaCO_2$ (mm Hg) | | | | |
| $P(A-a)O_2$ (mm Hg) | | | | |
| $P(a-ET)CO_2$ (mm Hg) | | | | |
| $V_D/V_T$ (%) | | | | |
| **MUSCLE METABOLISM** | **REST** | **EXERCISE (4 min)** | **RECOVERY (2 min)** | **PEAK VALUE (mM or μM)** |
| Lactate (mg·dl$^{-1}$) | | | | |
| Ammonia (μg·dl$^{-1}$) | | | | |
| Creatine kinase (U·l$^{-1}$) | | | | |
| | **REFERENCE** | **OBSERVED** | | |
| RQmus ($\delta\dot{V}CO_2/\delta\dot{V}O_2$) | 0.95 | | | |
| **SYMPTOM PERCEPTION** | **REST** | **EXERCISE (max)** | | **COMMENT** |
| Effort (observer impression) | | | | |
| Symptoms (subjective) | | | | |
| Perceived exertion (Borg scale/20) | | | | |
| Breathlessness (VAS scale/100) | | | | |

# Appendix E Frequently asked questions

## 1. What is the best protocol for patients with chronic disease?

Regardless of subject characteristics with respect to health or disease, the ideal exercise test protocol includes the following:

(a) a work rate increment that will allow the test to terminate in 8–12 min (see Chapter 3).

(b) selection of a mode of exercise, e.g., cycle, treadmill, or arm ergometer that is specific to the goals of the test (see Chapter 2).

## 2. What will cause resting *R* to differ from 0.80?

It is appropriate for resting $R$ to range between 0.70 and 1.00 and an $R$ of 0.80 is not atypical for rest. If its measurement truly represents resting conditions with appropriate prior fasting and avoidance of activity, an $R$ value of 0.8 suggests a substrate mix that is approximately 33% carbohydrate and 67% fat. Protein contributes little to resting energy production. Not unusually, an $R$ value of $> 1.00$ may be observed during the resting period prior to an exercise test. This is often due to hyperventilation which itself may be confirmed by examining $P_{ET}O_2$ and $P_{ET}CO_2$. Under more unusual circumstances, such as alcoholism or chronic starvation, $R$ may be lower than 0.70. Improper calibration of the gas analyzer(s) may also provide an explanation for $R$ outside the expected range.

## 3. What does MET stand for?

The MET is an abbreviation for resting metabolic rate. One MET is defined as a $\dot{V}O_2$ of $3.5\,ml \cdot kg^{-1} \cdot min^{-1}$. This value is considered by many to represent the average resting oxygen uptake rate per kilogram body weight for most people.

## 4. What is the best way to determine the metabolic threshold?

The most direct approach is to obtain serial arterial lactate samples in at least 1-min intervals throughout the exercise test. This invasive, time-consuming, and technically demanding method is not necessary when the integrative XT is performed. In this case, first examine the $\dot{V}_E$ versus $\dot{V}CO_2$ plot in order to identify the ventilatory threshold and remove that point from consideration as the metabolic threshold ($\dot{V}O_2\theta$). Next, examine the $\dot{V}CO_2$ vs $\dot{V}CO_2$ plot following the guidelines provided in Chapter 4. Assign a confidence value (e.g., using a 1–3 scale for low, medium, or high confidence, respectively). Next, examine the plots of $\dot{V}_E/\dot{V}O_2$ vs time and $\dot{V}_E/\dot{V}CO_2$ vs time utilizing the "dual criteria" explained in Chapter 4. When the metabolic threshold is identified, assign a confidence value as described above. For added confirmation $P_{ET}O_2$ versus time and $P_{ET}CO_2$ versus time may be used to detect $\dot{V}O_2\theta$ in a way similar to that employed for the $\dot{V}_E/\dot{V}O_2$ and

$\dot{V}_E/\dot{V}CO_2$ "dual criteria" as described in Chapter 4. Ideally, a second member of the lab staff should perform independent assessments. A meeting and discussion should resolve discrepancies.

## 5. How accurate are the autodetection methods of the metabolic threshold provided in some metabolic measurement systems?

Depending on the algorithms used to detect the metabolic threshold, automated or semiautomated detection schemes can have reasonable accuracy. However, the prudent individual will always overread the automated detection, even if the semiautomated scheme required some human input. This may be likened to the cardiologist overreading automated interpretation of the ECG.

## 6. How do some automated measurement systems calculate $V_D/V_T$?

One should interpret these estimations of $V_D/V_T$ cautiously. Calculation of $V_D/V_T$ requires use of the Bohr equation and measurement of arterial carbon dioxide partial pressure ($P_{a}CO_2$) by arterial blood gas analysis. Unless these measurements are made, use of equations that approximate $P_{a}CO_2$ from $P_{ET}CO_2$ can lead to erroneous $V_D/V_T$ estimations, particularly in patients with lung disease.

## 7. What might explain the discrepancy in results between $\dot{V}O_2$ calculated using the Douglas bag technique versus values obtained from an automated metabolic measurement system?

First, there is a need to establish what constitutes a meaningful discrepancy. Under ideal conditions with excellent technique, differences in $\dot{V}O_2$ of ±2–3% may be expected. Some believe that differences of up to 5% are acceptable. Second, differences may not be due to the automated system, but rather to poor Douglas bag technique. If the Douglas bag technique is good, one must then look to the individual elements responsible for the calculation of $\dot{V}O_2$. These include $\dot{V}_E$, $F_{\bar{E}}O_2$, $F_{\bar{E}}CO_2$, $F_IO_2$, $F_ICO_2$, $P_B$, and $T_E$. As shown in Appendix D (Table D8), small errors in some variables (i.e., $\dot{V}_E$ and $F_{\bar{E}}O_2$) can result in large errors in $\dot{V}O_2$. It would be disconcerting to observe a reasonably "accurate" $\dot{V}O_2$ with offsetting errors in $\dot{V}_E$ and $F_{\bar{E}}O_2$. That is, a $\dot{V}_E$ error that is 8% high and an $F_{\bar{E}}O_2$ error that is 8% low.

## 8. What are the advantages of performing exercise testing using breath-by-breath technology versus the mixing chamber method? Is one method better?

Both methods should yield identical data when averaged over comparable time periods. The advantage of breath-by-breath measurements is chiefly seen in increased data density. This provides the opportunity to observe rapid changes in gas transients such as $\tau\dot{V}O_2$ occurring during the onset of exercise. Breath-by-breath sampling might provide 20 data points in the first minute of exercise (assuming $f_R$ of 20 min$^{-1}$) to characterize the $\dot{V}O_2$ response curve, whereas even 10-s averaging from a mixing chamber system would yield only 6 data points.

## 9. What causes the variation seen in breath-by-breath $\dot{V}O_2$ data? How do you deal with this variability in choosing $\dot{V}O_{2max}$?

Assuming that the digital algorithms used to calculate $\dot{V}O_2$ are accurate from the integration of flow and gas concentration measurements, the correct accounting for water vapor, and corrections for barometric pressure and temperature, some breath-to-breath fluctuations are normal, but may be exaggerated by coughing or swallowing. Many automated breath-by-breath systems employ criteria to reject grossly aberrant breaths. The chief component affecting $\dot{V}O_2$ is ventilation. Changes in pedal frequency, becoming startled during an XT, pain, or sudden excess movements may all result in increasing ventilation, even if only for one breath. This is seen as breath-to-breath fluctuation.

Choosing $\dot{V}O_{2max}$ must be standardized at least within a given laboratory. Use of a single highest breath is not recommended. Rather, use of an averaging scheme is more appropriate (see Chapter 4).

## 10. How should we handle physically weak patients?

The first consideration is choosing the appropriate protocol, as indicated in the answer to question 1 above. The cycle ergometer may be a better choice for this patient group because of its lower initial work rate, extrinsic work rate control, and improved stability with decreased risk of falling. If the mouthpiece and noseclip present an uncomfortable patient interface, the mask may be considered provided that it has been previously evaluated for loss of accuracy in measuring $\dot{V}_E$ due to leaks. When cycle exercise is not possible, the treadmill test must be carefully conducted at very low speeds and grades, again providing the likelihood that the XT will continue for 8–12 min. Although handrail holding is generally to be discouraged, some handrail use may be necessary in the very weak for balance and confidence.

## 11. How do you diagnose the difference between a disease versus poor conditioning, especially if the patient has stopped because of leg fatigue?

Poor conditioning may be viewed as mild disease on the health–disease continuum. In the global case of ''cardiovascular diseases,'' a deconditioned person will have a low $\dot{V}O_{2max}$ and metabolic threshold (but not below the lower 95% confidence limit: see Appendix C, Reference Values for $\dot{V}O_{2max}$ and $\dot{V}O_2\theta$). The $f_C$–$\dot{V}O_2$ slope will be somewhat steeper than expected, but not as steep as in a person with heart disease.

# Index

Note: an asterisk marks a parameter whose definition may be found in the *glossary* pages 204–210


acetyl-CoA, formation 3
acidosis, chronic metabolic, ventilatory threshold, respiratory compensation point reduction 127–128
adenosine triphosphate (ATP) regeneration
  aerobic metabolic pathways 6
  cellular energy deprivation 5
  $NH_3$ derivation 144
aerobic capacity, submaximal testing 51
aerobic metabolism, exercise physiology 5–6
aerobic performance
  data analysis 154
    four-panel displays 159
African males/females, nomograms of lung function 229
AIDS, XT relative contraindication 88
Allen test, modified, arterial blood sampling 49
alveolar air equation 138
alveolar slope, $P_{ET}O_2$, and $P_{ET}CO_2$ 137, 138, 140
alveolar–arterial oxygen partial pressure difference ($P_{(A\text{-}a)}O_2$) 138–139
  definition, derivation, equation, and measurement units 138, 205
  normal/abnormal response 138–139
American Heart Association, ECG specifications 46
American Heart Association/American College of Sports Medicine (ACSM)
  Exercise Specialist certification 83
  *pro forma*, preparticipation screening for XT 253
  XT supervision 83
ammonia ($NH_3$) 144
  arterial blood sampling 48
  definition, derivation, and measurement units 144
  myopathy evaluation 73
  normal/abnormal response 144
anaerobic metabolism, exercise physiology 5–6
anaerobic threshold *see* metabolic threshold
anemia, impaired oxygen delivery 168
aneurysms, XT relative contraindication 87–88
angina
  CXT 73
  XT termination 88–89, 89
anxiety
  cardiovascular response pattern abnormalities 165, 167
  diagnosis 11, 12
  exercise prescription 12
  rapid shallow breathing association 173
  sinus tachycardia 113
  symptom perception abnormalities 178
aortic aneurysm, XT contraindication 87
*appendices* 204–263
arm ergometers 31–32
  calibration, accuracy, and precision 31
  maintenance 32
  maximal incremental work rate 82
  oxygen cost 212
  settings 78
  submaximal incremental work rate 64–65
arterial blood gas tensions ($Pa\text{O}_2$, and $Pa\text{CO}_2$) 135–137
  oxygen tension, defined 207
arterial blood sampling 48–50
  arterial catheter 49, 71
  calibration, accuracy, and precision 49–50
  description, and operational principles 48–49
  double arterial puncture 49
  laboratory tests 71
  maintenance 50
  modified Allen test 49
  oxygen saturation ($Sp\text{O}_2$), pulse oximetry 47
  $Pa\text{CO}_2$ determination, hyperventilation, and dead space increase 135
arterial pressure *see* blood pressure
arterial–end-tidal carbon dioxide partial pressure difference ($P_{(a\text{-}ET)}CO_2$) 139–141
  defined 207
  definition, derivation, and measurement units 139–140
  normal/abnormal responses 140–141
arteriovenous difference in oxygen content*
  definition, derivation, and measurement units 115–116, 205
  normal/abnormal response 116
arthritis, symptom perception abnormalities 178

assessment
  *case studies*
    for exercise program 185–7
    for pulmonary rehabilitation 191–195
asthma
  *case study* 181–5
  exercise-induced (EIA), CXT 71–73
  ventilatory flow limitation 134
  ventilatory limitation 169
  *see also* pulmonary disease
Åstrand–Ryhming cycling test 65
Åstrand–Ryhming nomogram of lung function 227
ataxia, XT termination 88–89, 89
ATP *see* adenosine triphosphate
atrial contractions *see* premature atrial contractions
atrial fibrillation
  cardiovascular response pattern abnormalities 167
  ECG 113, 114
  XT termination 89

Balke treadmill protocol 64, 78–79, 214, 241–242
basic life support (BLS), training, and certification 89
beta-sympathomimetic antagonists
  cardiovascular response pattern abnormalities 167
  $f_{Cmax}$ reduction 109
biological variability, means 140, 150
biomechanical efficiency, physical training 151
blood doping, oxygen delivery increase 168
blood pressure (BP)
  diastolic, XT termination 88–89
  mean, equation 119
  measurement
    intraarterial 47
    procedures 244
    resting 76
    sphygmomanometry 44–47
  monitor 84
  systemic arterial pressure 119–121
    defined 206
    definition, derivation, and measurement units 119–120
    normal/abnormal response 120–121
    oxygen uptake relationship 120
  systolic, XT termination 88–89
BLS *see* basic life support
"blue bloaters", lung disease 125–126
Bohr equation 2, 124
  $V_D/V_T$ 141
Borg scale for perceived exertion (psychometric scale) 256
bradycardia, sinus, ECG 113
breath-by-breath systems 45–46
  averaging method 97–98
  calibration, accuracy, and precision 45
  description, and operational principles 45
  maintenance 45–46
breathing, rapid shallow, ventilatory control abnormalities 173
breathlessness* 146–147
  definition, derivation, and measurement units 146, 205
  exertional, *case study* 187–191
  normal/abnormal response 146–147
  visual analog scale 146, 258
bronchitis, chronic
  ventilatory flow limitation 134, 169
  *see also* pulmonary disease
bronchoconstriction test 71–73
bronchospasm, exercise-induced (EIB), CXT 71–73
Bruce treadmill protocol 78–79, 214–215, 242
  cardiac exercise testing 73
  data table 64

CABG (coronary artery bypass grafting) 11, 13
calcium channel antagonists
  cardiovascular response pattern abnormalities 167
  $f_{Cmax}$ reduction 109
*calculations* 211–219
calibration, measurement concepts 16
calibration curve, mathematical adjustments 16
calibration data 16
carbohydrate
  respiratory quotient 7
  RQ value 106
  slope of ventilatory response increase 125
  ventilatory response pattern abnormalities 171
carbon dioxide
  analyzers 42
    calibration, accuracy, and precision 42
    maintenance 42
  production, defined 96–97
  tension, arterial, regulation 2
  *see also* arterial blood gas tensions; end-tidal gas tensions; pulmonary gas exchange
carbon dioxide output*
  calculation 216
  defined 96–97, 208
  ventilatory coupling 2
carboxyhemoglobinemia, impaired oxygen delivery 168
cardiac failure
  oscillating ventilation 173
  *see also* congestive heart failure
cardiac glycosides, cardiovascular response pattern abnormalities 167
cardiac output* 116–118
  cardiovascular coupling 2
  definition, derivation, and measurement units 116–117
  instantaneous oxygen uptake equation 117
  normal/abnormal response 117–118
cardiac rhythm

ECG abnormalities 114
XT termination 88–89
cardiac stroke volume (SV) 118–119
calculation 118
cardiac output, and $f_C$ association 2
defined 208
definition, derivation, and measurement units 118
estimation
incremental exercise 111
maximal exercise 112
normal/abnormal response 118–119
cardiac XT 73
cardiomyopathy
differential diagnosis 11
impaired oxygen delivery 169
SV reduction 118
cardiopulmonary coupling, external work rate 2
cardiopulmonary XT, supervision 83
cardiorespiratory fitness
classification 230–238
*see also* oxygen uptake, maximum
cardiovascular disease
cardiovascular limitation 164
cardiovascular response pattern abnormalities 164–166
differential diagnosis 9–10
disease progression/regression assessment 151–152
exercise prescription 12
impaired oxygen delivery 168–169
NYHA classification 99–100, 112
oxygen pulse response patterns 112
oxygen uptake, prolonged 105
shunt abnormalities
arterial blood gas tension abnormalities 136
gas exchange abnormalities 175
valvular
slope of cardiovascular response 111
SV reduction 118
XT relative contraindication 88
Weber classification 99–100
SV values 119
cardiovascular efficiency
oxygen pulse 111–112
slope of cardiovascular response 110–111
cardiovascular limitation 8, 10
data analysis 154
four-panel displays 159–161
nine-panel displays 159
diagnostic response patterns 162–167
cardiovascular response
abnormalities, diagnostic response patterns 164–167
four-panel display 159, 161
slope 110–111
carnitine palmitoyl transferase (CPT) deficiency, muscle metabolism abnormalities 176
*case studies*
assessment in preparation for exercise program 185–187
assessment for pulmonary rehabilitation 191–195
asthma 181–5
muscle fatigue, and exertional breathlessness 187–191, 199–203
occupational exposure to solvents 195–199
catheter, arterial, arterial blood sampling 49, 71
cellular energy generation
equations 3
metabolic substrates 7
cellular respiration coupling, external work rate 1–2
central nervous system symptoms, XT termination 89
chest wall compliance, reduced, ventilatory capacity reduction 124
chronic fatigue syndrome, muscle metabolism abnormalities 176–177
chronic obstructive pulmonary disease
6-minute walking test 95
abnormal symptom perception 177–178
*case study* 191–195
diagnostic XT 58
stair-climb 70
chronometers 19–20
chronotropic incompetence
cardiovascular response pattern abnormalities 165, 167
$f_{Cmax}$ reduction 109–110
citric acid cycle *see* Krebs cycle
clammy skin, XT termination 88–89
clinical exercise testing (CXT) 6–8, 67–74
defined 204
field tests 68–70
laboratory tests 70–74
physician supervision 83
purposes, setting, and protocols 51, 52
submaximal testing 51
ventilatory capacity determination 76
*see also* diagnostic XT
clinical medical history questionnaire 253
clocks *see* chronometers
cold skin, XT termination 88–89
collection bags *see* gas collection bags
confidence interval, standard deviation of the mean 150
confusion, XT termination 88–89, 89
congenital heart disease, SV reduction 9–10
congestive heart failure
slope of cardiovascular response 111
XT contraindication 87
consent, informed 74–75, 250
contractile coupling 2
contraindications to XT 87–91
absolute 88
relative absolute 88
*conversion constants* 217–219

Cooper distance measurements
walking and running tests 237–238
1.5-mile run 237
3-mile walk 238
Cooper tests 56, 57, 60
estimation of maximum oxygen uptake 213, 239
fitness categories 230, 232–233
coronary artery bypass grafting (CABG) 11, 13
coronary artery disease
impaired oxygen delivery 169
screening 11
slope of cardiovascular response 111
SV reduction 118
*see also* cardiovascular disease
counters 20
CPT *see* carnitine palmitoyl transferase
CR10 scale 145
crash cart, detailed contents 247–248
CWR *see* work rate tests, constant
CXT *see* clinical exercise testing
cyanosis, XT termination 88–89
cycle ergometers 21–27
calibration, pre-XT 78
concerns 23–25
description and operational principles 21–25
electrically braked 23
calibration, accuracy, and precision 27
maintenance 27
PWC170 test 23
field exercise testing (FXT) 60, 234–235
friction-braked 23
leg, advantages and disadvantages 25
maximal tests, work rate increments 79–80
mechanically braked 21–23
calibration, accuracy, and precision 25–27
counters 20
maintenance 27
r.p.m. error effects 22–23
Monark, calibration 245
oxygen cost 211
protocol *pro forma* 254
settings 77–78
Storer cycle test, estimation of maximum oxygen uptake 214
submaximal constant work rate tests, Åstrand–Ryhming test 65
submaximal incremental work rate tests 61–63
branching protocol 61
$f_C$, blood pressure, and RPE timing 61, 63
YMCA multistage 61, 63
Wingate test 25

data integration and interpretation 85–87, 149–179
data displays 152–162
graphical
four-panel 159–161
nine-panel 158, 168
recommended 78, 79
sequential, trending phenomena 161–162, 165
tabular 155–157, 168
multiple data
diagnostic response patterns 162–179
reduction and display 152–162
single variables
reference value comparison 149–150
serial measurements 151–152
technical factors 152–154
dead space
calculation, CXT 71
gas exchange abnormalities 173
$P_{(a-ET)}CO_2$ increases 140
$P_{ET}O_2$ and $P_{ET}CO_2$ influence 137–138
ventilatory equivalents 135
dead space–tidal volume ratio ($V_D/V_T$) 2, 141–142
age effects 142
Bohr equation 141
defined 208
definition, derivation, and measurement units 141–142
normal/abnormal response 142
ventilatory requirement 126
definitions, *glossary* 205–210
denial, symptom perception abnormalities 178
diabetes mellitus, XT relative contraindication 88
diagnostic exercise test (CXT: diagnostic) 8, 68
*case studies*
asthma 181–185
breathlesness and fatigue 187–191, 199–203
chronic obstructive pulmonary disease 58, 191–195
progress monitoring 68
termination 89
dietary recommendations, lung disease 126
differential diagnosis 9–11
diffusion impairment, $P_{(A-a)}O_2$ 139
digoxin
cardiovascular response pattern abnormalities 167
$f_{Cmax}$ reduction 109
diltiazem, $f_{Cmax}$ reduction 109
disability evaluation 9, 11, 12
Douglas bag technique, gas collection 32–35, 43
$d_{W6}$ *see* walking and running tests (6-minute walking distance)
dynamic hyperinflation, tidal flow–volume loop 134
dyspnea *see* breathlessness
dysrhythmias
cardiovascular response pattern abnormalities 165–167
CXT risk assessment 68
ECG 114, 115
exercise prescription 12
XT termination 89

ECG *see* electrocardiography
effort
  suboptimal
    conscious/subconscious 179
    data analysis, nine-panel display 156–157, 179
    definition and identification 178–179
EIA *see* asthma, exercise-induced
EIB *see* bronchospasm, exercise-induced
EILV *see* end-inspiratory lung volume
electrocardiogram (ECG) 46
  American Heart Association specifications 46
  calibration, accuracy and precision 46
  definition, derivation, and measurement units 112–113, 205
  dysrhythmias 114–115
  maintenance 46
  monitoring failure, XT termination 89
  normal response 113–114
  resting 12-lead 75
    electrode placement 75, 76
    skin preparation 75
  technician 84
electrochemical or fuel cell analyzers, oxygen analyzers 39
electron transport chain *see* mitochondrial pathway
Ellestad protocol, cardiac exercise testing 73
Embden–Meyerhof pathway 3–4
emergency procedures 89–91
  crash cart
    detailed contents 247–248
    drugs 248
  emergency response board 90
  resuscitation equipment 90–91
emphysema 13
  cardiovascular response pattern abnormalities 166
  gas exchange abnormalities 173–174
  *see also* pulmonary disease
end-inspiratory lung volume (EILV), $V_T$ relationship 133
end-tidal gas tensions ($P_{ET}O_2$ and $P_{ET}CO_2$) 137–138
  alveolar slope 137, 138, 140
  data analysis 154–155
  dead space influence 137–138
  definition, derivation, and measurement units 137
  normal/abnormal responses 137–138
endurance time (*t*)
  abnormal response 94
  definition, derivation, units of measurement 93, 208
  normal response 93–94
energetics and substrate utilization, exercise physiology 7
energy, *conversion constants* 217
equipment failure, XT termination 88–89
ergogenic drugs 11, 13
ergometers 21–32
  familiarization pretest 77
  recommendations 23
  settings 77–78
  *see also* arm; cycle; treadmill ergometers
errors, random and systematic 17–18
*errors in measurement of primary variables* 249
exercise endurance, CWR tests 65
exercise physiology 1–7
  aerobic and anaerobic metabolism 5–6
  cardiopulmonary coupling, external work 2
  cellular respiration coupling, external work 1–2
  data acquisition 85–86
  energetics and substrate utilization 7
  metabolic pathways 3–5
  threshold concepts 6–7
exercise prescription 11, 12
  cardiopulmonary rehabilitation 12
  CWR 74
  PXT 8, 53–55
exercise response variables 93–148
  6-minute walking distance 94–95
  arteriovenous difference in oxygen content 115–116
  cardiac output 116–118
  cardiac stroke volume 118–119
  ECG 112–115
  endurance time 93–94
  evaluation 8–9
  heart rate, maximum ($f_{Cmax}$) 109–110
  maximum minute ventilation 122–124
  metabolic, gas exchange, or lactic acid threshold 101–103
  muscle respiratory quotient 107–109
  oxygen pulse 111–112
  oxygen uptake
    maximum 96–100
    time constant 103–105
  pulmonary arterial pressure 121–122
  respiratory exchange ratio (*R*) 105–107
  respiratory rate 129–130
  shuttle test speed 95–96
  slope of cardiovascular response 110–111
  slope of the ventilatory response 124–126
  systemic arterial pressure 119–121
  tidal volume 128–129
  ventilatory threshold, respiratory compensation point 126–128
  walking and running distance 94
  work efficiency 100–101
Exercise Specialist certification, American College of Sports Medicine (ACSM) 83
exercise testing (XT)
  classification 7–8, 204
  contraindications 87–90
  differential diagnosis of disease 9–13
  emergency procedures 89–91
  equipment failure, XT termination 88–89
  equipment preparation 77–78
  explanation pretest 76–77

exercise testing (XT) (*cont.*)
  methods 51–92
    maximal vs submaximal 51–54
  nomenclature 7–8
  optimal protocol selection 78–83
  personnel recommendations 83–85
  physical fitness assessment 8–9
  preparation, *pro forma* 254
  preparticipation screening 253
  purpose 1–14
  report generation 86
  response variables 93–148
  safety considerations 87–91
  sequence, flow chart 84
  subject preparation 74–77
  termination indications 88
  *see also* clinical exercise testing (CXT); performance exercise testing (PXT)
exercise tolerance, evaluation 9
exertional breathlessness, *case studies* 187–191, 199–203
expiratory flow–volume relationships*
  defined 206
  *see also* inspiratory/expiratory flow
external work* 1–2

fat, RQ value 7, 106
fatigue
  XT termination 88–89
  *see also* chronic fatigue syndrome
$f_C$ *see* heart rate
$f_{Cmax}$ *see* heart rate, maximum
Fick equation 2, 110, 111
field exercise testing (FXT)
  CXT 68–70
  cycle test 60, 235
  defined 4
  PXT 55–60
  run tests 56–58
  step tests 58–60
  swim test 60, 236
  walking tests 55–56
fitness assessment
  categories, AHA, Åstrand and Cooper tests 232–235, 238–239
  CWR tests 65
  field tests 55–60
  laboratory tests 62
  *see also* performance exercise testing (PXT)
flow and volume transducers 36–38
  calibration, accuracy and precision 38
  description and operational principles 36–38
  hot-wire anemometer 38
  maintenance 38
  Pitot tube 37–38
  pneumotachograph 37
  turbine transducer 38
force, *conversion constants* 217
forced expired volume in 1 second ($FEV_1$) 35
  nomograms 228–229
  ventilatory capacity estimation 123, 124
$f_R$ *see* respiratory rate

gait problems, XT termination 89
gas analyzers 39–43
  blood sampling 49–50
  carbon dioxide analyzers 42
  mass spectrometry 42–43
  oxygen analyzers 39–42
  water vapor pressure 41
gas collection bags 32–35
  Douglas bag technique 32–35
  maintenance 34–35
  meteorological balloons 32, 34
gas exchange
  data analysis 154–155, 159
    four-panel displays 160–161, 163
    nine-panel displays 158, 173
  disorders, differential diagnosis 117
  impaired
    data analysis, nine-panel display 156–157, 173
    diagnostic response patterns 173–175
  mechanisms, $P_{(A-a)}O_2$ 139
gas exchange threshold *see* metabolic threshold
gas volumes, standardized, calculation 215–216
gasometers *see* spirometers and gasometers
general gas law 215
*glossary*
  exercise testing 204
  physiological variables 205–210
glycolysis, anaerobic 3–4

Haldane equation 128
Harbor–UCLA Medical Center, nine-panel graphical displays 157–158
heart block, ECG 114
heart rate ($f_C$)
  age-related decline 109
  cardiovascular response 2
  defined 205
  medication 166–167
  oxygen uptake relationship 110
  RPE relationship 145
  treadmill and cycle exercise comparisons 24
heart rate, maximum ($f_{Cmax}$) 109–110
  definition, derivation, and measurement units 109
  equation 109
  normal/abnormal response 109–110
  standard deviation 150

heart transplantation 11, 13
Henderson–Hasselbalch equation, bicarbonate calculation 135
hepatitis, XT relative contraindication 88
high-energy phosphates 2
hot-wire anemometer, flow and volume transducers 38
hypertension
  arterial systolic pressure increase relationship 120
  cardiovascular response pattern abnormalities 164–166
  CXT risk assessment 68
  exercise prescription 12
  pulmonary
    gas exchange abnormalities 174–175
    *Ppa* increase 121
hyperthyroidism, cardiovascular response pattern abnormalities 167
hyperventilation
  acute, ventilatory control abnormalities 172
  diagnosis 11, 12
  extreme, ventilatory limitation 170
  $f_R$ increase 130
  *R* adverse factor 107
  ventilatory equivalents 135
  $V_T$ abnormal responses 129
hyperventilation syndrome 11
  ventilatory control abnormalities 172
hypokalemia, XT relative contraindication 88
hypomagnesemia, XT relative contraindication 88
hypotension, exercise prescription 12
hypoventilation, ventilatory control abnormalities 172–173
hypoxemia
  CXT risk assessment 68
  exercise prescription 12
  oxygen uptake kinetics, cardiovascular and pulmonary disease 105
  *Ppa* increase 121–122

*I/E* ratio *see* ratio of inspiratory to expiratory time ($T_I/T_E$)
ILD *see* interstitial lung disease
illustrative cases and reports 181–203
incremental exercise protocols 66–67
indoor courses 18
infection
  acute, XT contraindication 87
  chronic, XT relative contraindication 88
informed consent 240
  pretest subject preparation 74–75
inspiratory/expiratory flow–volume relationships* 133–134
  defined 206
  definition, derivation, and measurement units 133
  normal/abnormal response 133–134
inspiratory/expiratory time ratio ($T_I/T_E$) 131–133
  definition, derivation, and measurement units 131, 207
  normal/abnormal response 131–133
instrumentation 15–50
interstitial lung disease (ILD), gas exchange abnormalities 173–174
isowork analysis, physical training 151

Joint Commission for the Accreditation of Hospital Organizations (JCAHO), clinical standards 87

Korotkoff sounds, tonal quality and interpretation 119
Krebs cycle 3–4

LA *see* lactate
laboratory exercise testing (LXT) 60–67
  CXT 70–74
    with/without arterial blood sampling 70–71
  defined 204
  fitness assessment 62
  PXT 60–67
  work rate tests
    maximal incremental 66–67
    submaximal constant 65–66
    submaximal incremental 61–65
lactate (La) 142–144
  arterial blood gas tensions 136
  blood concentrations, treadmill and cycle exercise comparisons 24
  definition, derivation, and measurement units 142–143
  metabolic threshold 143
  metabolism
    arterial blood sampling 48
    exercise prescription 12
    myopathy evaluation 73
  normal/abnormal response 143–144
  ventilatory control abnormalities 128
laser diode absorption spectroscopy (LDAS), oxygen analyzers 40
LED *see* light-emitting diode
leg cycle ergometers *see* cycle ergometers, leg
leg cycling, oxygen cost 211
lifestyle modifications 12, 13
  PXT 8
light-emitting diode (LED), pulse oximetry 47
lightheadedness, XT termination 88–89
lung function, nomograms 123, 150, 228–229
lung volume reduction surgery (LVRS) 11, 13
LVRS *see* lung volume reduction surgery

McArdle's syndrome
  La levels 143
  metabolic threshold, abnormal response 103
  muscle metabolism abnormalities 175–176
  *R* values 107
malingering
  diagnosis 11, 12
    symptom perception abnormalities 178

mass spectrometry 42–43
  calibration, accuracy and precision 42
  description and operational principles 42
  maintenance 43
maximum minute ventilation (MMV)* 122–124
  definition, derivation, and measurement units 122–123
  $f_C$ changes 2
  normal/abnormal response 123–124
maximum oxygen uptake *see* oxygen uptake, maximum*
maximum voluntary ventilation (MVV)*
  defined 206
  measurement 35, 123
measured courses 18–19
  indoor 18
  outdoor 19
measurement concepts 15–18
  accuracy 16
  calibration 16
  error 17–18
  precision 16
  validation 16
mechanical coupling 2
medical history
  multiple data analysis 152–153
  questionnaire, pretest preparation 74
medication
  cardiovascular limitation effects 164
  cardiovascular response pattern abnormalities 165–167
  ergogenic drugs 11, 13
metabolic cart operator 85
metabolic disease, XT relative contraindication 88
metabolic measurement systems 43–46
  breath-by-breath method 45–46
  mixing chamber method 43–45
metabolic pathways 3–4
  ATP regeneration 6
  exercise physiology 3–5
metabolic substrates, energetic properties 7
metabolic threshold*
  data analysis 159
  definition, derivation, measurement units 101–102
  equations 230–231
  lactate accumulation 143
  normal response 102–103
  interpretation 102–103
  oxygen and carbon dioxide uptake relationship 103
  physical fitness assessment 8–9
  terminology 102
  ventilatory equivalents and end-tidal gas tension relationships 103–104
metabolism
  aerobic and anaerobic 5–6
  muscle, data analysis 155
meteorological balloons
  gas collection 32
    calibration 34
metoprolol, $f_{C\max}$ reduction 109
metronomes 20–21
mitochondrial myopathy, $NH_3$ increase 144
mitochondrial pathway
  oxidative phosphorylation 3–5
  schematic representation 5
mixing chambers
  calibration, accuracy and precision 44
  maintenance 45
  metabolic measurement 43–45
Monark cycle ergometer, calibration 245
mononucleosis, XT relative contraindication 88
muscle diseases, differential diagnosis 11
muscle fatigue and exertional breathlessness, *case studies* 187–191, 199–203
muscle metabolism
  abnormalities, diagnostic response patterns 175–177
  data analysis 155
    definition and identification 175
    nine-panel display 156–157
muscle oxygen consumption*, oxygen delivery effectiveness 1–2
muscle respiratory quotient ($RQ_{mus}$) 107–109
  calculation 108
  definition, derivation, and measurement units 107–108, 207
  normal/abnormal response 108–109
    oxygen–carbon dioxide uptake relationship 108
muscle work*, conversion, external work 2
musculoskeletal disease, symptom perception abnormalities 178
musculoskeletal disorders, XT relative contraindication 88
musculoskeletal limitations 8, 10
MVV *see* maximum voluntary ventilation
myalgia, differential diagnosis 11
myoadenylate deaminase deficiency
  muscle metabolism abnormalities 176
  $NH_3$ levels 144
myocardial dysfunction, slope of cardiovascular response 111
myocardial infarction
  XT contraindication 87
  XT termination 89
myocardial ischemia
  CXT 73
  CXT risk assessment 68
  ECG 114–115, 116
  exercise prescription 12
  treadmill protocols 9
myocarditis, XT contraindication 87
myopathy 203
  cardiac output 117–118
  CXT evaluation 73

differential diagnosis 11
mitochondrial, muscle metabolism abnormalities 176
$NH_3$ increase 144
slope of cardiovascular response 111
myophosphorylase deficiency
metabolic threshold, abnormal response 103
*R* values 107
myxedema, XT relative contraindication 88

Naughton protocol, cardiac exercise testing 73
nausea, XT termination 88–89
neurological symptoms, XT termination 89
neuromuscular disorders, XT relative contraindication 88
New York Heart Association (NYHA)
cardiovascular disease classification 99–100
SV values 119
$NH_3$ *see* ammonia
nitrogen concentration, expired, equation 128
noise, random errors 17
nomograms
$FEV_1$ estimation 123
lung function 228–229
prediction values 150
nutrition
modifications 11, 13
*see also* carbohydrate

obesity, maximum oxygen uptake complications 99–100
occupational exposure to solvents, *case study* 195–199
Ohio spirometer 36
operative risk, assessment by exercise testing 240
outdoor courses 19
oxygen, *see also* arterial blood gas tensions; end-tidal gas tensions; gas exchange; pulmonary gas exchange
oxygen analyzers 39–42
calibration, accuracy and precision 40–41
Scholander procedure 40
water vapor 41
description and operational principle 39–40
electrochemical or fuel cell 39
laser diode absorption spectroscopy (LDAS) 40
maintenance 41–42
paramagnetic 39
zirconium oxide 39–40
oxygen breath* 130–131
definition, derivation, and measurement units 130, 209
equation 130
normal/abnormal responses 130–131
oxygen consumption
defined 96–97
muscle* 1–2
oxygen content *see* arteriovenous difference in oxygen content
oxygen cost of exercise 211–213
oxygen delivery
impaired
data analysis, nine-panel display 156–157, 168
definition and identification 167–168
diagnostic patterns 167–169
oxygen partial pressure
alveolar, increase 138
mixed venous, reduction 138
reference values, arterial blood and alveolar–arterial difference 139
oxygen pulse* 111–112
definition, derivation, and measurement units 111–112, 209
equation 111
normal/abnormal response 112
oxygen therapy 11, 13
oxygen uptake
alveolar, measurement 1–2
calculation 215–216
CWR tests 66
effect of errors in r.p.m. (cadence) 240
external work rate coupling 1–2
maximum*, cardiorespiratory fitness 230–233
peak 210
respiratory exchange ratio 2
r.p.m. error effects 22, 240
systemic arterial pressure relationship 120
time constant* 103–105
calculation 104
CWR tests 65–66
definition, derivation, and measurement units 103–104
normal/abnormal response 104–105, 106
treadmill and cycle exercise comparisons 24
*see also* breath-by-breath systems
oxygen uptake kinetics*, time constant, physical fitness assessment 8–9
oxygen uptake, maximum*
abnormal responses 99–100
cardiovascular disease classification 99–100
measured values 99
obesity complications 99–100
athletes 98
categories, AHA, Åstrand and Cooper tests 232–235, 238–239
definition, derivation, and measurement units 96–98, 209
estimation from predictive tests 211–215
incremental XT relationship 99
normal responses 98–99
physical fitness assessment 8–9
reference values 220–240
terminology 96–98
oxygenation, arterial, pulse oximetry 47–48

pacemaker, fixed-rate, XT relative contraindication 88
pallor, XT termination 88–89, 89
$Pa\text{O}_2$ and $Pa\text{CO}_2$ *see* arterial blood gas tensions

paramagnetic analyzers, oxygen analyzers 39
paresthesia, XT termination 89
patient interface 78
pedal revolution counters *see* counters
performance exercise testing (PXT: fitness assessment) 6–9, 53–67
  *case study* 185–191
  defined 204
  exercise prescription 53–54
  field tests 55–60
  fitness assessment 53
  laboratory tests 60–67
  maximal testing 66–67
  progress monitoring 54–55, 54–55
  purposes, setting and protocols 51, 52
  submaximal testing 51, 52
pericarditis, XT contraindication 87
peripheral measuring devices 46–50
  electrocardiography 46
  pulse oximetry 47–50
  sphygmomanometry 46–47
peripheral vascular disease 168
personnel
  assignment 83–84
  BP monitor 84
  ECG technician 84
  experience and qualifications 83
  metabolic cart operator 85
  supervision level 83
  test administrator 84
pharmacological interventions 11, 13
pharmacotherapy, CXT progress monitoring 68
phosphate compounds, high-energy, production 2
phosphorylation coupling 2
physical activity readiness, protocol *pro forma* 252
physical deconditioning, cardiovascular response pattern abnormalities 165–166
physical training
  assessment/preparation, *case study* 185–7
  biomechanical efficiency 151
  blood doping 168
  cardiovascular limitation 163–164
  data analysis, sequential graphing 162, 165
  exercise prescription 11, 12
  isowork analysis 151
  oxygen pulse response patterns 112
  response, PXT 8
  response measurements 151
  running economy 151
  sinus bradycardia 113
physiological variables, *glossary* 205–210
"pink puffers", lung disease 125
Pitot tube, flow and volume transducers 37–38
pneumotachograph, flow and volume transducers 37
power, *conversion constants* 217
power output, cycle ergometers 22
*Ppa see* pulmonary arterial pressure
predicted normal values *see* reference values
prediction equations, reference values 150
pregnancy
  XT guidelines 82–83
  XT relative contraindication 88
premature atrial contractions (PACs), ECG 113
preoperative risk assessment, CXT 73
preparation for exercise program, *case study* 185–187
pressure, *conversion constants* 217
progress monitoring
  CXT 68
  PXT 54–55
propranolol, $f_{C\max}$ reduction 109
protein, respiratory quotient 7
protocol *pro forma*
  cycle ergometers 254
  physical activity readiness 252
  preparation for exercise testing 251
  preparticipation screening for exercise testing 253
  treadmill ergometers 255
*protocols and supplemental materials* 241–260
psychological disorders
  differential diagnosis 11
  symptom perception abnormalities 178
  XT contraindication 87
psychometric scales
  Borg scale for perceived exertion 256
  CXT 71
  symptomatic evaluation, data analysis 155
$P_{(a\text{-}ET)}CO_2$ *see* arterial–end-tidal carbon dioxide partial pressure difference
$P_{ET}O_2$ and $P_{ET}CO_2$ *see* end-tidal gas tensions
pulmonary arterial pressure (*Ppa*) 121–122
  definition, derivation, equation, and measurement units 121, 207
  normal/abnormal response 121–122
pulmonary capillary transit time (*Tpc*), oxygen diffusion, alveolar–capillary membrane 138
pulmonary disease 11
  arterial blood gas tension abnormalities 136
  "blue bloaters"/"pink puffers" 125–126
  breathlessness scores 147
  cardiovascular response abnormalities 165–166
  chronic, oxygen uptake, prolonged 105
  dietary recommendations 126
  differential diagnosis 11
  exercise prescription 12
  $f_R$ values 130
  interstitial 11
  oxygen breath decrease 131
  $Pa\text{O}_2$ and $Pa\text{CO}_2$ increases 140

progression/regression assessment 151–152
$P_{(A\text{-}a)}O_2$ widening 139
restrictive, ventilatory capacity reduction 124
symptom perception abnormalities 127–128, 177–178
$T_I/T_E$ 131, 133
vascular disease 11
ventilatory control abnormalities 173
ventilatory equivalents 135
ventilatory limitation 169
ventilatory response pattern abnormalities 170–171
$V_T$ values 128–129
*see also* chronic obstructive pulmonary disease; *specific diseases*
pulmonary embolism, XT contraindication 87
pulmonary rehabilitation
initial assessment, *case study* 191–195
response 151
pulse oximetry
arterial blood sampling 48–50
calibration, accuracy and precision 48
confounding factors 48
description and operational principles 47–48
maintenance 48
PWC170 test, electrically braked ergometers 23
PXT *see* performance exercise testing

Queen's College single-stage step test 58–59, 214
*questions, frequent* 261–263

*R see* respiratory exchange ratio
ramp test 67
rating of perceived exertion (RPE) 144–146
Borg (psychometric) scale 144–146
definition, derivation, and measurement units 144–145, 207
$f_C$ relationship 145
interpretations 146
normal/abnormal response 145–146
recovery phase, data acquisition 86
*reference values* 220–240
reference values
defined 149
prediction equations 150
single variable comparison 149–152
regression equation 16
rehabilitation
CXT progress monitoring 68
response measurements 151
respiratory chain *see* mitochondrial pathway
respiratory compensation point* 126–128
respiratory exchange ratio (*R*) 2, 105–107
calculation 216
carbon dioxide output and oxygen uptake relationship 2
measurement 105
definition, derivation, and measurement units 105–106, 207
normal/abnormal responses 106–107
time relationship 107
terminology 105–106
respiratory muscle weakness, ventilatory limitation 124, 169–171
respiratory quotient (RQ)
defined 106
substrates 7
respiratory rate ($f_R$) 129–130
definition, derivation, and measurement units 129, 206
normal/abnormal response 129–130
resting phase, data acquisition 85
resuscitation equipment 90–91
crash cart 90–91
rheumatoid disorders, XT relative contraindication 88
risk assessment
CXT 8, 68
preoperative 11, 13
Rockport walking test 55–56
estimation of maximum oxygen uptake 213–214
RPE *see* rating of perceived exertion
r.p.m. (cadence)
*conversion constants* 217
effect of errors on mechanically braked, cycle ergometers 22–23
effect of errors on work rate and oxygen uptake 240
indicators *see* counters
RQ *see* respiratory quotient
$RQ_{mus}$ *see* muscle respiratory quotient
running tests *see* walking and running tests

safety considerations 87–91
contraindications 87–90
JCAHO standards 87
Scholander procedure, calibration gas accuracy 40
shunt
intracardiac, gas exchange abnormalities 175
physiological
gas exchange abnormalities 173
$P_{(A\text{-}a)}O_2$ increase 139
shuttle test
10-meter 69–70
20-meter 57–58
course 19
speed
definition, derivation, and measurement units 95–96
normal/abnormal responses 96
time intervals and estimated oxygen uptake
10-meter 69–70
20-meter 59
Siconolfi multistage step test 59–60, 212
sinus arrhythmias, ECG 113
sinus bradycardia 113
sinus tachycardia 113

six-minute walking distance ($d_{W6}$) *see* walking and running tests
skin symptoms, XT termination 88–89
slope, alveolar 137, 138, 140
slope of cardiovascular response*
  definition, derivation, and measurement units 110–111, 205
  Fick equation 110
  normal/abnormal response 111
slope of ventilatory response* 123, 124–126
  definition, derivation, and measurement units 124, 205
  equation 124
  normal/abnormal response 125–126
smoking cessation 11, 13
solvents, occupational exposure, *case study* 195–199
speed, *conversion constants* 218
sphygmomanometry 46–47
  description and operational principles 46–47
  intraarterial blood pressure measurement 47
  Korotkoff sounds, tonal quality and interpretation 119
spirometers and gasometers 35–36
  calibration, accuracy and precision 36
  description and operational principles 35–36
  dry gasometers 36
  dry rolling-seal 36
  maintenance 36
  Ohio spirometer 36
  Tissot spirometer 32
    leak tests 34
  water-sealed 35–36
sports medicine, ergometers 21
*Spo*$_2$ *see* arterial oxygen saturation
stair-climb, chronic obstructive pulmonary disease 70
stair-step incremental work rate tests 67, 80–82
  Bruce and Balke treadmill protocols 64, 73, 78–79, 214–215
standard deviation of the mean
  confidence interval 150
  variability degree 140, 150
standardized gas volumes 215–216
step tests 58–60
  oxygen cost 211–213
  Queen's College single-stage step test 58–59, 214
  Siconolfi multistage step test 59–60, 214
  stair-step incremental work rate tests 67, 80–82
stoicism, symptom perception abnormalities 178
stopwatches *see* chronometers
Storer cycle test, estimation of maximum oxygen uptake 214
suboptimal effort 156–7, 178–9
*supplemental materials* 241–260
surgery 11, 13
  CXT progress monitoring 68
SV *see* cardiac stroke volume
swim test 60, 236
symptom perception
  abnormalities 127–128, 177–178
    definition and identification 177
  data analysis 155
  rating of perceived exertion (RPE) 144–146, 207, 256
systemic arterial pressure 206

*t see* endurance time
tachometer 20
  *see also* counters
tachycardia
  sinus, ECG 113
  supraventricular
    cardiovascular response pattern abnormalities 167
    ECG 113
  ventricular, ECG dysrhythmias 115
  XT termination 89
TCA *see* Krebs cycle
testing methods *see* exercise testing (XT)
therapeutic interventions, evaluation 11, 13
thoracotomy, preoperative risk assessment, CXT 73
thromboembolic disease
  cardiovascular response pattern abnormalities 166
  XT contraindication 87
  *see also* pulmonary disease
thrombus, intracardiac, XT contraindication 87
thyrotoxicosis
  cardiovascular response pattern abnormalities 165
  XT relative contraindication 88
tidal volume ($V_T$) 128–129
  definition, derivation, and measurement units 128, 210
  equation 128
  normal/abnormal response 128–129
  $V_E$ relationship 128, 129
timing devices 19–21
  chronometers 19–20
  counters 20
  metronomes 20–21
Tissot spirometer 32, 34
total lung capacity (TLC), inspiratory and expiratory flow–volume relationships 133–134
*Tpc see* pulmonary capillary transit time
transplantation, heart 11, 13
treadmill ergometers
  advantages and disadvantages 25
  calculation of grade increment 249
  calibration
    accuracy and precision 28–30
    pre-XT 78
  description and operational principles 27–28
    grading 28–29
    speed 29–30
  grading, angle relationship 29–30
  maintenance 30

maximal incremental work rate 80–82
oxygen cost
running 212
walking 211–212
walking and running tests 211–212
protocol *pro forma* 255
safety 30–31
settings 78
submaximal constant work rate 65
submaximal incremental work rate 63–64
Balke protocol 64, 214
Bruce protocol, data table 64, 214–215
tricarboxylic acid (TCA) cycle *see* Krebs cycle
$T_I/T_E$ *see* inspiratory/expiratory time
turbine transducer, flow and volume transducers 38

vascular disease
peripheral, impaired oxygen delivery 168
pulmonary 11
ventilation
oscillating, ventilatory control abnormalities 173
treadmill and cycle exercise comparisons 24
*see also* hyperventilation; maximum minute ventilation; maximum voluntary ventilation
ventilation disorders, differential diagnosis 10–11
ventilatory capacity
defined 208
determination pretest 76
spirometry 35
ventilatory capacity measurement, MVV 123
ventilatory control abnormalities
data analysis, nine-panel display 156–157, 172
definition and identification 171–172
diagnostic patterns 171–173
ventilatory equivalents* 134–135
definition, derivation, and measurement units 134, 208
equations 134
normal/abnormal response 134–135
ventilatory failure, ventilatory control abnormalities 172–173
ventilatory limitation 8, 10
data analysis 154, 159, 169–170
four-panel displays 160, 162
nine-panel display 156–157, 158, 169
definition and identification 124, 169
diagnostic patterns 169–170
ventilatory response pattern abnormalities
data analysis, nine-panel display 156–157, 170
diagnostic patterns 159, 170–171
ventilatory threshold
physical fitness assessment 9
respiratory compensation point*
definition, derivation, and measurement units 126–127
normal/abnormal response 127–128
terminology 126–127
ventricular aneurysm, XT relative contraindication 88
ventricular contractions
ECG dysrhythmias 115
premature (PVCs), ECG 113
XT termination 89
ventricular fibrillation, ECG dysrhythmias 115
verapamil, $f_{Cmax}$ reduction 109
vertigo, XT termination 89
visual analog scale for breathlessness 146, 258
visual disturbance, XT termination 89
vital capacity (VC), nomograms 228–229
volume, *conversion constants* 218
volume transducers *see* flow and volume transducers
volume-measuring devices 32–43
desirable qualities 32
flow and volume transducers 36–35
gas collection bags 32–36
spirometers and gasometers 35–38
$V_T$ *see* tidal volume
$V_D/V_T$ *see* dead space–tidal volume ratio

walking and running tests
6- and 12-minute 69
6-minute walking test
definition, derivation, measurement units 94
equations 231
normal/abnormal responses 95
protocol 243
Cooper distance measurements 56–57, 237–239
1.5-mile run 237
3-mile walk 238
data analysis, sequential graphing 161–162
distance
definition, derivation, measurement units 94, 205
normal/abnormal responses 94
endurance time, normal/abnormal 93–94
oxygen cost, treadmill ergometers 211–212
Rockport 55–56
Shuttle 2-meter 57–58
timed 55–58
physical fitness assessment 9
*see also* treadmill ergometers
warm-up phase, data acquisition 85
water vapor pressure
gas analyzers 41
oxygen analyzers, calibration 41
water vapor pressure ($P_{H20}$) 246
Weber classification, cardiovascular disease 99–100
weight, *conversion constants* 218–219
Wingate test, cycle ergometers 25
work, *conversion constants* 219
work efficiency*
calculation 100

work efficiency (*cont.*)
definition, derivation, measurement units 100, 206
incremental exercise, oxygen uptake and work rate relationship calculation 100
muscle work conversion 2
normal/abnormal response 100–101
physical fitness assessment 8–9
XT response variables 100–101
work rate increment 210
work rate and oxygen uptake, effect of errors in r.p.m. (cadence) 240
work rate tests
constant (CWR)
CXT 73–74
oxygen uptake time constant 65–66
*t*, normal/abnormal responses 93, 94
$f_{Cmax}$ and $f_C$/work rate relationship 51, 52
incremental
arterial blood gas tensions 135, 136
cardiac output 117–118
$f_R$ responses 129–130
maximal 66–67
maximum oxygen uptake relationship 99
minute ventilation and oxygen uptake relationship 123
$P_{(A-a)}O_2$ changes 139, 140
*t*, normal/abnormal responses 93, 94
ventilatory equivalents 134–135
laboratory tests 66–67
oxygen uptake coupling 1–2
variable, *t*, normal/abnormal responses 93–94
*see also* arm ergometers; cycle ergometers; treadmill ergometers; walking and running tests
work rate *(W)*, defined 210

XT *see* exercise testing

YMCA cycle ergometer test 61

zirconium oxide analyzers, oxygen analyzers 39–40